KEY ASPECTS OF ELDER CARE

Managing Falls, Incontinence, and Cognitive Impairment

Sandra G. Funk, Ph.D., is Professor and Director of the Research Support Center (RSC) at the School of Nursing, the University of North Carolina at Chapel Hill. A faculty member of the School of Nursing for over 15 years, she served as coordinator of the graduate research sequence, teaching graduate research methods, statistics, and computer applications for 9 years, and has been Director of the RSC for the past 6. She has served as research and statistical advisor to nursing faculty and graduate students in several universities, and for 5 years was research advisor to the Robert Wood Johnson fellows in general pediatrics at Duke University. She has served as principal and co-investigator of numerous grants and has published in the areas of preschool developmental screening, research utilization, decision making, scaling, and cluster analysis.

Elizabeth M. Tornquist, M.A., has been a member of the faculty of the School of Nursing at the University of North Carolina at Chapel Hill for 15 years, where she teaches scientific writing to graduate students and serves as editor in residence. Ms. Tornquist is also on the faculty of the Curriculum of Public Health Nursing at the School of Public Health, the University of North Carolina at Chapel Hill. She is a former journalist and freelance writer and is the author of *From Proposal to Publication: An Informal Guide to Writing about Nursing Research* as well as numerous articles on writing.

Mary T. Champagne, Ph.D., R.N., is Associate Professor and Dean at the School of Nursing, Duke University; Associate Director of Nursing Services, Duke University Hospital; and Senior Fellow at the Duke University Center for the Study of Aging and Human Development, Durham, NC. She is co-principal investigator of a 5-year study that is testing interventions to prevent the development of acute confusion in hospitalized elderly patients. She is currently the National Nurse Advisor for Humana Heart Institute International in Louisville, KY.

Ruth A. Wiese, M.S.N., R.N., a former faculty member of the University of Nebraska College of Nursing and an in-service instructor and coordinator of staff development in a clinical setting, is currently a Research Instructor at the School of Nursing, the University of North Carolina at Chapel Hill, and Project Coordinator for "Moving New Nursing Knowledge into Practice: A CE Program."

KEY ASPECTS OF ELDER CARE

Managing Falls, Incontinence, and Cognitive Impairment

Sandra G. Funk, Ph.D.

Elizabeth M. Tornquist, M.A.

Mary T. Champagne, Ph.D., R.N.

Ruth A. Wiese, M.S.N., R.N.

Editors

SPRINGER PUBLISHING COMPANY
New York

Springer Publishing Company, Inc.
536 Broadway
New York, NY 10012-3955

92 93 94 95 96 / 5 4 3 2 1

Library of Congress Cataloging-in-Publication Data

Key aspects of elder care: managing falls, incontinence, and
    cognitive impairment / Sandra G. Funk . . . [et al.], editors
        p.   cm.
    Includes bibliographical references and index.
    ISBN 0-8261-7720-4
    1. Geriatric nursing.   2. Falls (Accidents) in old age.
3. Urinary incontinence in old age.   4. Cognition disorders in old
age.   I. Funk, Sandra G.
    RC954 · K49   1992
    618 · 97—dc20   92–7827
                                                             CIP

Printed in the United States of America

Moving New Nursing Knowledge into Practice: A CE Program

ADVISORY COMMITTEE

Chair:

Carolyn A. Williams, Ph.D., R.N., F.A.A.N.
Professor and Dean, School of Nursing
University of Kentucky

Members:

Linda R. Cronenwett, Ph.D., R.N., F.A.A.N.
Director of Nursing Research
Dartmouth-Hitchcock Medical Center

Cynthia M. Freund, Ph.D., R.N., F.A.A.N.
Associate Professor and Acting Dean
School of Nursing
The University of North Carolina at Chapel Hill

PROJECT TEAM

Project
Director:

Sandra G. Funk, Ph.D.
Professor and Director, Research Support Center
School of Nursing
The University of North Carolina at Chapel Hill

Co-Project
Director:

Elizabeth M. Tornquist, M.A.
Lecturer, School of Nursing
The University of North Carolina at Chapel Hill

Clinical Nursing
Research
Specialist:

Mary T. Champagne, Ph.D., R.N.
Associate Professor and Dean, School of Nursing
Duke University, Durham, NC

Project
Coordinator:

Ruth A. Wiese, M.S.N., R.N.
Research Instructor, School of Nursing
The University of North Carolina at Chapel Hill

Administration
Specialist:

Sheila P. Englebardt, M.Ed., R.N., C.N.A.
Clinical Assistant Professor, School of Nursing
The University of North Carolina at Chapel Hill

General
Advisor:

Laurel Archer Copp, Ph.D., R.N., F.A.A.N.
Professor, School of Nursing
The University of North Carolina at Chapel Hill

"Moving New Nursing Knowledge into Practice: A CE Program" is funded by the Division of Nursing, DHHS, Grant #1 D10 NU24318-01.

Contents

Part IV. Managing Cognitive Impairment

Acknowledgments

As noted in Chapter 1, this volume emanates from a project that is designed to improve the dissemination of nursing research to practicing clinicians. The success of the effort stems from the energy, minds, and talents of many people—certainly the investigators whose research you will be reading and the clinicians who interpret and use it. Less visible but no less important is the team behind the project—the team that puts on the conferences, teaches the workshops, provides consultation through the information center, and edits the books: Elizabeth Tornquist, project co-director and editor; Ruth Wiese, project coordinator; Mary Champagne, clinical nursing research specialist; and Sheila Englebardt, administration specialist. It is the extraordinary commitment and talent of these folks that has enabled the project to so successfully move research into the hands of clinicians. Of particular note in the editing of this volume and those that preceded it is the work of Elizabeth Tornquist. Elizabeth has been a driving force behind many aspects of the project, but especially in helping researchers to clearly present their thoughts and research to others. Her work is not just editing words; it is also helping the writer with logic and flow, with expression, and even with thinking. The ease with which you will read this volume owes much to Elizabeth's input. To recognize her contributions, I would have preferred to name Elizabeth first editor of this volume, but we were advised against changing the order of names. I hope this note will serve to alert readers to the extraordinary contributions of Elizabeth and all our team members.

Support for this project was provided by a special projects grant (#1 D10 NU24318-01), "Moving New Nursing Knowledge into Practice: A CE Program," awarded to the School of Nursing, The University of North Carolina at Chapel Hill, from the Division of Nursing, Bureau of Health Professions, Department of Health and Human Services. We are most appreciative of the support provided by the Division of Nursing for this project and of the thoughtful direction and guidance provided by our Advisory Committee: Dr. Carolyn A. Williams, Dr. Linda R. Cronenwett, and Dr. Cynthia M. Freund. For this volume and the conference it reports, Dr. Carol C. Hogue, Associate Professor at The University of North Carolina at Chapel Hill; Dr. Jean F. Wyman, Associate Professor, Medical College of Virginia, Virginia Commonwealth University; and Dr. Virginia J. Neelon, Associate Professor, The University of North Carolina at Chapel Hill, provided content expertise in the areas of managing falls, incontinence, and cognitive impairment, respectively; we are grateful for their contributions. Heartfelt thanks are extended to our project secretary, Frances G. Hoffman, for her work on this volume, and to Brian Neelon and Michael Terry, who worked with the editors in developing conference materials and preparing this volume.

For those wishing to contact our information center or receive copies of the newsletter, *Nursing Research/Nursing Practice Connection*, call or write: Ruth Wiese, Project Coordinator, School of Nursing, CB# 7460 Carrington Hall, The University of North Carolina at Chapel Hill, Chapel Hill, NC 27599-7460; telephone: (919) 966-2263.

S.G.F.

Contributors

Patricia G. Archbold, D.N.Sc., R.N., F.A.A.N.
Professor, Department of Family Nursing, School of Nursing, Oregon Health
  Sciences University, Portland

Barbara M. Bates-Jenson, R.N., N.N., C.E.T.N.
Clinical Nurse Specialist and Project Coordinator, Borun Center for Gerontological Research, University of California, Los Angeles

Cornelia Beck, Ph.D., R.N.
Professor and Associate Dean for Research and Evaluation, College of Nursing,
  University of Arkansas for Medical Sciences, Little Rock

Leigh A. Bertholf, M.S., R.N.
Instructor, College of Nursing, University of Nebraska Medical Center, Kearney
  Division

Kevin R. Bishop, M.S.N., A.R.N.P.
Clinical Associate, Labor and Delivery, Shands Teaching Hospital, Gainesville,
  FL

Carol A. Brink, M.P.H., R.N.
Associate Professor of Clinical Nursing, School of Nursing, University of
  Rochester, NY

Louis D. Burgio, Ph.D.
Research Professor of Medicine, School of Medicine, University of Pittsburgh,
  PA

Emily Campbell, M.S., R.N.
Professor, School of Nursing, University of Wisconsin, Madison

John Carlson, M.A.
Research Instructor, School of Nursing, The University of North Carolina at
  Chapel Hill

Marcia Casselman, M.S.
Research Assistant, Textiles and Clothing, Iowa State University, Ames

Brenda L. Cleary, Ph.D.
Associate Professor and Associate Dean, School of Nursing (Permian Basin), Texas Technical University Health Sciences Center, Odessa

Sandra D. Clements, M.N., R.N., C.S.
Project Coordinator/FICSIT, Department of Rehabilitation Medicine, School of Medicine, Emory University, Atlanta, GA

Joyce Colling, Ph.D., R.N., F.A.A.N.
Professor and Chair, Community Health Care Systems, School of Nursing, Oregon Health Sciences University, Portland

Linda R. Cronenwett, Ph.D., R.N., F.A.A.N.
Director of Nursing Research, Dartmouth-Hitchcock Medical Center, Hanover, NH

Jeanette Daly, M.A.
Research Assistant, College of Nursing, The University of Iowa, Iowa City

Nancy E. Dayhoff, Ed.D., R.N.
Associate Professor, School of Nursing, Indiana University, Indianapolis

Ananias C. Diokno, M.D.
Clinical Professor, School of Medicine, University of Michigan, Ann Arbor

Molly C. Dougherty, Ph.D., A.R.N.P.
Professor and Research Coordinator, College of Nursing, University of Florida, Gainesville

Joan Eisch, M.S., R.N., F.N.P.
Lecturer, Decker School of Nursing, State University of New York at Binghamton

Lois K. Evans, D.N.Sc., R.N., F.A.A.N.
Associate Professor, School of Nursing, University of Pennsylvania, Philadelphia

Marquis D. Foreman, Ph.D., R.N.
Assistant Professor, College of Nursing, University of Illinois at Chicago

Corre J. Garrett, Ed.D., R.N., C.C.R.N.
Assistant Professor, School of Nursing, East Carolina University, Greenville, NC (deceased)

Phyllis A. Gimotty, Ph.D.
Chief, Biostatistics, Michigan Cancer Foundation, Detroit

Merwyn R. Greenlick, Ph.D.
Professor and Acting Chair, Department of Public Health and Preventive Medicine, School of Medicine, Oregon Health Sciences University, Portland

Teresa A. Gyldenvard, M.A., O.C.N.
Family Therapist, Human Development and Family Studies, Iowa State University, Ames

Betty Jo Hadley, Ph.D., R.N.
Professor and Assistant Dean for Academic Development and Research, College of Nursing and Health, University of Cincinnati, OH

Theresa A. Harvath, Ph.D., R.N.
Assistant Professor, Department of Family Nursing, School of Nursing, Oregon Health Sciences University, Portland

Patricia Heacock, Ph.D., R.N.
Associate Professor, College of Nursing, University of Arkansas for Medical Sciences, Little Rock

Marta Heffner, M.S.
Research Assistant, College of Nursing, The University of Iowa, Iowa City

Ann L. Hendrich, M.S.N., R.N.
Clinical Research Nurse, Methodist Hospital of Indiana, Inc., Indianapolis

Virginia Henderson, A.M., R.N., F.A.A.N., F.R.C.N.
Research Associate Emeritus, School of Nursing, Yale University, New Haven, CT

Kathleen Heslin, M.Sc.N.
Director of Nursing Medical Services, Saint Joseph's Health Centre, London, Ontario, Canada

Carol C. Hogue, Ph.D., R.N., F.A.A.N.
Associate Professor, School of Nursing, The University of North Carolina at Chapel Hill

Linda M. Hollinger, Ph.D., R.N.
Associate Professor and Assistant Chairperson for Education, Department of Medical Nursing, College of Nursing, Rush–Presbyterian–St. Luke's Medical Center, Chicago, IL

Jeffrey C. Huston, Ph.D., P.E.
Professor, Biomedical Engineering, Iowa State University, Ames

Mario Jacques, R.N.
Nurse Manager, Emergency, Saint Joseph's Health Centre, London, Ontario, Canada

Thomas A. Kippenbrock, Ed.D., R.N.
Assistant Professor, Department of Nursing Administration and Teacher Education, School of Nursing, Indiana University, Indianapolis

Thomas Kruckeberg, M.S.
Systems Programmer II, College of Nursing, The University of Iowa, Iowa City

Carolyn J. Kundel, Ph.D., C.H.E.
Associate Professor, College of Family and Consumer Sciences, Iowa State University, Ames

Janice M. Larson, M.S.N., R.N.
President, Extended Family, Inc., Oshkosh, WI, and Part-time Faculty, University of Wisconsin–Oshkosh

Colleen Leckie, R.N.
Nurse Manager, Surgery, Saint Joseph's Health Centre, London, Ontario, Canada

Colleen M. Lucas, M.N., R.N., C.S.
Clinical Nurse Specialist, Good Samaritan Hospital and Medical Center, Portland, OR

Robert Mayer, M.D.
Assistant Professor, Department of Urology, School of Medicine, University of Rochester, NY

Meridean L. Maas, Ph.D., R.N., F.A.A.N.
Associate Professor and Chair, Department of Organizations and Systems, College of Nursing, The University of Iowa, Iowa City

Eleanor McConnell, M.S.N., R.N.
Clinical Nurse Specialist, Department of Veterans' Affairs Medical Center, Durham, NC

B. Joan McDowell, Ph.D., C.R.N.P.
Assistant Professor, Schools of Medicine and Nursing, University of Pittsburgh, PA

Elizabeth McNeely, Ph.D., C.G.N.P.
Assistant Professor, Nell Hodgson Woodruff School of Nursing, Emory University, Atlanta, GA

M. Patrick McNees, Ph.D.
President, North Rim Systems, Anchorage, AK

Susan Mercer, D.S.W.
Professor, Graduate School of Social Work, University of Arkansas for Health Sciences, Little Rock

Judy Miller, Ph.D., R.N., C.
Assistant Professor, Department of Adult and Geriatric Health, School of Nursing, The University of North Carolina at Chapel Hill

Lati Modarressi, M.A.
Data Base Manager, Department of Psychiatry, College of Medicine, The University of Iowa, Iowa City

Ruth A. Mooney, Ph.D., M.E.D., A.R.N.P., C.
Visiting Assistant Professor, College of Nursing, University of Florida, Gainesville

Joyce Mullin, B.Sc.N., R.N.
Nurse Educator, Saint Joseph's Health Centre, London, Ontario, Canada

Virginia J. Neelon, Ph.D., R.N.
Associate Professor and Director, Biobehavioral Laboratory, School of Nursing, The University of North Carolina at Chapel Hill

Annette H. Newman, M.S., R.N.
Nursing Instructor, Family and Health Careers, Lane Community College, Eugene, OR

Daniel R. Newman, B.A.
Department of Psychology, Middle Tennessee State University, Murfreesboro

Diane Kaschak Newman, M.S.N., R.N.C., C.R.N.P.
Nurse Practitioner, Golden Horizons, Newtown Square, PA

Allen Nyhuis, M.S.
Biostatistician, Methodist Hospital of Indiana, Inc., Indianapolis

Joseph G. Ouslander, M.D.
Medical Director, Jewish Homes for the Aging of Greater Los Angeles, Reseda, CA

Patricia A. Patterson, M.S., R.N., C.C.R.N.
Assistant Administrator, Director of Nursing, Good Shepherd Hospital, Barrington, IL

Betty D. Pearson, Ph.D., R.N., C.A.
Associate Professor, Foundations of Nursing Department, University of Wisconsin–Milwaukee

Karen Perkin, B.Sc.N., R.N.
Quality Assurance Coordinator, Saint Joseph's Health Centre, London, Ontario, Canada

Sue Popkess-Vawter, Ph.D., R.N.
Professor, School of Nursing, University of Kansas Medical Center, Kansas City

Betty J. Reynolds, Ed.D., R.N., C.A.N.P., G.G.N.P.
Associate Professor and Director, RN Access Program, School of Nursing, The University of North Carolina at Wilmington

Jo Ellen Rude Ross, M.A.
Project Director, Department of Preventive Medicine, College of Medicine, The University of Iowa, Iowa City

Carolyn M. Sampselle, Ph.D., R.N.
Assistant Professor, School of Nursing, University of Michigan, Ann Arbor

John F. Schnelle, Ph.D., A.B.
Associate Director, Borun Center for Gerontological Research and Professor in Residence, Department of Medicine and Gerontology, School of Medicine, University of California, Los Angeles

Michael S. Sellberg, B.S.
Research Assistant, Biomedical Engineering and Engineering Mechanics, Iowa State University, Ames

Georgene C. Siemsen, M.S., R.N.C.
Clinical Nurse Specialist, University Hospital, Oregon Health Sciences University, Portland

Rebecca A. Sisson, Ph.D., R.N.
Assistant Professor, College of Nursing, University of South Florida, Tampa

Diane A. Smith, M.S.N., R.N., C.R.N.P.
Nurse Practitioner, Golden Horizons, Newtown Square, PA

J. Christopher Smith, M.A.
Research Assistant, The University of Iowa, Iowa City

Mary E. Soja, M.S.N., R.N.
Assistant Professor, Department of Nursing Administration and Teacher Education, School of Nursing, Indiana University, Indianapolis

Barbara J. Stewart, Ph.D.
Professor, Department of Family Nursing, School of Nursing, Oregon Health Sciences University, Portland

Neville E. Strumpf, Ph.D., R.N., C., F.A.A.N.
Associate Professor, School of Nursing, University of Pennsylvania, Philadelphia

Heather Thornton-Lawrence, R.N.
Staff Nurse, Surgery, Saint Joseph's Health Centre, London, Ontario, Canada

Jayne Towers, R.N.
Clinical Coordinator, Medicine, Saint Joseph's Health Centre, London, Ontario, Canada

Patricia Tunink, M.A.
Research Assistant, The University of Iowa, Iowa City

Patricia E. Hadley Vermeersch, Ph.D., R.N.
Assistant Professor, College of Nursing, University of North Dakota, Grand Forks

Chris Walton, M.N.Sc., R.N.
Project Director, College of Nursing, University of Arkansas for Medical Sciences, Little Rock

Thelma J. Wells, Ph.D., R.N., F.A.A.N., F.R.C.N.
Professor, School of Nursing, University of Rochester, NY

Marilyn White, B.S.N., R.N.
Graduate Student, School of Nursing, Vanderbilt University, Nashville, TN

Lynn Wick, R.N.
Staff Nurse, Rehabilitation, Saint Joseph's Health Centre, London, Ontario, Canada

Bradford Williams, M.D.
Chairman, Department of Obstetrics and Gynecology, Alachua General Hospital; and Director, Women's Clinic, University of Florida Student Infirmary, Gainesville

Steven L. Wolf, Ph.D., F.A.P.T.A.
Professor, Department of Rehabilitation Medicine, and Associate Professor, Department of Anatomy and Cell Biology, School of Medicine, Emory University, Atlanta, GA

Paul J. Woodward, Ph.D.
Statistical and Psychometric Consultant, Iowa City, IA

George Woodworth, Ph.D.
Statistical Consultant, Department of Statistics, The University of Iowa, Iowa City

Jean F. Wyman, Ph.D., R.N., C.S.
Associate Professor, School of Nursing, Medical College of Virginia, Virginia Commonwealth University, Richmond

Part I

INTRODUCTION

[1]

Elder Care: From Research to Practice

Sandra G. Funk and Elizabeth M. Tornquist

WARNING[1]

When I am an old woman I shall wear purple
With a red hat which doesn't go, and doesn't suit me.
And I shall spend my pension on brandy and summer gloves
and satin sandals, and say we've no money for butter.
I shall sit down on the pavement when I'm tired
And gobble up samples in shops and press alarm bells
And run my stick along the public railings
And make up for the sobriety of my youth.
I shall go out in my slippers in the rain
And pick the flowers in other people's gardens
And learn to spit.

You can wear terrible shirts and grow more fat
And eat three pounds of sausages at a go
Or only bread and pickle for a week
And hoard pens and pencils and beermats and things in boxes.

But now we must have clothes that keep us dry
And pay our rent and not swear in the street
And set a good example for the children.
We must have friends to dinner and read the papers.

But maybe I ought to practice a little now?
So people who know me are not too shocked and surprised
When suddenly I am old, and start to wear purple.

                                                              Jenny Joseph

To wear only purple, or eat only bread and pickles; to live as one likes, with dignity—these are goals for all, including the elderly. But the abilities of elderly people to live with independence and dignity are threatened when their health and functioning are compromised, as they are with a hip injury from a fall, or the loss of cognitive abilities, or from the limitations imposed by incontinence. Today the independence and functioning of the elderly are also threatened by a deteriorating health care system. In the opening chapter of this volume, Virginia Henderson—the world's best known and best loved nurse—gives a powerful analysis of current problems in health care delivery in the U.S. and the role of nurses in improving the system. Her opening chapter presents an overarching framework for efforts to improve care of all people, both young and old.

Within that framework of need for open, accessible, humane care, this volume looks at three particular areas of concern for the elderly—falls, incontinence, and cognitive impairment. These are key problems for the elderly in acute and long-term care settings and at home. Any of them threatens the elderly's independence and quality of life; together they represent major obstacles to continued functioning.

The nurse plays a crucial role in caring for the elderly and assisting them with living—whether in the home, in a nursing home, or in an acute care setting. As Virginia Henderson (1978) said in her classic description, the nurse's role is "to help people, sick or well, in the performance of those activities contributing to health or its recovery (or to a peaceful death) that they would perform unaided if they had the necessary strength, will, or knowledge" (p. 34). By helping the elderly to maximize functional abilities and to minimize the effects of chronic impairments, the nurse can make an enormous contribution to the quality and longevity of the elder's life.

Research can offer guidance to the nurse who is caring for the elderly patient. It can identify major problem areas, ways to assess them, and effective interventions for their alleviation. It can suggest strategies for promoting function and provide a better understanding of the patient's perspective on the experience. While much about elder care remains to be studied, critical and important studies are available to guide clinicians. Unfortunately, in this area as in many other areas of nursing, there is a sizable gap between research and practice (Brett, 1987; Kirchhoff, 1982). The purpose of this volume is to share with practicing nurses the latest nursing research on key aspects of caring for the elderly—to move the ideas and findings of the research into the practice setting.

This book is one part of a multifaceted approach to improving the dissemination of nursing research and, ultimately, the use of research in nursing practice. There are four major components to the approach:

1. Carefully structured topic-focused conferences present nursing research findings that are ready for practice in a form that is easy to understand and that emphasizes usefulness in the clinical setting.
2. Pre- and postconference workshops assist clinicians and administrators in selecting research-based innovations appropriate for use in their settings and assist them in identifying suitable implementation strategies.
3. Carefully edited books based on the conference research presentations and discussions are published to ensure that the research is broadly disseminated.
4. An information center and newsletter provide consultation and a communication mechanism for clinicians and administrators during the implementation of the innovations. (See Funk, Tornquist, & Champagne, 1989a, for a fuller explanation of this approach.)

Topics for the conferences are selected based on their importance to the practice of nursing, their applicability to a broad range of settings, the availability of ongoing research in the area, the ability of nurses to control interventions, and the perceived gap between knowledge and practice. Researchers are invited through a national call to submit their research for presentation at the conference, and submissions are reviewed by a panel of individuals with practice and research expertise in the topic area, or with methodological or statistical expertise. Papers are selected based on scientific merit, significance, and readiness for practice. The conference is structured to include information on the current bases for practice, the selected research papers, discussions led by clinicians and researchers that focus on moving the research into practice, discussion of strategies for implementation, and demonstration sessions. Extensive consultation is provided to researchers to assist them with the preparation of research presentations that are scientifically sound, clear, and practice oriented.

Two previous conferences using this approach to dissemination of nursing research focused on comfort—management of pain, fatigue, and nausea—and recovery—improving nutrition, rest, and mobility. These conferences were attended by hundreds of nurses from five countries, and the majority were employed in clinical settings. Evaluations of the conference conveyed the participants' excitement and enthusiasm for improving their practice based on the research they had heard (Funk, Tornquist, & Champagne, 1989b). Springer Publishing Company has published the books that are companion to the conferences (Funk, Tornquist, Champagne, Copp, & Wiese, 1989, 1990), and both of them have been awarded American Journal of Nursing Book of the Year awards.

The third conference was equally successful. Held in April of 1991, it focused on key aspects of elder care—managing falls, incontinence, and cognitive impairment. This volume stems from the 1991 conference; its purpose is to provide a wider audience of practicing nurses with the most current research on caring for the elderly—research that describes falls, why they occur, how they can be predicted, and what can be done to prevent them; research that tests promising nursing-based interventions for reducing incontinence and its consequences; and research that helps us to better understand confusion in the elderly, to better assess its presence and fluctuation, and to better assist the confused elderly with activities of daily living. Since the purpose of the volume is to present the latest in nursing research, the selected papers necessarily reflect the scope and focus of research today. Negative findings are included when they are felt to illustrate an important point. Replicated findings were preferred, but unreplicated research is also included if aspects of the findings are ready for informal use or clinical trials, point to important factors that should be considered in practice, or alert the reader to important future research in a new area. Collectively, these works provide the clinician with the knowledge and means to enhance practice and improve patient functioning.

Each chapter has been edited extensively with the clinical audience in mind. Each study is presented as a full research report, but technical language is minimized, only directly relevant literature is cited, research methods are presented directly and simply, results sections focus on describing the major findings rather than the statistics, and discussion sections detail implications for practice. Introductory papers describe strategies for using research in practice and the current bases for nursing practice in the areas of falls, incontinence, and cognitive impairment. New research studies follow. A discussion of this new research, emphasizing implications for practice and directions for further research, concludes each section.

This book represents an effort to effectively communicate research findings that are relevant and ready for use, in a form that is understandable to practicing nurses, with suggestions for implementation and further clinical evaluation. The book is only one—though we think crucial—step in the process of moving from the conduct of research to its use in practice. As outlined in the chapter on improving practice through research utilization, it is hoped that the clinician reading this book will take note of particularly relevant findings and begin to use the new knowledge in practice—whether informally through viewing elderly patients in a new light or formally through making changes in patient care. Always, the clinician should evaluate the impact of such changes.

To assist clinicians with this process, to allow them to share their implementation experiences with one another, and to afford clinicians and researchers an opportunity for dialogue, we have established an information center and a newsletter, *Nursing Research/Nursing Practice Connection*, which will provide a mechanism for such communication. Clinicians are invited and encouraged to share their implementation experiences with others through the center and its newsletter; researchers are invited to share their latest findings and updates of research on falls, incontinence, and cognitive impairment. Through an ongoing exchange of ideas and experiences of researchers and clinicians, patient care will truly be enhanced.

REFERENCES

Brett, J. L. (1987). Use of nursing practice research findings. *Nursing Research, 36,* 344–349.

Funk, S. G., Tornquist, E. M., & Champagne, M. T. (1989a). A model for improving the dissemination of nursing research. *Western Journal of Nursing Research, 11,* 359–365.

Funk, S. G., Tornquist, E. M., & Champagne, M. T. (1989b). Application and evaluation of the dissemination model. *Western Journal of Nursing Research, 11,* 486–491.

Funk, S. G., Tornquist, E. M., Champagne, M. T., Copp, L. A., & Wiese, R. A. (Eds.). (1989). *Key aspects of comfort: Management of pain, fatigue, and nausea.* New York: Springer.

Funk, S. G., Tornquist, E. M., Champagne, M. T., Copp, L. A., & Wiese, R. A. (Eds.). (1990). *Key aspects of recovery: Improving nutrition, rest, and mobility.* New York: Springer.

Henderson, V., & Nite, G. (1978). *Principles and practice of nursing.* New York: Macmillan.

Joseph, J. (1987). Warning. In S. Martz (Ed.), *When I am an old woman I shall wear purple.* Watsonville, CA: Papier Maché Press.

Kirchhoff, K. T. (1982). A diffusion survey of coronary precautions. *Nursing Research, 31,* 196–201.

[2]

Excerpts from a Conversation with Virginia Henderson

Virginia Henderson

I don't lecture because if I have to give a lecture, I don't sleep from the time I've said I'll give the lecture until I give it! And then I get up and talk about things that I think are important but that the audience may not think are important at all. So I think, why should I stay awake for the rest of my life, when all I've got to do is let you ask me questions about things that you're interested in and that you think I might have some opinion on that would be worth listening to. Besides, we have the example of Donahue and a few others who get up every morning and get a roomful of people to talk. I don't see why we shouldn't do that ourselves! So just imagine that you're at Donahue's show. Now I can't run up those steps the way he does and hold a microphone to you, but I'm open for almost any question that you want to pose to health care providers. I want to stress that term "health care providers." I am not just interested in nursing. I'm interested in seeing for our people a decent health care system. I think what nurses do is a tremendously important part of that health care system. At present, however, I do not think we are free to give the kind of care we are capable of giving, or provide the health services that this country deserves.

I'm going to say a great many indiscreet things. That's just the beginning. But it's perfectly fair to start out with my thinking. The most dangerous thing I'll say is that I think our health care system . . . um, I don't like to use bad words, is no damned good!

8

Q: What would you propose that we do as nurses to help change or improve the health care system?

VH: Maybe we ought to have some sort of an injection that you can give people that gives them courage to say what they think and take the consequences. That doesn't mean being rude to anybody, but it's up to us, I think, who spend the time with people, sick and well, struggling to help them with their health care problems, to be open and frank about what their needs are. People don't like you for doing that. If you bring about change, they may be grateful to you when it happens, but it's not a popular stand. I'm saying that we must be willing to put ourselves in a position to be resented. Now that's just a beginning.

Q: Do you see progress in nursing?

VH: I see tremendous progress, and I think nursing is on an upswing. I think the world appreciates nurses more than they ever have. Of course in wartime, we are always popular.[1] It's too bad we have to have a war for people to be nice to nurses. In the First World War, when we were student nurses in our army nurse uniforms, we could go anywhere, and in a little while, we'd find that some man over in the corner of the room had called our waiter and said, "I'd like to pay for dinner for those girls over there." I'm not saying we should work for free dinners, but I do think it's nice to be valued. There have been some comprehensive studies recently of the public's attitude toward nurses and doctors, and our image comes off very well.

The public have come to expect health care. I think that they are on the verge of a revolution, which I wish would come—it should have come sooner. The public should be demanding health care. The strange thing is that the public expects the government to provide an education for them—you don't hesitate to say you expect to be educated at the expense of tax dollars, yet people often say to me, "Oh, you believe in socialized medicine." I reply that I believe in tax-supported health care, then I ask them where they've been to school, and it turns out they've been to public schools all their lives. So I say, "And you believe in socialized education, don't you?" We do! There's no difference; but we have been infected by this virus that makes all of us afraid to be associated with socialized medicine.

[1]This conversation took place during the Persian Gulf Conflict in spring 1991.

Q: Some people say the Department of Veterans' Affairs is a form
       of socialized medicine. Can you comment on that?

VH: Notice that I speak of tax-supported health care, because of this
       prejudice against the term "socialized medicine." But the De-
       partment of Veterans' Affairs *is* socialized medicine: the mili-
       tary services have free health care. The interesting thing is that
       in military medicine, health care providers are all salaried—it's
       not a fee-for-service system. People in the military, as well as
       many other employees of government agencies, have tax-
       supported health care. We should all be informed about how
       available tax-supported health care is for many, many groups in
       this country. It's a minority who don't have it. But for some
       reason or other, that minority, and the providers for those
       people who are willing to pay for health care, have dominated
       this country. As I said, a very large proportion of our citizens
       have tax-supported health care, and that is socialized medicine.
       What's more, almost all of these people are given copies of their
       health record, whereas the people who go to private physicians
       and hospitals can't get hold of their records. That record tells
       you more about your health than you could possibly learn in
       any other way. And it's withheld from you. It's very hard to
       understand this. We all ought to have a copy of our health
       record.
       I can tell you an interesting thing that's happening in Japan.
       If you are employed in Japan, you get wonderful health care
       through the health services set up for workers. Since it is
       common for women who get married in Japan to not work
       afterwards, many women live at home with their families. The
       government of Japan has decided that those people deserve
       better health care than they've been getting. So they have made
       a provision that doctors and nurses have to go together to see
       these women in their homes on a routine basis, and must mail
       the women a copy of their health record. There are wonderful
       things happening all over this world that we ought to know
       about and imitate. Of course, just as education is faulty every-
       where, so is health care, and it'll never cease to be a problem as
       to how to keep it adequate. It's going to be a long time before
       every country is entirely satisfied with the health care they get,
       but certainly the people of Canada, for instance, who have
       recently acquired a universally available health service, are very
       happy about it; they are very proud of it.

Q: I'd like to know how you would propose that we structure a
      tax-supported health care system. I'm a pediatric nurse and am
      very familiar with our high infant mortality rate, and the cost of
      having children in the neonatal intensive care unit. I'd like you
      to talk a bit about what a tax-supported health care system
      would support and how it would take the limited resources that
      we have and put them to best use. Should we support neonatal
      intensive care units and organ transplantation, or should we
      support prevention? Where should the money go?

VH: We should support all types of health care that are essential to
      the human race. Of course you pay for preventive care, and of
      course you pay for sick babies in the neonatal intensive care
      unit. Preventive care is not as dramatic as care when somebody
      is terribly sick. It's harder to sell it to people. But if we had
      preventive care, it would be much cheaper than curing people
      of all these terrible diseases or keeping them in a bed some-
      where for the rest of their lives with people running around
      waiting on them. It goes without saying that preventive care
      must be provided; then we provide care to people who get sick
      in spite of good preventive care.
         We have come to a point where the percentage of the gross
      national product spent on health care in this country is 11%. In
      Japan, it is about 5%. I can't give the figures for Canada,
      England, and Germany, but they are in between those figures.
      We are spending more money on health care in this country
      than any other country, and our health statistics are none too
      good. They live longer in Japan than we do here. And their
      maternal and infant statistics are better. In many places in this
      country, we cannot get doctors to allow us to practice nurse
      midwifery. The countries where nurse midwives can practice
      have far better statistics than we do in maternal and infant
      health. We like to blame somebody else, but it's my fault, it's
      your fault, it's all our faults. I know it's maddening when I say
      these things. But I think I'm telling you the truth.
         I say that if no doctor is present, and somebody needs help, it
      is up to the nurse to diagnose and treat the patient. And that's
      what they're doing, all over the world. So let's admit it, and
      let's prepare people to do it. I think you'll find that Canadian
      nurses go into the far reaches of Canada where doctors don't
      want to live and can't make too much money—they go and take
      care of people, and that's what they do: they diagnose and
      treat. Plenty of us live in communities where we are the best

prepared people to help others with their health problems. Also, I say if a person cannot get well, it's up to us to help them die well. Now, when you get to be my age, you'll realize that this is quite an interesting problem.

Q: Could you comment on third-party reimbursement for nurses' services?

VH: Well, I don't know why we want to get in deeper trouble than we're already in. We're in this trouble because doctors have insisted on fee for service. And what has that brought us?

Q: But nurses can only practice if they are provided with a salary—or if they look for, let's say, patients who are elderly and who are mainly on Medicare reimbursement. Otherwise, we have to work for someone, and that does not seem to promote independence in practice.

VH: I'm not saying we should be paid by anybody at all. I'm saying we must be salaried and that salaries must come as teachers' salaries do—from taxes. That's what I'm saying. I'm not sure whether this fee for service is good anyway. Let me just put it in very psychological and hateful language. If you are paid to see patients as long as they are sick, it pays you to keep them sick. It's as simple as that. I went to a doctor not very long ago because I had a rash on my arm, and he said, "Miss Henderson, I haven't the faintest idea what's the matter with you, but come back next week if you aren't better." And I thought to myself, why should I go back next week, and pay him another fee, to tell me that he hasn't any idea what's wrong with me? So I went to another doctor, and he looked at me, and he said, "Miss Henderson, that's ticks." Well, I know a tick or two and I knew it wasn't ticks, but he prescribed $32 worth of medicine not knowing what was wrong with me. Well, I have a very intelligent cousin who looked in the *Encyclopedia Britannica* and found this thing that we all get—we're very likely to get it in the country—Scabies, that's what I had. But the specialist in skin disease and the other doctor who seemed very intelligent gave me no help. Maybe if they had realized that they weren't going to get paid unless they found out what was wrong with me, they would have diagnosed it immediately.

We must walk that hard road of putting the welfare of the patient ahead of our own, taking unpopular views and positions, and changing things. We've got to assume more responsibility for changing health care in this country than we have. We've let other people tell us what we can do. That's what I think. I'm not stating a fact, it's an opinion.

Q: I work in a research-oriented institution, and our nursing practices are primarily based on medical research. What can I do to get my nurses to base their practice more on nursing research?

VH: How can we make nursing research interesting and attractive to nurses? I did my bit years ago. I was at Teachers College for 15 or 20 years; when I went there, I worked as an assistant to Martha Ruth Smith, who later became Dean of the School of Nursing at Boston University. She taught a very practical course that introduced nurses to research.

We divided the classes up into groups of four, and every group had to decide to study a particular procedure in nursing. They then divided into two subgroups, and presented two different ways of doing the procedure. That was easy, because almost all the hospitals they represented liked their own way of doing things and had perpetuated their own system for many years; so they were proud to show their way of doing it. The class as a whole was invited to raise questions about those two methods. After a while, it was evident that both methods were very open to questions and criticism. And so, from the discussions we collected a lot of clinical problems. For the rest of the course, each student did a little research on one of the problems.

From then on, I began thinking that all our work should have research applied to it. I no longer took any method for granted as the best. I think all those people who took this course really got excited about research; one student met me in the hall one day, waving something, and she'd gotten so excited that she had taken her research to Johnson & Johnson, and she'd gotten a response, and she was nearly dead with excitement—she felt she was on the verge of changing the whole practice of nursing. We were—hundreds of us, finally I suppose thousands—terribly excited about research.

Widespread interest in nursing research really began about midcentury. During that time, I went to about three fourths of the states and asked three questions of people: What research have you done on nursing? What research do you know about that we should know about? And if you had the resources, what problem would you study? What I discovered was that at least half of the studies being done had to do with the education of students. Everybody was interested in that. A large proportion of the studies done by nurses were not on the practice of nursing, but on the education of nurses. Now I wondered why in the world that was, and one of the guesses I hazarded was this: The people who should have been interested in helping us with the problems of how to help people were our most closely associated health workers—doctors. (You may be surprised when I say this. But doctors are the people who know most about the medical science underlying our practice.) They didn't come to help us with this job of making our practice research-based. Their practice is research-based, but the doctors didn't come to help us. The fact that doctors didn't want to help threw us on the mercy of the social scientists, and all nursing schools began to employ sociologists, anthropologists, and psychologists to help our students conduct research. They had to advise the students how to study problems; and it didn't take them ten minutes to persuade nurses to study something that belonged in the social science field rather than in the field of nursing, because they didn't know how to go into the clinical units and work with students on patient-centered problems. We should be grateful to the social scientists; they helped us the best they could, but actually we did ourselves a great disservice in giving up on the doctors and leaving them alone. They didn't want to help us; so we said, "All right, you go play your own game and we'll take care of ourselves." And for years, we have been turning out studies of problems that are not primarily the problems that nurses, in my opinion, should be concerned with.

Nursing still seems determined to go it alone. Nurses seem to be trying to take away from all other groups the help that they have been getting from those other groups. I don't like this. I don't like the competitive relationship between doctors and nurses. Who suffers from it? The public. Until we learn to be friends with doctors and work with doctors on the problems of patients, we are, in my opinion, going to be doing a disservice to humanity. Now I'm not telling you it's easy. It's hard, but let's stop being afraid of doctors, for one thing.

I'll tell you a little story. When I started teaching in Norfolk, Virginia, I was in my late 20s, I suppose, and a new group of students was coming. The Director of Nurses was named Miss Brickhouse. (I tried to help her a little bit by calling her "Brukus" but she didn't like that.) She was a tall, beautiful, blond woman, and she and I were partners in running this school. I said we ought to have a party for the students, and she said,

"Well, if you want to stick your neck out and ask Mr. Pender for money for a party you can, but I'm not going to do it." Well, I was foolish enough to stick my neck out, and Mr. Pender gave me a few dollars, I don't remember how much, and I had a party for the incoming students. I got a solarium fixed up like a cabaret, and I sent out an invitation announcing the opening of a cabaret at such and such an address, and I invited all the doctors, and asked them to come in their tuxedos, and when they came in their tuxedos I hung towels over their arms and told them they were the waiters. And they loved it, believe it or not. From then on, they began giving parties for the nurses. If I was anything at that place, I was a friend of the doctors. They knew I was going to give them trouble every now and then, but they were a wonderful support in trying to change things. The hospital was staffed entirely by nurses who had graduated from that school and who didn't want to change anything. They wanted to keep it the way it was, in its pristine glory. I realized that if I was going to do anything for the patients and for the students in that school, I would have to have the friendship of the doctors.

I do not think that nursing and medicine are so different. I think what makes us different is that nurses have assumed responsibility for 24-hour service, and doctors have not. Therefore, we know a lot more about the patient than they do, and we have many more opportunities to meet the patient's needs than the doctors do. But I think we share many tasks and many responsibilities, and the sooner we learn to work with doctors as partners, the better for the human race.

Q: Sometimes when we focus on independent practice, we focus on physician replacement rather than looking at what nurses can do: promoting health, identifying self-care needs in the patients, and providing health education. We have a lot to offer as nurses. There is a lot of pressure to be independent, but is it independent to do physician-related work?

VH: I take it you're arguing for greater separation of medicine and nursing than I'm advocating. You are suggesting that a nurse and a physician are two entirely different things. And I don't believe that. I believe that we are two related health workers trying to meet the health needs of the people. I wish we could get some different names for nurses and doctors, so that we could get rid of the idea that this is a doctor's task and that is a nurse's task. I would like to point to the nurse midwife as a pattern that we should be imitating in every field. By the way, I'll tell you an interesting thing about nurse midwives. Judith Kraus, Dean of the School of Nursing at Yale, was married to a Lutheran minister. And she got him so interested in her work, when she came home talking about it, that he decided to give up the ministry and be a nurse. And guess what kind of a nurse he has chosen to be? A nurse midwife. How do you like that? It's clear to me that the nurse midwife and obstetrician do the same thing. But the nurse midwife knows that in some cases, there are surgical procedures in connection with the birth of a child that he or she can't do. Now I think all of us ought to work toward this kind of a relationship with the physician in whatever clinical field we find ourselves in. I think it is a myth that the work of the doctor and the nurse are different. I don't see how the nurses in northern Canada, where there are no doctors, can say that what they're doing is doctor's work. It isn't doctor's work at all. It's the work of nurses who are trying to help people with their health problems. And if there are no doctors around to help them with these problems, what do you do? Just wash your hands of them? Or do you try to help them? Well, I think it's humane to try to help them. That's what nurses who work in the upper regions of Canada are doing. And that's what they're prepared to do. If you want to believe that doctors and nurses are different and their work is different, I cannot persuade you, but if there was anything I could do that would persuade you, I'd do it.

Q: Now that nursing faculty have to do research and write papers, what effect has that had on their teaching, or on them as teachers?

VH: Well, doctors have been doing that all these years. They've had to be involved in research and to teach and practice; and as a matter of fact, if you're really interested in health care in this country, I don't know how you can avoid getting involved in all three things—research, teaching, and practice.

Q: You have commented on the need for nursing to move in the direction of physicians and to become more research-based in practice, which we all agree we need to do. You said that physicians had done it all along, and they have. But sometimes physicians are viewed as not caring for patients, because they're involved in doing research. How can nurses become more involved in research without losing the caring that makes our profession stand out?

VH: If nurses believe that the welfare of the patient comes first, they can make the choice to give their time to patients. On the other hand, medicine is where it is today—technically effective in a great many areas—because of the research that doctors have done. I don't believe that the answer is to ask nurses to give up research. There are all kinds of ways we make decisions in this world—based on our intuition, based on practice that we observe, based on some authority who tells us what to do, and based on research. There's nothing mystical about "research." What research does is to supply observations and measurement of the results of what is done, and I don't see how we can give it up. It's imbedded in our thinking and in our practice.

    I have spent my life trying to validate what we do, looking for material, information, measurements, tests, to give us more confidence in what we're doing. So it has been a revelation to me, and in fact a blow to my professional pride, to see what nursing research has turned into. I see volumes coming out now that are reports of research, one after the other, and when I read them, or go and hear research reports, I'm deeply discouraged, because I can't stay awake!

Q: As a clinician in long-term care, I'm interested in your opinion of the care of the elderly now, and how you've seen that change over the years.

VH: I don't suppose anything has changed more than the care of the elderly, which has changed because Medicare has paid doctors to take care of old people. However, Medicare has been so abused that it's no longer meeting the needs of the elderly as we thought it would. I condemn this abuse, but I don't know how to stop it. I think it's wonderful that we have tax funds available to help old people; this has put them in a better position than the average middle-aged person. We also have Medicaid, which is supposed to help the indigent, but that's been abused, too. We seem to seesaw between groups who are getting more and less attention. What we want is a system that enables everybody to get what they need, but we must work for it. It's a hard life that we've chosen to lead, but terribly interesting.

Q: What are your thoughts about ambulatory care nursing today?

VH: We have made care in hospitals so expensive, with our DRG's, that we are now attempting to correct that by sending people home as soon as possible, or by treating people in ambulatory services. This too is being abused; often people who need institutionalized care are not getting it. I don't know any easy formulas to give you for accomplishing the things that seem to me to be needed. But I don't believe that the system of diagnostic related groups has settled the question of how long a person should stay in a hospital. People are being sent home now when they're very ill. I know a person who was sent home hemorrhaging. I know the person was hemorrhaging because I went to see her in the hospital and there was a great big spot of blood on the sheet, but before I knew it, she was being discharged. That's just one example, but I know that it's not rare these days. Of course I believe in home care, but I believe in fair, judicious use of institutions, too.

Q: I'm interested in your comments about the role that sociologists and psychologists have played in nursing. I know that we went through a period when our language was ambiguous; I can remember very well, for example, charting that "the patient apparently has ceased to breathe." It seems to me that we have continued that ambiguity in the development of nursing diagnoses, and I would like to have your comments on its use.

VH: My view of nursing diagnosis is so well known and so unpopular that I've been congratulating myself that I haven't gotten a question on it. I think it's one of the ways we are wasting most of our time. (Every time I say that, I get applause from the audience, so I must strike a familiar chord.) Nursing diagnosis is one of the most unfortunate things that's happened to us. Again, it is the nurse pulling away from the doctor, doing something different, establishing our own territory. If you are the patient, think how it must strike you to see the nurses working on something they think is wrong with you, while the doctors are working on something that they think is wrong with you but they're using different language to express it. I think it's perfectly absurd, so I advocate the work of a man named Lawrence Weed. He had the most beautiful system of medical care that I have seen. We stressed it in our book *Principles and Practices of Nursing*, and I advocate this for everybody. Weed had a questionnaire that he gave the patient—it contained hundreds of multiple-choice questions, and the patient answered on a computer. So he began with a tremendous amount of information about the patient. Now that's the first plus. Then he and the nurses worked together as a team—there was none of this nursing diagnosis and medical diagnosis; they worked together on what was wrong, the problems the patient faced. And they both had equal access to the patient's record. I don't know whether he gave the patient a copy of the record, but I would suspect he did. I have the greatest respect for Dr. Weed, and I marvel that there are many people who have never heard of him, because what he did would change the whole picture.

Q: You are such a wonderful role model for living one's elderly years, and I wondered if you could share the secrets of how we as nurses can live happy and productive elderly years as you have done.

VH: Thank you for the compliment; I wish that I felt I deserved it, but to myself I'm a physical wreck, so it's very hard for me to advise you to do what I've done. I can't possibly share my success with you, because I don't feel as if I've been so successful. You can see, I have to take a cane to walk and I fall down at the drop of a hat.

Audience: That certainly is the one thing that everyone in this room disagrees with you on.

VH: Thank you all, you've been a wonderful group to talk with, and I've enjoyed it very much. Good luck to everybody.

[3]

Managing Falls, Incontinence, and Cognitive Impairment: Nursing Research

Thelma J. Wells

Growing old is expected. It's the natural order, the ripening of the individual through the seasons of life. Most people want to grow old, though with the proviso that their lives be of quality and their deaths meaningful. It is the privilege of gerontological nursing to work with the elderly in their quest for quality and meaning.

Since 1900, the percentage of Americans age 65 or older has tripled. Currently, about 12.5% of the total population in this country is in this age group, and the projection for the year 2030 is that the elderly will make up 22% of Americans (American Association of Retired Persons, 1990). It is important to note that the elderly population is composed of different chronological age groups: the young-old (those between 65 and 84 years of age), and the old-old (those 85 and over). This latter group, the 85-plus group, is the fastest growing subset of the old. Between 1960 and 1990, the growth rate for the old-old was three times the overall elderly population growth. Within the 85-plus group are the centenarians, a special subset that has increased more than tenfold since 1950 (Spencer, Goldstein, & Taeuber, 1987). The age wave is on us and rising.

Examination of the gender and race variables contributing to life expectancy at birth and at age 65 highlights the dynamics of the old population. According to 1988 data, women outlive men, having a longer life expectancy both at birth and at age 65 (U. S. Department of Health and Human Services [DHHS], 1990). Since the elderly population is composed mainly of women, gerontology is and will continue to be principally about women. So strong is the gender factor that it outweighs the significant socioeconomic variance imbedded in race, placing the life expectancy of black females (73.4 years) ahead of that for white males (72.3 years) (in 1988, white females had the longest life expectancy at birth—78.9 years, while black males had the lowest, 64.9 years). Projections for the years 2000 to 2050 estimate about a one-year increase in life expectancy at birth for males, but a six-year increase for females.

There are also gender differences in the living conditions of the elderly (Schick, 1986). Most of the old population live in private households, but men are more likely to be living with a spouse whereas women are more likely to live alone. While only 5% of the old are in nursing homes, the risk of institutionalization increases with age (DHHS, 1981). The typical nursing home resident is a white female in her late 80s.

The majority of the old are active community members and consider themselves to be in good to excellent health (DHHS, 1990). However, there are racial differences in health self-assessment, with more blacks than whites reporting themselves in fair to poor health.

Two major problems of the elderly are chronic conditions and dependence. Arthritis is the most common chronic condition in the old, followed by hypertension, hearing impairment, heart disease, and cataracts (National Center for Health Statistics, 1990). It is important to note that chronic disease develops across the life span but displays its long-term outcomes during old age. For example, arthritis progresses through multiple stages over 55 or more years, beginning as early as age 20. Lifestyle factors interact with this progression; for example, lifestyle may contribute to weight gain, a factor accentuating the disease process. Nurses should play an active role in promoting healthy lifestyles across the life span, for educating people about healthy behaviors can delay chronic disease and limit its eventual impact.

Dependence, or reliance on someone else for support or aid, increases with age (National Center for Health Statistics, 1990). Within the nursing home population, the level of dependence is measured as the degree of need for assistance with activities of daily living. The level of need is greater than in the community but follows similar patterns (DHHS, 1989). Of foremost importance is the fact that all activities of daily living are environmentally interactive—that is, the design of equipment, clothing, furniture, and space affects dependence. For example, bathing dependence is related to ease of getting in and out of a tub, while dressing dependence is related to size and location of buttons and zippers. Thus, some environmental change might reduce dependence.

Factors such as type of chairs, whether beds are height adjustable, availability of commodes, and distances to toilets have a great impact on dependence.

Elder care requires an understanding of complex interactions with multiple potential intervention points: normal aging involves a gradual mix of physiological, social, and psychological changes within a nonspecific time frame and with individual variance. The sum of this normal aging defines the old. Superimposed on normal aging is life-style, which exists on a continuum from very healthy to very unhealthy. Also superimposed is chronic illness—that is, disease acquired at earlier life stages and brought into old age. Further, there is always the potential for acute illness, especially infectious processes and sudden traumas. And there are always life crises such as the death of significant others, and common life stresses such as problems related to finances or housing. The environment—space, objects, and people—has a mix of positive and negative impacts. The bottom line is function: the ability to do the things a person needs to do such as eating and toileting, and also the ability to do the things a person wants to do such as smelling the flowers and visiting friends. Function is the pulse beat of gerontological nursing. Mobility, urine control, and cognition are considered the three functional areas of major concern.

The changes in mobility that occur with aging include a wider base of support (i.e., the feet are placed wider apart as a result of an altered center of gravity due to height reductions); shorter steps and reduced compensatory arm movements due to decreased hip and spine flexibility; and increased postural sway due to neurological and musculoskeletal decrement (Bottomley et al., 1990).

Rather than focus on immobility, gerontological nurses now direct their energy to mobility and falls. This is a mark of great progress. It demonstrates a belief in mobility for elderly patients and a desire to understand the possible consequence of mobility—falls. In the not too distant past, institutional falls were considered an oddity and a reflection of poor care, since the elderly were supposed to be bedfast or chairfast. Lack of institutional falls is now an oddity, suggesting a poor rehabilitation program.

The issue of falls in the elderly is complex. First, one must consider the normal consequences of age. Perceptual loss is a significant factor; the elderly often need help to see where they are walking. And even when standing still, a situation in which the person actually sways, decreased vision increases the magnitude of sway. Mobility changes plus environmental effects, such as foot–floor friction, combine to increase the risk of falling with age.

To complicate matters, falls can also be a sign of disease, either an initial presentation of a disease or a result of its treatment. For example, it is not uncommon to find that a fractured hip results from cardiac arrhythmia. That is, the arrhythmia triggers a transient cerebral ischemia, which in turn causes a fall, resulting in fracture. Or pharmacologic treatment may include a host of drugs that potentially contribute to falls. Often, multiple factors interact to cause falls.

Falls may also be a symptom of related functional problems: toenails must be kept short; ingrown nails and corns are problematic; shoes must be adequate. Pain from a dysfunctional foot or joint can be a contributory factor. In addition, confused people may misjudge their ability to discern their surroundings, thus increasing the potential for falls. Urinary frequency, especially nocturia and urgency, are associated risks since they cause old people to rush to the toilet. Further, floors wet with urine increase environmental risk.

To date, nursing research related to falls has been primarily descriptive. In this early phase of research, key factors are being noticed and relationships explored. There has been some work done to identify risk profiles of non-fallers, fallers, and repeat fallers in an effort to develop assessment tools that are predictive of falls. This descriptive base is also providing a beginning basis for developing effective preventive actions.

The second major area of concern for the gerontological nurse is urinary control. The significant changes in urine control that occur with age include decreased bladder capacity and voiding delay, increased postvoid residual, and uninhibited contractions (Resnick & Wells, 1990). It should be emphasized that there is nothing inherent in the aging process that causes incontinence as a normal outcome: the changes generally suggest a neurological decrement and are influenced by many factors.

Urinary incontinence may be a simple, transient problem—the consequence of fluid intake, such as drinking large amounts of caffeinated beverages; the result of medication, such as a muscle relaxant that affects the external urethral sphincter; a side effect of drugs that alter the sensorium; or a result of diuretic agents. Urinary tract infection probably plays a secondary rather than a primary role; infection typically makes an incontinence problem worse. Usually its resolution improves, but does not cure, the incontinence. Other transient causes include fecal impaction, improperly positioned pessaries, and associated urethritis. Basically, transient causes are fairly simple to evaluate and treat.

Complex, established incontinence problems can arise from varied etiologies. The most common etiologies in the aged are (1) stress, particularly among women, which causes leakage on exertion, such as laughing or coughing; (2) urge, which is experienced by both sexes, especially among the old-old, and is experienced as urine loss with strong urgency and little warning; (3) mixed causes seen in females as combined stress and urge incontinence; and (4) overflow, or urine loss as a constant dribble made worse by exertion, as in male benign prostatic hypertrophy, but also arising from neurologic causes in both sexes. A diagnosis is usually based on a careful review of the medical history and a thorough physical examination that includes postvoid residual and simplified bladder testing. Reasonable referral criteria have been developed to detect individuals who need further evaluation. There are many treatment options, including behavioral, pharmacologic, and surgical intervention.

There are two common conditions underlying the classification "functional incontinence," a term applied to those who, on evaluation, have no simple or complex cause for incontinence but do exhibit some other behavioral reason for wetting. These behavioral reasons include confusion—difficulty in finding the toilet, difficulty knowing what to do in the toilet, or even difficulty in recognizing bladder signals as the precursor to toileting; and immobility—whether from pain, paralysis, or restraint—which clearly prevents responsive, self-initiated toileting. Some elderly have dysfunctional voiding; that is, they do not wet themselves but they toilet frequently, voiding as often as three times an hour. While technically not incontinent, they constitute an important subset of people with urine-control problems.

As with falls, the primary focus of nursing research on urinary incontinence was until recently descriptive, with some attention given to assessment tools. But there is now a growing body of work on behavioral treatments being evaluated in clinical trials. Research is needed on risk profiles, prevention, and chronic-care settings.

A final area of concern in the functioning of the elderly is cognition. Cognitive changes in aging are generally agreed to be decremental (Feldman & Lopez, 1982). Memory can be viewed as a three-level information storage system—primary brief coding, very short-term sensory storage, and long-term secondary storage. The greatest changes occur in the short- and long-term storage levels, with less change at the primary brief coding level. Sensorimotor and cognitive speed, as well as problem solving, also decrease with age.

The research findings on cognitive changes need to be viewed with considerable caution. First, there is great individual variance, which raises important questions about any conclusions drawn about cognitive changes with age. Second, multiple interrelated factors are known to affect cognitive outcomes, such as state of health, motivation, pacing, and practice. Studies of the multiple factors are particularly useful because the information can be used to guide development of teaching strategies. Third, and perhaps most important, age-related decrements in cognition are of modest magnitude. Most elders find that taking a few minutes longer to recall a memory or complete a jigsaw puzzle does not affect lifestyle.

The major type of cognitive impairment seen in the elderly is termed "confusion," meaning that the observer perceives the behavior or speech of another as inappropriate. It is important to bear in mind that initially, it may be the observer who is confused, who has mis-interpreted or failed to understand. When I am the observer, I com-monly say, "I'm confused. You said ___, but I think ___. Can you straighten me out?" And sometimes the situation is clarified, and no one is confused. At other times the confusion shifts away from me, the observer, and becomes more clearly a problem of the person I observe.

Confusion may be simple and transient, such as that arising from sensory misperception. Decreased vision due to common visual field abnormalities or diminished lens accommodation, increased lens opac-ity, or slower light/dark adaptation can significantly reduce sensory input. Commonly, high-frequency hearing loss creates disrupted hear-ing, making it easy to misinterpret conversations. These sensory changes, combined with the stress of illness and strange environments, create a high probability for perceptual confusion.

Sometimes, confusion-like symptoms can result from a short-term affective disorder, such as depression. Depression is a common reaction to cumulative loss and to the acknowledgment of an unpleasant reality; it may also be more complex and profound. In either case, depressed old people may simply not be interested in playing reality-testing games or in attending to usual and expected behaviors. Thus, depression can mask itself as confusion.

Confusion can also be a symptom of a related problem. For example, there is a report of an elderly man who presented in a confused state due to sleep deprivation caused by urinary frequency (Kelly & Feigenbaum, 1982). Acute head injury after a fall can also present as confusion if a slow cerebral bleed accumulates to a critical threshold.

Acute confusion is also a likely outcome of physiological instability. Transient physiological stress, arising from dehydration, drug effects, or metabolic imbalance, can create a massive assault on cerebral homeosta-sis in the old. These physiological crises are so common that one should wonder why more old people in grave physiological distress are not confused, rather than why so many are.

All of these transient confusion problems are by definition short-term, reversible states. But they are very frightening to the old, are alarming to their families, and frequently initiate repressive and inappropriate care on the part of uninformed caregivers. Therefore it is important for the nurse to view them very seriously.

Complex chronic cognitive impairment problems are those arising from diagnosed progressive dementias or other nonreversible processes that are destructive to the central nervous system. Fears of these tragic diseases haunt the old. Such fears are justified among the old-old since the prevalence of these disorders increases markedly in the 85-and-over age group.

As one might expect, nursing research on cognitive impairment has been primarily descriptive, noting key factors and relationships among patients in acute care settings. While the data base in general is limited, it may now be adequate for intervention studies. Researchers have also begun to examine chronic care settings as sites for clinical studies.

I hope that we are at last moving forward in the struggle to provide quality care to elders. I believe that practice directs research and research directs education. That is, questions arising from practice should direct our research. Knowledge gained in research should provide the educational bases for curriculum. New knowledge tested and used in practice will generate further questions. And so the spiral moves upward, tracing a path to quality nursing care.

REFERENCES

American Association of Retired Persons. (1990). *A profile of older Americans.* Washington, DC: American Association of Retired Persons.

Bottomley, J. M., Blakeney, B., O'Malley, T., Satin, D. G., Smith, H., & Howe, M. C. (1990). Rehabilitation and mobility of older persons: An interdisciplinary perspective. In S. Brody & L. Pawlson (Eds.), *Aging and rehabilitation II* (pp. 77–94). New York: Springer.

Feldman, H. S., & Lopez, M. A. (1982). *Developmental psychology for the health care professions, Part 2: Adulthood and aging.* Boulder CO: Westview Press.

Kelly, J., & Feigenbaum, L. (1982). Another cure for reversible dementia: Sleep deprivation due to prostatism. *Journal of the American Geriatrics Society, 30,* 645–646.

National Center for Health Statistics. (1990). *Current estimates from the National Interview Survey, 1989* (Centers for Disease Control, Series 10, No. 176). Hyattsville, MD: U. S. Government Printing Office.

Resnick, N. M., & Wells, T. J. (1990). Maintaining and restoring continence. In S. Brody & L. Pawlson (Eds.), *Aging and rehabilitation II* (pp. 211–230). New York: Springer.

Schick, F. L. (Ed). (1986). *Statistical handbook on aging Americans.* Phoenix, AZ: Oryx Press.

Spencer, G., Goldstein, A., & Taeuber, C. (1987). *America's centenarians.* Washington, DC: U. S. Department of Health and Human Services.

U. S. Department of Health and Human Services. (1989). *Nursing home utilization by current residents: United States, 1985* (Vital and Health Statistics, Series 13, No. 102) (DHHS Publication No. PHS 89-1763). Hyattsville, MD: U.S. Government Printing Office.

U. S. Department of Health and Human Services, The Federal Council on Aging. (1981). *The need for long term care.* Washington, DC: Office of Human Development Services.

U. S. Department of Health and Human Services, Public Health Service, Centers or Disease Control, National Center for Health Statistics. (1990). *Health United States, 1989* (DHHS Publication No. PHS 90-1232). Hyattsville, MD: U. S. Government Printing Office.

SUGGESTED ADDITIONAL READINGS

Falls

Gibson, M. J. (1987, April) Gerontology special supplement series, No. 4: The prevention of falls in later life [Focused issue]. *Danish Medical Bulletin, 34*(4).

Whedon, M. B., & Shedd, P. (1989). Prediction and prevention of patient falls. Image: *Journal of Nursing Scholarship, 22,* 108–114.

Woolarott, M. (Ed.). (1990, January). Balance and falls [Focused issue]. *Topics in Geriatrics Rehabilitation, 5*(2).

Urinary Incontinence

Diokno, A., & Kennedy, A. (Eds.). (1989, March). Gerontology special supplement series, No. 8: Management of urinary incontinence of the elderly [Focused issue]. *Danish Medical Bulletin, 36*(8).

Knebl, J. (Ed.). (1990). Urinary incontinence [Focused issue]. *Southwestern, 6*(2).

National Institutes of Health Consensus Development Conference on Urinary Incontinence. (1990). The October 1988 papers. *Journal of the American Geriatrics Society, 38,* 263–386.

Confusion

Abraham, J., Buckwalter, K., & Neundorfer, M. (Eds.). (1988, March). Alzheimer's Disease [Focused issue]. *The Nursing Clinics of North America, 23*(1).

Cohen, G. D. (1988). *The brain in human aging.* New York: Springer.

Foreman, M. D. (1986). Acute confusional states in hospitalized elderly: A research dilemma. *Nursing Research, 35,* 34–38.

[4]

Using Research in Practice

Linda R. Cronenwett

The ultimate purpose of nursing research is to improve nursing practice. You have the opportunity, in reading the research reports presented here, to consider whether or not the research is relevant and substantial enough to warrant changes in *your* practice. In this chapter, I will review the definitions of research use and suggest strategies that you might use to decide whether the findings are ready to move into practice.

DEFINITIONS OF RESEARCH USE

In other fields, experts in research utilization have delineated two forms of research use: decision-driven and knowledge-driven models (Caplan, 1979; Weiss, 1980). The decision-driven models are the form of research use we most commonly think of when we talk about integrating research and practice. The basic assumption is that research is used when new knowledge is used to formulate a policy, procedure, or program. The critical point here is that the review and integration of the scientific base lead to some decision, course of action, or outcome.

Many nurses have been exposed to decision-driven models of research use such as the Conduct and Utilization of Research in Nursing (CURN) Project (1983) and the videotapes from Horn Video Productions (1987, 1989). Using these models, a clinical problem is identified, the relevant literature is found and critiqued, and new protocols for practice are developed, implemented, and evaluated. This form of research use is crucial to our profession. It is also complex, involving political, organizational, and attitudinal components in addition to the existence of research that is relevant to practice.

The knowledge-driven or conceptual model of research use is characterized by the influence of research findings on *thinking*, as opposed to decisions or immediate actions. From this point of view, you use research when you attend a research conference or read a research journal. In the process, you expose yourself to new knowledge, not necessarily with a specific practice problem in mind, but to stay abreast of what questions are being asked in your field, what hypotheses are being generated by initial findings, and what innovations have been developed and tested. You might be stimulated by an assessment instrument or a new theory instead of feeling a need to apply the findings of a particular study. Weiss and her colleagues (1980) have referred to this view of research use as "knowledge creep." They propose that research is, in fact, "used," even when there is no immediate application to practice. The function of this form of research use is to keep you open to new information and ready to formulate new policies or question the assumptions of old programs.

As you read this book, you will certainly use research, looking at it from the knowledge-driven model point of view. You will become aware of the questions being asked about three areas of nursing practice. You may learn about some theory or approach that makes you think about other nursing problems in a new light. If you are not satisfied with the state of the science, you may decide to conduct a study yourself. On the other hand, maybe your current care plans, critical paths, or practice guidelines are soundly based on current knowledge, according to the studies presented. The effect of the book, then, may be for you to redouble your efforts to see that all patients receive the best standard of care. Any of these outcomes will be valuable.

Because this book includes a summary of the science on the three topics of interest—falls, incontinence, and cognitive impairment—and these summaries are presented along with the newest research, you have an excellent basis for determining whether you want to take some action to change practice in your setting. So let's proceed with a discussion about how to assess new knowledge for its applicability to your practice.

NEED FOR CHANGE IN YOUR SETTING

First of all, does anyone perceive a need for change in practice in your setting? To perceive such a need, someone must be open to the possibility of change. What is the culture among the nurses and managers with whom you work? Is there an openness to the idea of change based on scientific information?

When change is considered, who plans the change? Are the staff who will implement the change involved in the planning? Is anyone in your work group familiar with theoretical models of research utilization (such as those reviewed by Crane, 1985)? Have you talked about what models seem to work best among your colleagues: problem-solving models, linkage models, social interaction models, or research and development models? Have you experimented with research-use activities using guidelines from the CURN Project (1983), Stetler and Marram (1976) (or Stetler & DiMaggio, 1991), or Goode, Lovett, Hayes, and Butcher (1987)? If not, you may decide that the biggest need for change in your setting is the need to change the culture. You may want to pick one innovation and use it to create a model for research-based change in your setting. If so, consider choosing an innovation with these characteristics: a clear advantage over past practice, compatibility with current staff values and norms, low complexity, ease of experimentation on a limited basis, and highly visible outcomes (Rogers, 1983). Pick one important and sellable idea and begin the process of changing your culture.

If your colleagues are used to the idea of change, it will still enhance your ability to use research-based findings if there is some preexisting evidence of a need for change. Have you had a set of patient complaints that struck a common theme? Have your quality assessment activities uncovered a problem? Have you been achieving less than ideal outcomes from certain interventions or critical paths? Have some newly hired staff members mentioned that your approaches to certain practice problems differ from what they did in another setting? Have you been seeing an increase in problems such as falls, incontinence, or confusion, and thus may have an increased readiness among staff to try something new? Proposed practice changes are likely to be welcomed if a perceived need for change exists. You may want to focus initial planning efforts on activities that will heighten your colleagues' perceptions of the need for change.

READINESS OF THE RESEARCH FOR PRACTICE

The other critical component necessary for change in practice is the readiness of the science. Even if everyone agrees that current practice could be improved, you want to be sure that there is sufficient scientific evidence for any change you propose. How do you know when the scientific evidence provides a clear rationale for a change in practice?

You start formulating your opinion by reading what the investigators say in the opening and concluding sections of their reports. Do they summarize a group of studies from which findings converge to support a change in practice? Or do the investigators indicate that this was the first and only study with the reported findings? How similar are the characteristics of the people studied to the patients with whom you work? How similar is the study's environment to the setting in which you work? If several investigative teams have concluded that the evidence for a change in practice is fairly clear and if studies have been conducted with patients who resemble your own, in settings similar to your own, you have strong support for a change in your practice.

The extent of the evidence required for change may vary depending on the needs of your practice setting. Let's consider, for example, how the evaluation of the research base might differ, depending on whether you are trying to affect nurses' sensitivity to patient experiences, methods of assessment, or interventions.

Sensitivity to Patient Experiences

Healthy nurses may have no idea what it feels like to experience a particular illness or surgery, or to care for someone who has that experience. Even when the nurse is knowledgeable about the medical and nursing facts of the situation, he or she may know little about human responses to the illness experience, the symptoms or reactions with which the patient and family have to cope, or the resources available to assist recovery or adaptation. In the last 5–10 years, nurse researchers have studied the experiences of patients and their families using qualitative research methods. When you read these research reports, your practice changes in terms of sensitivity to patient cues, styles of assessment or teaching, and even intervention. In this book, you will see a report by Cleary of how caregivers experience the strain of caring for Alzheimer's patients and a report by Evans of what it feels like to be restrained.

There is rarely a large body of replicated work about patient experiences. But you *will* use what you read because the impact comes from reading the report. You see the actual words of patients and families, and these words lead you to do a better job of eliciting your own patients' experiences and perceptions. As a result, you will understand your patients and families better than you have in the past, and you will plan your nursing care differently—and thus change your practice. There are few risks to such use of research; and your increased sensitivity should benefit your practice.

Methods of Assessment

You will also see reports of studies whose primary aim was to establish the reliability and validity of various methods of assessment (for example, see the chapters by Neelon et al. and Vermeersch in this volume). Some instruments are developed solely for research purposes, but most are designed to serve clinical purposes. To assess the readiness of these instruments for use in practice, you need to know how to evaluate the reliability and validity of the instruments. The researchers give you that information in their reports; if you do not understand, write to the authors and ask whether and under what conditions the instrument is ready for clinical assessment purposes.

If you are interested in trying the instrument in practice, you can write and ask the researcher if further data are being collected or desired. Usually you can obtain a copy of the instrument and directions for its use in exchange for forwarding your data to the investigator. If you have a population of patients who differ from the sample used by the investigator, there would be benefits to collaboration for both of you. Perhaps the investigator would analyze your data using the same techniques as were used in the original studies. Both you and the investigator would then know whether the instrument works as well in your population and environment as it did with other patient samples.

A final issue regarding instruments is how much will be gained at what cost; that is, what are the relative benefits of making the assessment compared to the costs in patient and staff time that will be necessary to perform and document the assessment? One also has to ask if the assessment will affect some outcome. Data collected for data collection's sake alone will be unlikely to be worth the labor costs; however, if the assessment will lead to new interventions, and these interventions improve patient outcomes, the instrument can be considered ready for use in terms of its cost/benefit ratio.

Interventions

Generally, scientific findings that appear to provide a rationale for changing nursing interventions require the most careful critique and evaluation of the research base. Again, particular attention must be paid to the issues of fit between the settings and samples studied and the populations and settings in which the findings will be applied. In addition, you should consider the following questions (Stetler & Marram, 1976) as you decide the extent of further effort you can or must devote to evaluating the research base:

1. Do you have a theoretical or scientific basis for your current practice?
2. How effective is your current method of practice?
3. What degree of potential risk could be associated with the implementation of the new findings?

For example, let's consider the early findings of Holtzclaw (1990) about the effect on the shivering associated with a patient's chemotherapy of terrycloth wraps to the extremities. Certainly, her early report was unreplicated and pertained only to a small sample of patients. Should the results of such a study be used?

First, you could ask if there is a theoretical or scientific rationale for current methods of helping patients with the discomforts of shivering. Are nurses experimenting with comfort measures or providing only medications as ordered? If no interventions are currently being tried or if the current interventions are ineffective (that is, not diminishing the shivering), you can move to consideration of risk. What level of risk would be associated with wrapping a patient's arms and legs with terrycloth? If the risk is minimal, then it is reasonable to consider applying these research findings yourself and evaluating the results of your trial in the same way you would evaluate an idea that came from any other source or way of knowing, such as intuition, logic, or problem-solving.

Your ideas for research-based changes in practice will require significantly more evidence and evaluation if the current basis for practice is effective and risk-free and is believed to be based on scientific evidence. Recently, for example, multiple investigators have studied the relative effectiveness of heparinized saline versus saline as a flushing solution for intermittent infusion devices (Goode et al., 1991). Because providers believed that there was scientific evidence demonstrating the benefit of using heparinized saline and because there is always risk involved in a clogged line, nurses needed evidence to demonstrate the effectiveness of saline, even though the change would decrease both supply and labor costs. At this point, we even have the editor of a nursing research journal calling for this well-justified change in practice (Downs, 1991).

Depending on the characteristics of the change in practice you are considering, your need for evaluation of the research base may be accomplished by the work presented in this book. However, if your innovation is perceived as risky, if it involves withholding care that is currently considered standard practice, if implementation would require changes in policies or procedures, if new equipment or supplies would be required, or if implementation would be impossible without the support of other health care providers, then you are likely to have to expend greater effort to collect, evaluate, and make a case for the quality of the research base that supports your innovation.

Integrating a body of research literature into a coherent argument for a practice innovation is no small task. If you have had training to critique a research base as a part of your education and you have some flexibility regarding how you spend your work time, follow up on your ideas from this volume by conducting your own review and critique of the litera-ture. In our society in particular, nothing establishes expertise on a topic as well as an intimate familiarity with the research base. By reviewing the literature yourself, you also have the advantage of being exposed to other ideas, other nuances of the same idea, or other strategies or suggestions for practice that perhaps haven't yet occurred to you.

If you feel uncomfortable with your ability to find or critique a re-search base, does that mean you can't use your ideas for changing practice? No. Just choose different strategies for this phase of the pro-cess. Here are some ideas:

1. Find a colleague in your setting who *is* responsible for reviewing research and proposing research-based innovations—a clinical nurse specialist, a director of research, the chair of your practice or standards committee, a staff development instructor, or a nurse with advanced education who works on your unit. Share your ideas with this person and request help in the evaluation of the research base. Offer to call the investigators whose studies set you thinking about change and ask them to assist in the process of finding the studies that deserve consideration. Ask your colleague to lead a discussion of the articles with you and other nurses on your unit.

2. Contact a faculty member in your specialty at your local School of Nursing. See if you can set up a process whereby a student is assigned to assist in evaluating a specified research base as a part of fulfilling the requirements for a research course. If that's not possible, maybe the faculty member would do the evaluation for you in return for your giving one or two lectures to his or her students.

3. If you have no access to nursing colleagues who are able and willing to assist you in the review process, do the best job you can to collect all the pertinent articles related to the innovation, and then ask a colleague from another discipline to validate your understanding of the implications for practice to be derived from this research base.

Although this chapter includes a number of ideas about when and how to evaluate the research base for a change in practice, and although you are encouraged to try innovations that are low risk and do not compete with current practices that are effective and well supported by scientific findings, there is one caveat that must be considered. Practices once adopted are difficult to change (Dixon, 1990). You should be cautious about implementing an expensive intervention without a full evaluation of its effectiveness. Just as we are today reluctant to take the heparin out of flushing solutions, we might be reluctant someday to remove your innovation from practice.

SUMMARY

The challenge to you as you read the chapters of this book is to think broadly about your practice. As you read, make notes about all ideas that come to mind. Without a doubt, you will use research in at least one of the ways described in this chapter. Hopefully, you will evaluate the science base for one or more practice changes that you are willing to consider. When you complete your reading and evaluation of the science, you may be ready to make a specific practice change. For further reading on the "how to's" of research utilization, additional references are appended. Remember to keep notes on your experiences so that you can share the results with others. In the next decade, how we use research will be as important as the knowledge generation activities themselves.

REFERENCES

Caplan, N. (1979). The two-communities theory and knowledge utilization. *American Behavioral Scientist, 22,* 259–470.

Crane, J. (1986). Research utilization: Theoretical perspectives. *Western Journal of Nursing Research, 7,* 261–268.

CURN Project (Horsley, J. A., Crane, J., Crabtree, M. K., & Wood, D. J.) (1983). *Using research to improve nursing practice: A guide.* New York: Grune & Stratton.

Dixon, A. S. (1990). The evolution of clinical policies. *Medical Care, 28,* 201–220.

Downs, F. S. (1991). How to make a difference. *Nursing Research, 40,* 323.

Goode, C. J., Lovett, M. K., Hayes, J. E., & Butcher, L. A. (1987). Use of research-based knowledge in clinical practice. *Journal of Nursing Administration, 17*(12), 11–18.

Goode, C. J., Titler, M., Rakel, B., Ones, D. S., Kleiber, C., Small, S., & Triolo, P. K. (1991). A meta-analysis of effects of heparin flush and saline flush: Quality and cost implications. *Nursing Research, 40,* 324–330.

Holtzclaw, B. J. (1990). Effects of extremity wraps to control drug-induced shivering: A pilot study. *Nursing Research, 39,* 280–283.

Horn Video Productions. (1987). *Using research in clinical nursing practice* [film]. Ida Grove, IA: Horn Video Productions.

Horn Video Productions. (1989). *Research utilization: A process of organizational change* [film]. Ida Grove, IA: Horn Video Productions.

Rogers, E. M. (1983). *Diffusion of innovations.* New York: Free Press.

Stetler, C. B., & DiMaggio, G. (1991). Research utilization among clinical nurse specialists. *Clinical Nurse Specialist, 5* 151–155.

Stetler, C., & Marram, G. (1976). Evaluating research findings for applicability in practice. *Nursing Outlook, 24,* 559–563.

Weiss, C. H. (1980). Knowledge creep and decision accretion. *Knowledge: Creation, diffusion, utilization, 1,* 381–404

ADDITIONAL REFERENCES

ANA Commission on Nursing Research. (1981). *Guidelines for the investigative function of nurses.* Kansas City, MO: ANA.

Barnard, K. E. (1980). Knowledge for practice: Directions for the future. *Nursing Research, 29,* 208–212.

Beal, J. A., & Love, C. F. (Eds.). *Nursing Scan in Research.* Hagerstown, MD: J. B. Lippincott, (1988–present, bimonthly).

Brett, J. L. (1987). Use of nursing practice research findings. *Nursing Research, 36,* 344–349.

Brett, J. L. (1989). Organizational integrative mechanisms and adoption of innovations by nurses. *Nursing Research, 38,* 105–110.

Breu, C., & Dracup, K. (1985). Implementing nursing research in a critical care setting. *Journal of Nursing Administration, 6* (12), 14–17.

Buckwalter, K. C. (1985). Is nursing research used in practice? In J. C. McCloskey & H. K. Grace (Eds.), *Current issues in nursing* (2nd ed., pp. 110–123). London: Blackwell Scientific Publishers.

Burns, N., & Grove, S. K. (1987). *The practice of nursing research: Conduct, critique and utilization.* Philadelphia: W. B. Saunders.

Champion, V. L., & Leach, A. (1989). Variables related to research utilization for nursing: An empirical investigation. *Journal of Advanced Nursing, 14,* 705–710.

Connelly, C. E. (1986). Replication research in nursing. *International Journal of Nursing Studies, 23,* 71–77.

Coyle, L. A., & Sokop, A. G. (1990). Innovation adoption behavior among nurses. *Nursing Research, 39,* 176–180.

Crane, J. (1985). Research utilization—nursing models. *Western Journal of Nursing Research, 7,* 494–497.

Cronenwett, L. R. (1986). Research contributions of clinical nurse specialists. *Journal of Nursing Administration, 16*(6), 6–7.

Cronenwett, L. R. (1987). Research utilization in practice settings. *Journal of Nursing Administration, 17* (7–8), 9–10.

Cronenwett, L. R. (1988). Disseminating research to clinicians. *CNR* (Newsletter of the ANA Council of Nurse Researchers), *15* (1), 1,3.

Cronenwett, L. R. (1990). Improving practice through research utilization. In S. Funk, E. Tornquist, M. Champagne, L. Copp, & R. Wiese (Eds.), *Key aspects of recovery: Improving nutrition, rest, and mobility* (p. 7–22). New York: Springer.

Cruise, M. J., Alderman, M. C., & Gorenberg, B. D. (1989). Facilitating research utilization: A model for nurse managers. *Nursing Connections, 2,* 53–61.

Curlette, W. L., & Cannella, K. S. (1985). Going beyond the narrative summarization of research finding: The meta-analysis approach. *Research in Nursing & Health, 8,* 293–301.

Edwards-Beckett, J. (1990). Nursing research utilization techniques. *Journal of Nursing Administration, 20*(11), 25–30.

Fetter, M. S., Feetham, S. L., D'Apolito, K., Chaze, B. A., Fink, A., Frink, B. B., Hougart, M. K., & Rushton, C. H. (1989). Randomized clinical trials: Issues for researchers. *Nursing Research, 38,* 117–120.

Firlit, S. L., Kemp, M. G., & Walsh, M. (1986). Preparing master's students to develop clinical trials. *Western Journal of Nursing Research, 8,* 106–109.

Firlit, S. L., Kemp, M. G., & Walsh, M. (1987). Nursing research in practice: A survey of research utilization content in master's degree programs. *Western Journal of Nursing Research, 9,* 612–617.

Funk, S. G., Champagne, M. T., Wiese, R. A., & Tornquist, E. M. (1991). Barriers to using research findings in practice: The clinician's perspective. *Applied Nursing Research, 4,* 90–95.

Funk, S. G., Tornquist, E. M., & Champagne, M. T. (1989). A model for improving the dissemination of nursing research. *Western Journal of Nursing Research, 11,* 361–367.

Haller, K. B., Reynolds, M. A., & Horsley, J. A. (1979). Developing research-based innovation protocols: Process, criteria, and issues. *Research in Nursing and Health, 2,* 45–51.

Havelock, R. G. (1969). *Planning for innovation through dissemination and utilization of knowledge.* Ann Arbor: Center for Research on Utilization of Scientific Knowledge, ISR, University of Michigan.

Havelock, R. G. (1972). *Research-user linkage and social problem solving.* Ann Arbor: Center for Research of Utilization of Scientific Knowledge, ISR, University of Michigan.

Havelock, R. G. (1973). *The change agent's guide to innovation in education.* Englewood Cliffs, NJ: Education Technology Publications.

Horsley, J. A. (1985). Using research in practice: The current context. *Western Journal of Nursing Research, 7,* 135–139.

Horsely, J. A., & Crane, J. (1986). Factors associated with innovation in nursing practice. *Family and Community Health, 9,* 1–11.

Janken, J. K., Dufanlt, M. A., & Yeaw, E. M. S. (1988). Research roundtables: Increasing student/staff nurse awareness of the relevance of research to practice. *Journal of Professional Nursing, 4,* 186–191.

Ketefian, S. (1975). Application of selected nursing research findings into nursing practice: A pilot study. *Nursing Research, 34,* 89–92.

King, D., Barnard, K. E., & Hoehn, R. (1981). Disseminating the results of nursing research. *Nursing Outlook, 19,* 164–169.

Kirchhoff, K. T. (1982). A diffusion survey of coronary precautions. *Nursing Research, 31,* 196–201.

Kirchhoff, K. T. (1983). Should staff nurses be expected to use research? *Western Journal of Nursing Research, 5,* 245–247.

Kruger, J. C. (1978). Utilization of nursing research: The planning process. *Journal of Nursing Administration, 8*(1), 6–9.

Krueger, J. C., Nelson, A. H., & Wolanin, M. O. (1978). *Nursing research:*

Development, collaboration and utilization. Germantown, MD: Aspen Publishers, Inc.

Larson, E. (1989). Using the CURN project to teach research utilization in a baccalaureate program. *Western Journal of Nursing Research, 11,* 593–599.

Lindeman, C. A. (1988). Research in practice: The role of the staff nurse. *Applied Nursing Research, 1,* 5–7.

Lobiondo-Wood, G., & Haber, J. (1986). *Nursing research: Critical appraisal and utilization.* St. Louis: C. V. Mosby.

Loomis, M. E. (1985). Knowledge utilization and research utilization in nursing. *Image: Journal of Nursing Scholarship, 17,* 35–39.

Mallick, M. (1983). A constant comparative method for teaching research critiquing to baccalaureate nursing students. *Image: Journal of Nursing Scholarship, 15,* 120–123.

Massey, J., & Loomis, M. (1988). When should nurses use research findings? *Applied Nursing Research, 1,* 32–40.

Maurin, J. T. (1990). Research utilization in the social-political arena. *Applied Nursing Research, 3,* 48–51.

Miller, J. R., & Messenger, S. R. (1978). Obstacles to applying nursing research findings. *American Journal of Nursing, 78,* 632–634.

Phillips, L. R. F. (1986). *A clinician's guide to the critique and utilization of nursing research.* Norwalk, CT: Appleton-Century-Croft.

Roberts-Gray, C., & Gray, T. (1983). Implementing innovations: A model to bridge the gap between diffusion and utilization. *Knowledge: Creation, Diffusion, Utilization, 5,* 213–232.

Rothman, J. (1980). *Social R & D: Research and development in the human services.* Englewood Cliffs, NJ: Prentice Hall.

Stark, J. L. (1989). A multiple-strategy based research program for staff nurse involvement. *Journal of Nursing Administration, 19,* 7–8.

Stetler, C. B. (1985). Research utilization: Defining the concept. *Image: Journal of Nursing Scholarship, 17,* 40–44.

Stokes, J. E. (1981). Utilization of research findings by staff nurses. In S. D. Krampitz & N. Pavlovich (Eds.), *Readings for nursing research.* St. Louis: C. V. Mosby.

Tanner, C. A. (1987). Evaluating research for use in practice: Guidelines for the clinician. *Heart and Lung, 16,* 424–431.

Topham, D. L., & DeSilva, P. (1988). Evaluating congruency between steps in the research process: A critique guide for use in clinical nursing practice. *Clinical Nurse Specialist, 2,* 97–102.

Part II

MANAGING FALLS

[5]

Managing Falls: The Current Bases for Practice

Carol C. Hogue

Many frail elderly persons consider a fall the beginning of the end, the boundary marker between independence and dependence or death. Very fit elders also fall, usually in response to considerable external hazard. To make the best use of our clinical resources in preventing falls and supporting function in older adults, we need to understand who falls in what circumstances, how people fall, and what the consequences are. We need to frame our nursing actions to promote the greatest possible independence while we strive to provide safety for those entrusted to our care. At this time, there is little scientific evidence of the effectiveness of interventions to prevent falls, although research in progress now will bring us closer to the information we seek. We must, however, be shrewd in how we use the information currently at hand.

Some years ago Charlie Brown was having trouble sorting out his life and he "unloaded" on his psychiatrist, Lucy. After listening with full attention, she calmly replied, "You must remember, Charlie, life is like an ocean voyage. Most voyagers place their deck chairs at the stern of the vessel so they can while away the hours looking at where they have been. A few put their chairs in the front of the boat so they can observe where they are going. You must make up your mind, Charlie, where you want to put your deck chair."

"But Lucy," Charlie plaintively replied, "My problem is that I can't get my deck chair opened!"

There are several ways to interpret that metaphor; one interpretation related to falls is that while the research does not shout out clearly documented interventions to prevent falls, we know enough to open our deck chairs and put them in the front of the boat.

EPIDEMIOLOGY

Falls are a leading cause of injury, disability, and death among the elderly (Fife, 1987; Hogue, 1982a). Each year approximately one third of the population 65 years and older who are living at home will fall at least once, and over two thirds of persons living in nursing homes will fall (Campbell, Reinken, Allan, & Martinez, 1981; Prudham & Evans, 1981; Tinetti, 1987). We should emphasize five points: (1) Falls are not accidents. (2) Disability and death from falls increase with age. (3) Geriatric falls tend to have multiple causes. (4) Assessment is the key to prevention. (5) Many strategies and techniques can be used by health professionals and by older persons and their families to prevent falls and injuries from falls.

People of all ages fall; children fall as much as old people (Hogue, 1982b). Among elderly persons, even when no physical injury occurs (which is the case 90% of the time), a fall can lead to fear of falling, restriction of activity, loss of confidence, loss of mobility, and loss of independence (Gibson, 1987; Tinetti, Richman, & Powell, 1990; Vellas, Cayla, Bocquet, dePemille, & Albarede, 1987). Families of older fallers may feel guilty that they did not prevent the fall and react by imposing limits on independence. Deaths from falls increase in late life; while women fall more (until about age 85) and are hospitalized more, men have higher fall death rates (Hogue, 1982a). The proportion of falls resulting in fracture is low, probably only 5–6% (Gryfe, Amies, & Ashley, 1977; Tinetti, 1987); but the absolute number of fractures is high (Fife, Barancik, & Chatterjee, 1984a; Jacobsen et al., 1990). One particular fracture—hip fracture, which is the most common serious injury from falls in older persons, places heavy demands on the patient, the family, and the health care system. While other fractures, especially Colles or wrist fracture, and other injuries, mainly soft tissue injury, exceed hip fracture in numbers, they do not match the disability and death accompanying hip fracture (Melton, 1988; Miller, 1978; Mossey, Mutran, Knott, & Craik, 1989).

In the United States, there are 220,000 hip fractures a year among persons 65 and older (Kellie & Brody, 1990). The incidence rises sharply after age 50 and is highest among the very elderly. Beginning at about age 40, in white women, the incidence of hip fracture doubles every 5–6 years for the rest of life (Melton & Cummings, 1987). Among those who live to be 90, 33% of women and 17% of men will fracture their hips (Melton, 1988). The role of osteoporosis in hip fracture is well known, but somewhat less widely appreciated are factors such as orientation of the hip to the floor. Most of us fall forward on our hands and knees; very frail people are more likely to sit down hard when they fall, placing the end of the femur at impact. Protective responses tend to be weak or slow in falls that result in hip fracture, and local shock absorbers, the muscles, tend to be weak or atrophied (Cummings & Nevitt, 1989; Melton, Wahner, Richelson, O'Fallon, & Riggs, 1986). The economic cost of hip fracture is great: in this country, a few years ago, direct costs of hip fractures were estimated at seven billion dollars per year (Peck et al., 1988). The number of hip fractures in the oldest old will increase exponentially over the next 60 years unless we make major changes in the care of our older citizens. Death rates associated with hip fracture have improved; in-hospital mortality decreased from 11.3% in 1970 to 6.1% in 1983, but even now, 2–4 people of 10 with hip fracture die within the first 6 months (Rodriguez, Sattin, & Waxweiler, 1989).

INSTITUTIONAL FALLS

Repeated falls are a common reason for admission of previously independent people to long-term care institutions. While there are many frail elderly people in the community, in nursing homes there are very few fit elderly. It is not surprising, then, that the rate of falls in nursing homes is especially high: 1650 falls/1000 residents/year (Rubenstein et al., 1988). Hospital falls are also frequent. Mortality is higher among those who fall in institutions, because of the greater frailty of those fallers.

There are particular problems that make falls prevention both important and difficult in acute care institutions (Whedon & Shedd, 1989). Patients are acutely ill; cardiovascular disease, arthritis, and diabetes are prevalent; patients remain in bed, becoming deconditioned; oral intake tends to be low; high-risk medications are often started, sometimes in doses too great; the environment is new and sometimes fraught with new risk, if, for example, floors are slick and hard. What is counted as a fall in a hospital is evidently different from what is counted as a fall in noninstitutional settings. Because of concern about liability coupled with a long-standing tradition of viewing patient falls as "incidents" or errors, and because of the more or less continuous supervision of patients by health care workers, it is possible that more institutional falls are recorded than noninstitutional falls. Complicating the measurement of institutional falls is the common notion that some nursing staff underreport falls because of fear of criticism.

A major problem in hospital falls prevention is the short time for intervention. Further, while there is research evidence that restraints do not prevent falls (Evans & Strumpf, 1990; Innes & Turman, 1983; Werner, Cohen-Mansfield, Braun, & Marx, 1989), and that immobility inevitably leads to critical declines in multiple body systems in frail elders (Bortz, 1982; Harper & Lyles, 1988; Hogue, 1985), risk management officers in many institutions appear to be more devoted to traditional practices and reduction of liability than to scientific evidence.

To summarize, women fall more than men until the age of 85, but men who fall are more likely to die from falls. Children fall a lot, but they tend not to be injured. All falls in older adults have the potential of limiting activity and quality of life. Only 1–2% of falls to older adults result in hip fracture, but the consequences of hip fracture and the fact that we cannot consistently predict which fallers will fracture lead to the need to prevent falls. Institutional falls tend to occur in frail people, often with rapidly changing functional status, and usually with no dramatic external influence.

WAYS OF VIEWING FALLS

While falls have been noted since Biblical times (Ecclesiastes IV:9, 10) and the results of systematic inquiry into the etiology of falls have been known for more than 40 years (DeHaven, 1942), relatively little scientific or clinical attention was directed toward falls until very recently. Falls are common throughout life; that may be one reason their significance for elderly people has not been grasped by some. In addition, for many years, widespread misunderstanding of the causes of falls among both lay people and professionals limited progress in reducing falls and injury from falls (Hogue, 1991). Gradually, however, the unscientific term *accident* with its connotation of chance, fate, and unexpectedness is being replaced by the description of injuries and the situations in which they occur, making prevention of these situations easier. "Accident" refers to a random or chance event, yet existing data indicate that accidents, like diseases, are nonrandom events. In fact, falls can be predicted as well as myocardial infarction. The term accident also has the connotation of bad luck, carelessness, or even sinfulness. Thus, attitudes toward fallers still vary widely, from the belief held by some that falls are inevitable in the very old to overemphasis by others on the individual's personal responsibility to avoid hazards. Falling is not a part of normal aging; falls are not accidents; they are predictable; they are treatable. Efforts to reduce falls and injury from falls can be improved. Many or most interventions to prevent falls, however, are more appropriately carried out by health care providers and family members than by the person at risk for falling (Haddon, 1980; Hogue, 1980, 1982b).

Dynamics and Classification of Falling

Everyone knows what a fall is, yet details of the definition are difficult. A definition that has recently been identified by three major groups, the Kellog International Work Group on the Prevention of Falls (Gibson, 1987), the Institute of Medicine (Berg & Cassells, 1990), and the investigators of the eight cooperative agreement studies known as FICSIT (Frailty and Injuries, Cooperative Studies and Intervention Trials [Miller et al., in press]) is the following: a fall is an unintentional event that results in a person coming to rest on the ground or other lower level. For some, the definition ends there; for others, exceptions are displacements caused by sustaining a violent blow, loss of consciousness, stroke, or seizure.

The postural control system is dependent upon sensory input, central nervous system integration, and motor outputs. With increasing age and pathology, the system responds more slowly to displacement from the center of gravity (Horak, Shupert, & Mirka, 1989; Masdeu et al., 1989; Sloane, Baloh, & Honrubia, 1989; Stelmach & Worringham, 1985; Wolfson, Whipple, & Amerman, 1985; Woolacott, Shumway-Cook, & Nashner, 1982).

Think about how falls occur. Falls have phases; understanding those phases is a way of getting our deck chairs open; it sets the stage for planning interventions. Falls occur when the performance level of an individual is inadequate for the demands of environmental tasks, that is, when there is a mismatch. When environmental demands are great, even very fit individuals may be unable to recover from a sudden loss of balance in time to prevent a fall. On the other hand, if individuals are very frail, they may be unable to maintain postural control (prevent a fall) with virtually no external provocation. If at the point of impact the energy transfer exceeds the ability of the soft and bony structures to dissipate that energy, injury occurs.

The more frail people are, the more they depend on the environment for support, both before and after falls (Hogue, 1982b, 1991; Waller, 1978). The speed of emergency care and the appropriateness of early treatment and rehabilitation have profound effects on consequences (Waller, 1973). There is nothing about even a hip fracture that should be fatal or disabling. In very frail persons with very limited physiologic reserve, and in those with concurrent disease, factors related to treatment, decreased mobility, and changes in environment and nutrition may lead to disability or death after hip fracture (Buchner & Wagner, in press; Magaziner, Simonsick, Kashner, Hebel, & Kenzora, 1989; Siebens, 1990).

There is very little information on the social and behavioral factors that may predispose elderly persons to fall. Because psychosocial factors have been shown to influence gait, balance, and physical function (Maki, Holliday, & Topper, 1991) and mobility limitations are important predictors of falls (Harris & Kovar, 1991; Sudarsky & Ronthal, 1983), cognitive and emotional status may be associated with falls (Buchner & Larson, 1987; Mossey, 1985; Silverton & Tideiksaar, 1989). Research in that area is in progress. Fear of falling may cause some elderly persons to limit their activity; this activity limitation may further impair lower extremity strength and balance (Bhala, O'Donnell, & Thoppil, 1982; Maki et al., 1991; Murphy & Isaacs, 1982; Tinetti et al., 1990).

It is useful in planning prevention to think of types of falls. Isaacs classified falls according to the type of activity being pursued at the time of the fall. The Isaacs typology is hierarchical, with an increasingly smaller force responsible for the fall. Isaacs' six categories of falls include (1) imposed (contact with a major external hazard); (2) judgmental error (occurring during hurried activity); (3) perceptual error (contact with an object that could have been avoided); (4) posture change (moving from lying, sitting, standing, with no external hazard); (5) walking (occurring during normal, unhurried walking, with no external hazard); and (6) standing (occurring while standing quietly) (Isaacs, 1978).

The lesson to be learned from the Isaacs typology is that as internal impairments mount, less external force is needed for a fall to occur. Dichotomizing falls into "external falls" or "internal falls" is probably useful so long as one remembers that there is usually overlap between the categories in the middle of the continuum. That is, combinations of etiologic factors are more likely in people with some impairment. An occasional fall or "external" fall is one that is associated with major environmental provocation, a fall that could occur to any fit person of any age. Falls that occur with no apparent external hazard are sometimes called internal falls or geriatric falls. Geriatric falls are best divided into two categories: those related to a single major factor such as postural hypotension or syncope; and a much larger category of falls related to multiple factors, both intrinsic and external.

If a fall is due to a single intrinsic factor (syncope, postural hypotension, stroke), our efforts are directed toward that single cause. If the fall is related to a clearly hazardous activity, as is true for 5% of community residents' falls (Tinetti, Speechley, & Ginter, 1988), that hazardous activity can be addressed. The great majority of falls in old age, however, have multiple causes, usually including postural instability, and are precipitated by little external demand. These falls are likely to recur. Because those fallers are typically frail, they are likely to be injured and to recover poorly (Lipsitz, Jonsson, Kelley, & Koestner, 1991; Overstall, 1980; Tinetti et al., 1988; Tinetti, Williams, & Mayewski, 1986; Wild, Nayak, & Isaacs, 1981).

In the early period of our clinical science on falls prevention, we took a "laundry-list" approach to falls risk. That is, we made lists of factors observed in older people who fell, sometimes without looking at the *meaning* of those factors. Just as 40–50 years ago it was suggested that TV sets and, in rural areas, telephone poles were risk factors for myocardial infarction, there was a time (fairly recently in fact) when some considered "building type" and "retirement" to be risk factors for falls in older people. We know now that in the early days of television, ownership of a TV set was a marker of relative affluence but there is no direct relationship between TV sets and myocardial infarction, and we also know more now about real risk factors for falls. We can do better now; we can get our deck chairs open and take a logical view of risk factors for falls.

Falls Risk Factors

Risk factor intervention has been very effective in reducing cardiovascular disease; with falls, however, we have a larger set of risk factors and they tend to change. Many risk factors can be eliminated; some cannot. Nevertheless, if we can reduce some risk factors, we can reduce the risk, because the greater the number of risk factors, the greater the risk of falls (Nevitt, 1991; Tinetti et al., 1988).

There are four groups of risk factors that contribute to falls: age-related declines, acute and chronic diseases, medications, and environmental hazards. Declines in vision are contributors to falls. Visual acuity is important, but loss of ambient and peripheral vision and loss of contrast sensitivity are also important (Campbell et al., 1981; Horak et al., 1989; Nevitt, Cummings, Kidd, & Black, 1989). Two studies have found visual impairments predictive of falls in women, but not in men (Campbell, Borrie, & Spears, 1989; Felson et al., 1989). Decreases in muscle mass (Aniansson, Ljungberg, Rundgren, & Wetterquist, 1984), muscle strength (Aniansson & Zetterberg, 1984; Campbell et al., 1989; Nevitt et al., 1989; Tinetti et al., 1986; Whipple, Wolfson, & Amerman, 1987), walking speed (Campbell et al., 1989; Ims & Edholm, 1981; Nevitt et al., 1989; Wolfson, Whipple, Amerman, & Tobin, 1990), and the balance control system (Ring, Nayak, & Isaacs, 1988; Robbins et al., 1989; Tinetti, 1986; Tinetti et al., 1988; Wild et al., 1981), which are consequences of the sedentary behavior common in late life or consequences of disease, have all been shown to be more common among fallers than non-fallers. Declines in liver and kidney function may slow the metabolism of drugs, increasing their toxic effects. Increases in reaction time (Nevitt et al., 1989) and postural hypotension (Lipsitz, 1989) are functional deficits more common in late life and are associated with falls.

Acute and chronic disease, especially cardiovascular disorders (Lipsitz, 1985), diseases leading to poor gait (Tinetti, 1987), dizziness (Sloane et al., 1989), syncope (Lipsitz, 1985), musculoskeletal diseases that impair mobility skills and encourage sedentary behavior—which further impairs mobility—dementia and delirium (Buchner & Larson, 1987; Janken, Reynolds, & Swiech, 1986; Morse, Tylko, & Dixon, 1987; Nevitt et al., 1989) all increase the risk of falling. Although alcohol is thought to increase the risk of falling, and one controlled study (Waller, 1978) found that fallers who were seen at an emergency department had a higher rate of heavy drinking than did non-fallers, other studies (Campbell et al., 1989; Tinetti et al., 1988) have found little or no association between alcohol and falls. A common clinical observation is that those at highest risk for falls because of impairments related to disease, inactivity, or medications commonly stop drinking. Campbell et al. (1989) found that women who drank only small amounts and drank only infrequently were more likely to be fallers.

There are three groups of medications we particularly worry about: sedatives and hypnotics; tranquilizers, especially those with long half-life (Librium, Tranxene, Valium, and Dalmane); and antihypertensive drugs. Elderly persons taking tranquilizers with long half-life are 70% more likely to fracture hips than older persons on no psychotropic drug (Ray & Griffin, 1991; Ray, Griffin, & Downey, 1989).

Environmental hazards thought to be associated with falling, especially in frail elders, include low ambient lighting, glare, dangerous stairs, clutter, loose rugs, and slippery, uneven floors. Methods to study environments carefully and the rationale for observing particular aspects of the environment are not very well developed yet, so there are few firm data on the contribution of environmental factors to falling. Fallers seem more willing to attribute falls to external factors, while non-fallers may negotiate apparently hazardous environments with no difficulty. One woman's environmental risk factor may be another's unrisky environment; as abilities decline, the effect of environment increases (Rodriguez, Sattin, DeVito, & Wingo, 1991).

More controlled studies are needed to allow us to conclude which of these risk factors *cause* falls; in the meantime, clinical care can be strengthened by reducing the number of risk factors whenever possible, and by using the best information available at this time.

Managing Falls

Let us focus more sharply on clinical maneuvers to prevent falls and support function. Figure 5.1 is a typology of falls risk adapted from an Institute of Medicine review (Berg & Cassells, 1990). The factors on the right belong to the risk factor classes on the left; the factors listed are included because a statistically significant association with falls has been shown in multiple studies, at least two of which were prospective. Factors considered moderate, weak, or inconsistent because of lesser research findings are not included. All these factors are intrinsic.

We need a few more links in the chain. We were excited to learn in 1989 of the success of Fiatarone and colleagues (Fiatarone et al., 1990) in increasing lower extremity muscle strength and size in 90-year-old men in a nursing home. What neither they nor anyone else has shown yet is whether such increases in muscle strength can be maintained after the intensive training program, whether those increases make a difference in everyday functional abilities, and whether they prevent falls. My own group is presently piloting an intervention directed at those practical, long-term outcomes.

Here is my suggestion for a quick screen for falls risk in older adults. Those who are over 75, who use a walking aid or have had a prior fall with little or moderate external demand, or who are disoriented are at high risk. You can identify those people very quickly. If any of these factors are present, you assess and modify risk factors, evaluate mobil-

FIGURE 5.1. Intrinsic risk factors for falls. Adapted from: R. L. Berg & J. S. Cassells. (1990).

RISK FACTOR CLASS	RISK FACTOR
Demographic	Age ≥80, men
General health, function	ADL/IADL, mobility impairment, incontinence History of falls
Medical diagnosis	Dementia, Parkinson's
Musculoskeletal, neuromuscular	▼Hip, knee, ankle strength, ▼grip strength
Sensory	▼Visual acuity
Gait, balance, physical performance	Gait abnormalities, ▼Walking speed Impaired dynamic balance Difficulty rising from chair
Cognitive, psychological	▼ Mental status test score, depression
Medication use	Sedatives, hypnotics, anxiolytics Number of medications

FIGURE 5.2. Functional risk factors for falls.

RISK FACTOR	ASSESSMENT TECHNIQUE
Sitting balance poor	▪ Sit up straight for 60" (arms on chest) ▪ Sitting reach
Lower extremity weakness	▪ Rise from chair (arms on chest)
Standing balance poor	▪ Pick up object on floor ▪ Standing reach
Gait impaired	▪ Walk

ity, assess the safety of the environment, and learn the details of prior falls.

Figure 5.2 gives a short list of risk factors with simple assessment techniques; this functional mobility assessment has been shown to be highly predictive of falls (Hogue, Studenski, & Duncan, 1990). Simplify that a little more and you have the "Get up and go test," which requires the person being assessed to rise from a straight chair, walk 3 meters (about 10 feet), turn around, return to the chair and sit down (Mathias, Nyak, & Isaacs, 1986; Podsiadlo & Richardson 1991). While the test can be scored on a 4-point scale, "pass/fail" is more appropriate clinically. That is, anyone whose performance is uncertain should be further assessed.

Any intervention that requires behavior change, that is, behavior change in a staff nurse, a family caregiver, or a patient, must be accompanied by an effective behavioral strategy to achieve the investment of the person who needs to change. We must not take that for granted. To engage in health promoting behaviors, a person needs information, skills, a sense of potential accomplishment, a regimen that fits the person, an effective relationship with health care providers, and social support from family or friends (Becker, 1990; Dishman & Ickes, 1981; Martin & Dubbert, 1984). Staff members who are asked to change behaviors also need the support of others and a behavioral strategy to help them.

Home hazards should be modified whenever possible. Assessment of environments is not as easy to do well as one might think, but here are some suggestions. Determine how people get from one place to another;

ask them to show you how they care for themselves in a usual day. Observe the older person moving in his or her own environment, and ascertain how frequently hazards are encountered. A cluttered room that a frail older person never enters might not merit comment. A systematic review should include how people get in and out of their homes: access, doorway, threshold; and in all rooms, lighting, flooring, furniture, storage, cords, and clutter. Height of stored objects and ease of reaching light switches should be noted. Stairs should be observed for lighting, railing, surface, and rise height. Bathrooms should have rubber tub mats, grab bars, and nonskid floor mats. While it may not always be feasible to renovate homes that have hazards for frail elderly persons, suggestions can usually be made to make environments less demanding and more forgiving, and to provide human help to lessen task demand.

For those who have fallen, it is important to learn the history of the fall and to determine, if possible, the type of fall. If the fall was "external," counseling avoidance of the hazard is likely to be appropriate. If the fall was predominantly internal, or a geriatric fall, up to 20% of the time a single major cause—hypotension, psychotropic drug, neurologic disease, or loss of consciousness—can be identified by taking a fall history. Multiple factors are involved at least 80% of the time; they can be deduced from the fall history and other information. A fall history should ask, "Where were you? What were you doing? Did you know you were going to fall? Did you pass out? How did you get up?"

We must consider geriatric falls as sentinel events: that is, the fall may be a signal of new underlying illness. So we must do a thorough examination and have a high level of suspicion while encouraging resumption of prior function and encouraging independence. Treatment for the very-high-risk person might include physical training, a home alarm system, help with chores, encouragement from family or friends, and modification of home hazards. Physical training might include teaching the person how to walk safely, teaching transfer skills for nonambulatory persons, increasing muscle strength, improving balance, coaching on how to reach objects, and coaching on how to fall and on how to get up from the floor.

Our suggestions for managing falls in institutional settings include the techniques for quick screening and mobility assessment as well as the interventions noted above. In addition, in institutions, priorities should be set. High-risk patients should be identified and staffing considered in relation to the ability to observe those at high risk, anticipate need for moving, and respond promptly to requests. Call lights need to be within easy reach. Patients should be monitored more closely on admission or transfer, during acute illness, and after a fall. Changes in physical vigor should be noted and used to raise the index of suspicion. Thoughtful monitoring of drugs and prevention of delirium may reduce falls and injury. Whenever possible, patients should be dressed in their own clothing and shoes. Environmental hazards, including equipment for care, slippery floors, and the like must be considered.

The use of restraints has been considered in this country in a new light in recent years. Restraints and side rails do not prevent falls; they seem to encourage falls and, by limiting activity, lead to deconditioning, which brings on muscle weakness. In several studies, patients who have been restrained in bed or chair have had high rates of falls (Evans & Strumpf, 1990; Innes & Turman, 1983). Of course, beds should be low when care is not being given.

In general, to reduce the risk of falling and injury we should think broadly about strategies in four categories: considering the phases of falls, changing the environment, decreasing task demand, and strengthening individuals. All strategies must support autonomy, independence, and mobility as much as possible. Also, there are things we should encourage for all frail older people and for those who hope to avoid frailty: limit psychotropic and antihypertensive drugs, maintain physical activity, strengthen emotional and social well-being, promote general health, and create safe environments. Assessment is the key to prevention, and there are many strategies and techniques that can be used by health professionals and by older persons and their families to prevent falls and injuries from falls.

REFERENCES

Aniansson, A., Ljungberg, P., Rundgren, A., & Wetterquist, H. (1984). Effect of a training program for pensioners on condition and muscular strength. *Archives of Gerontology and Geriatrics, 3,* 229–241.

Aniansson, A., & Zetterberg, C. (1984). Impaired muscle function with aging: A background factor in the incidence of fractures of the proximal end of the femur. *Clinical Orthopedics, 191,* 193–201.

Becker, M. H. (1990). Theoretical models of adherence and strategies for improving adherence. In S. A. Shumaker, E. B. Schron, & J. K. Ockene (Eds.), *The handbook of health behavior change* (pp. 5–43). New York: Springer.

Berg, R. L., & Cassells, J. S. (Eds.). (1990). Falls in older persons. Risk factors and prevention. In *The second fifty years. Promoting health and preventing disability* (pp. 263–289). Washington, DC: National Academy Press.

Bhala, R. P., O'Donnell, J., & Thoppil, E. (1982). Ptophobia: Phobic fear of falling and its clinical management. *Physical Therapy, 62,* 187–190.

Bortz, W. M. (1982). Disuse and aging. *Journal of the American Medical Association, 248,* 1203–1208.

Buchner, D. M., & Larson, E. B. (1987). Falls and fractures in patients with Alzheimer's type dementia. *Journal of the American Medical Association, 257,* 1492–1495.

Buchner, D., & Wagner, E. H. (in press). Can frail health be prevented? *Clinics in Geriatric Medicine*.

Campbell, A., Borrie, M. J., & Spears, G. F. (1989). Risk factors for falls in a community-based prospective study of people 70 years and older. *Journal of Gerontology, 44*, 112–117.

Campbell, A., Reinken, J., Allan, B., & Martinez, G. S. (1981). Falls in old age: A study of frequency and related clinical features. *Age and Ageing, 10*, 264–270.

Cummings, S. R., & Nevitt, M. C. (1989). A hypothesis: The causes of hip fractures. *Journal of Gerontology, 44*, 107–111.

De Haven, H. M. (1942). Mechanical analysis of survival in falls from heights of fifty to one hundred and fifty feet. *War Medicine, 2*, 586–596.

Dishman, R. K., & Ickes, W. (1981). Self-motivation and adherence to therapeutic exercise. *Journal of Behavioral Medicine, 4*, 421–438.

Evans, L. K., & Strumpf, N. E. (1990). Myths about elder restraint. *Image: Journal of Nursing Scholarship, 22*, 124–128.

Felson, D. T., Anderson, J. J., Hannan, M. T., Milton, R. C., Wilson, P. W. F., & Kiel, D. P. (1989). Impaired vision and hip fracture. The Framingham study. *Journal of the American Geriatrics Society, 37*, 495–500.

Fiatarone, M. A., Marks, E. C., Ryan, N. D., Meredith, C. N., Lipsitz, L. A., & Evans, W. J. (1990). High-intensity strength training in nonagenarians. Effects on skeletal muscle. *Journal of the American Medical Association, 263*, 3029–3034.

Fife, D. (1987). Injuries and deaths among elderly persons. *American Journal of Epidemiology, 126*, 936–941.

Fife, D., Barancik, J. I., & Chatterjee, M. S. (1984). Northeastern Ohio Trauma Study: Injury rates by age, sex, and cause. *American Journal of Public Health, 74*, 473–478.

Gibson, M. J. (1987). The prevention of falls in later life. *Danish Medical Bulletin, 34*, 1–24.

Gryfe, C., Amies, A., & Ashley, M. (1977). A longitudinal study of falls in an elderly population: Incidence and morbidity. *Age and Ageing, 6*, 201–210.

Haddon, W., Jr. (1980). Advances in the epidemiology of injuries as a basis for public policy. *Public Health Reports, 95*, 411–421.

Harper, C. M., & Lyles, Y. M. (1988). Physiology and complications of bed rest. *Journal of the American Geriatrics Society, 36*, 1047–1054.

Harris, T., & Kovar, M. G. (1991). National statistics on the functional status of older persons. In R. Weindruch & M. Ory (Eds.), *Frailty reconsidered: Reducing frailty and fall-related injuries in the elderly* (pp. 15–28). Springfield, IL: Charles C Thomas.

Hogue, C. C. (1980). Epidemiology of injury in older age. In S. G. Haynes & M. Feinlieb (Eds.), *Epidemiology of aging* (pp. 127–138). Bethesda: National Institutes of Health.

Hogue, C. C. (1982a). Injury in late life. Part 1. Epidemiology. *Journal of the American Geriatrics Society, 30*, 183–190.

Hogue, C. C. (1982b). Injury in late life. Part 2. Prevention. *Journal of the American Geriatrics Society, 30*, 276–280.

Hogue, C. C. (1985). Mobility. In E. L. Schneider, C. J. Wendlend, A. W. Zimmer, N. List, & M. Ory (Eds.), *The teaching nursing home. A new approach to geriatric research, education, and clinical care* (pp. 231–244). New York: Raven Press.

Hogue, C. C. (1991). A person–environment model for understanding fall risk. In R. Weindruch & M. Ory (Eds.), *Frailty reconsidered: Reducing frailty and fall-related injuries in the elderly* (pp. 96–105). Springfield, IL: Charles C. Thomas.

Hogue, C. C., Studenski, S., & Duncan, P. (1990). Assessing mobility: The first step in preventing falls. In S. G. Funk, E. M. Tornquist, M. T. Champagne, L. A. Copp, & R. A. Wiese (Eds.), *Key aspects of recovery. Improving nutrition, rest, and mobility* (pp. 275–280). New York: Springer.

Horak, F. G., Shupert, C. L., & Mirka, A. (1989). Components of postural dyscontrol in the elderly: A review. *Neurobiology of Aging, 10,* 727–738.

Ims, F., & Edholm, O. (1981). Studies of gait and mobility in the elderly. *Age and Ageing, 10,* 147–156.

Innes, E. M., & Turman, W. G. (1983). Evolution of patient falls. *Quality Review Bulletin, 9,* 30–35.

Isaacs, B. (1978). Are falls a manifestation of brain failure? *Age and Ageing, 7,* 97–111.

Jacobsen, S. J., Goldberg, J., Miles, T. P., Brody, J. A., Stiers, W., & Rimm, A. A. (1990). Hip fracture incidence among the old and the very old: A population-based study of 745,435 cases. *American Journal of Public Health, 80,* 871–873.

Janken, J. K., Reynolds, B. A., & Swiech, K. (1986). Patient falls in the acute care setting: Identifying risk factors. *Nursing Research, 35,* 215–219.

Kellie, S. E., & Brody, J. A. (1990). Sex-specific and race-specific hip fracture rates. *American Journal of Public Health, 80,* 326–328.

Lipsitz, L. A. (1985). Abnormalities in blood pressure homeostasis that contribute to falls in the elderly. *Clinics in Geriatric Medicine, 1,* 637–648.

Lipsitz, L. A. (1989). Orthostatic hypotension in the elderly. *New England Journal of Medicine, 321,* 952–957.

Lipsitz, L. A., Jonsson, P. V., Kelley, M. M., & Koestner, J. S. (1991). Causes and correlates of recurrent falls in ambulatory frail elderly. *Journal of Gerontology: Medical Sciences, 46,* M114–122.

Magaziner, J., Simonsick, E. M., Kashner, M., Hebel, J. R., & Kenzora, J. E. (1989). Survival experience of aged hip fracture patients. *American Journal of Public Health, 79,* 272–278.

Maki, B. E., Holliday, P. J., & Topper, A. K. (1991). Fear of falling and postural performance in the elderly. *Journal of Gerontology: Medical Sciences, 46,* M123–131.

Martin, J. E., & Dubbert, P. M. (1984). Behavioral management strategies for improving health and fitness. *Journal of Cardiac Rehabilitation, 4,* 200–208.

Masdeu, J. C., Wolfson, L., Lantos, G., Tobin, J. N., Grober, E., Whipple, R., & Amerman, P. (1989). Brain white-matter changes in the elderly prone to falling. *Archives of Neurology, 46,* 1292–1296.

Mathias, S., Nayak, U. S. L., & Isaacs, B. (1986). Balance in elderly patients: The "get-up and go test." *Archives of Physical Medicine and Rehabilitation, 67,* 387–389.

Melton, L. J., III. (1988). Epidemiology of fractures. In B. L. Riggs & L. J. Melton, III (Eds.), *Osteoporosis: Etiology, diagnosis, and management* (pp. 133–154). New York: Raven Press.

Melton, L. J., III, & Cummings, S. R. (1987). Heterogeneity of age-related fractures: Implications for epidemiology. *Bone and Mineral, 2,* 321–331.

Melton, L. J., III, Wahner, H. W., Richelson, L. S., O'Fallon, W. M., & Riggs, B. L. (1986). Osteoporosis and the risk of hip fracture. *American Journal of Epidemiology, 124,* 254–261.

Miller, C. W. (1978). Survival and ambulation following hip fracture. *Journal of Bone and Joint Surgery, 60,* 930–934.

Miller, J. P., Schechtman, K., Province, M., Arken, C., Smith, D., Mulrow, C., Ory, M., Weiss, S., Hadley, E. & the FICSIT Study Group. (in press). Preplanned metaanalysis in a clinical trial aimed at reducing frailty and injuries in older person. *Controlled Clinical Trials.*

Morse, J. M., Tylko, S. J., & Dixon, H. A. (1987). Characteristics of the fall-prone patient. *Gerontologist, 27,* 516–522.

Mossey, J. M. (1985). Social and psychologic factors related to falls among the elderly. *Clinics in Geriatric Medicine, 1,* 541–544.

Mossey, J. M., Mutran, E., Knott, K., & Craik, R. (1989). Determinants of recovery 12 months after hip fracture: The importance of psychosocial factors. *American Journal of Public Health, 79,* 279–286.

Murphy, J., & Isaacs, B. (1982). The post-fall syndrome: A study of thirty-six elderly patients. *Gerontology, 28,* 265–270.

Nevitt, M. C. (1991). Ascertainment and description of falls. In R. Weindruch & M. Ory (Eds.), *Frailty reconsidered: Reducing frailty and fall-related injuries in the elderly* (pp. 476–495). Springfield, IL: Charles C Thomas.

Nevitt, M. C., Cummings, S. R., Kidd, S., & Black, D. (1989). Risk factors for recurrent nonsyncopal falls: A prospective study. *Journal of the American Medical Association, 261,* 2663–2668.

Overstall, P. W. (1980). Prevention of falls in the elderly. *Journal of the American Geriatrics Society, 28,* 481–484.

Peck, W. A., Riggs, B. L., Bell, N. H., Wallace, R. B., Johnston, C. C., Jr., Gordon, S. L., & Shulman, L. E. (1988). Research directions in osteoporosis. *American Journal of Medicine, 84,* 275–282.

Podsiadlo, D., & Richardson, S. (1991). The timed "Up & Go": A test of basic functional mobility for frail elderly persons. *Journal of the American Geriatrics Society, 39,* 142–148.

Prudham, D., & Evans, J. (1981). Factors associated with falls in the elderly: A community study. *Age and Ageing, 10,* 141–146.

Ray, W. A., & Griffin, M. R. (1991). Prescribed medications, falling, and fall-related injuries. In R. Weindruch & M. Ory (Eds.), *Frailty reconsidered: Reducing frailty and fall-related injuries in the elderly* (pp. 76–89). Springfield, IL: Charles C. Thomas.

Ray, W. A., Griffin, M., & Downey, W.. (1989). Benzodiazepines of long and short elimination half-life and the risk of hip fracture. *Journal of the American Medical Association, 262,* 3303–3307.

Ring, C., Nayak, U. S. L., & Isaacs, B. (1988). Balance function in elderly people who have and have not fallen. *Archives of Physical Medicine and Rehabilitation, 69,* 261–264.

Robbins, A. S., Rubenstein, L. Z., Josephson, K. R., Schulman, B. L., Osterweil, D., & Fine, G. (1989). Predictors of falls among elderly people: Results of two population-based studies. *Archives of Internal Medicine, 194,* 1628–1633.

Rodriguez, J. G., Sattin, R. W., DeVito, C. A., Wingo, P. A., & the Study to Assess Falls Among the Elderly Group. (1991). Developing an environmental hazards assessment instrument for falls among the elderly. In R. Weindruch & M. Ory (Eds.), *Frailty reconsidered: Reducing frailty and fall-related injuries in the elderly* (pp. 76–89). Springfield, IL: Charles C. Thomas.

Rodriguez, J. G., Sattin, R. W., & Waxweiler, R. J. (1989). Incidence of hip fractures, United States, 1970–1983. *American Journal of Preventive Medicine, 5,* 175–181.

Rubenstein, L. Z., Robbins, A. S., Schulman, B. L., Rosado, J., Osterweil, D., & Josephson, K. R. (1988). Falls and instability in the elderly. *Journal of the American Geriatrics Society, 36,* 266–278.

Siebens, H. (1990). Deconditioning. In B. Kemp, K. Brummel-Smith, & J. W. Ramsdell (Eds.), *Geriatric rehabilitation* (pp. 177–191). Boston: Little, Brown.

Silverton, R., & Tideiksaar, R. (1989). Psychosocial aspects of falls. In R. Tideiksaar (Ed.). *Falling in old age: its prevention and treatment* (pp. 87–110). New York: Springer.

Sloane, P. D., Baloh, R. W., & Honrubia, V. (1989). Components of postural dyscontrol in the elderly: Clinical implications. *American Journal of Otolaryngology, 10,* 422–429.

Stelmach, G. E., & Worthington, C. J. (1985). Sensorimotor deficits related to postural stability: Implications for falling in the elderly. *Clinics in Geriatric Medicine, 1,* 679–694.

Sudarsky, L., & Ronthal, M. (1983). Gait disorders among elderly patients. *Archives of Neurology, 40,* 740–743.

Tinetti, M. E. (1987). Factors associated with serious injury during falls by ambulatory nursing home residents. *Journal of the American Geriatrics Society, 35,* 644–648.

Tinetti, M. E., Richman, D., & Powell, L. (1990). Falls efficacy as a measure of fear of falling. *Journal of Gerontology, 45,* P239–243.

Tinetti, M. E., Speechley, M., & Ginter, S. F. (1988). Risk factors for falls among elderly persons living in the community. *New England Journal of Medicine, 319,* 1701–1707.

Tinetti, M. E., Williams, T. F., & Mayewski, R. (1986). Fall risk index for elderly patients based on number of chronic disabilities. *American Journal of Medicine, 80,* 429–434.

Vellas, B., Cayla, F., Bocquet, H., dePemille, F., & Albarede, J. L. (1987). Prospective study of restriction of activity in old people after falls. *Age and Ageing, 16,* 189–193.

Waller, J. A. (1973). Emergency care from fatalities from injury and illness in the nonhighway setting. *Journal of Trauma, 13,* 54–60.

Waller, J. A. (1978). Falls among the elderly—Human and environmental factors. *Accident Analysis and Prevention, 10,* 21–33.

Werner, P., Cohen-Mansfield, J., Braun, J., & Marx, M. S. (1989). Physical restraints and agitation in nursing home residents. *Journal of the American Geriatrics Society, 37,* 1122–1126.

Whedon, M. B., & Shedd, P. (1989). Prediction and prevention of patient falls. *Image: Journal of Nursing Scholarship, 21,* 108–114.

Whipple, R. H., Wolfson, L. J., & Amerman, P. M. (1987). The relationship of knee and ankle weakness to falls in nursing home residents: An isokinetic study. *Journal of the American Geriatrics Society, 35,* 13–20.

Wild, D., Nayak, U. S. L., & Isaacs, B. (1981). How dangerous are falls in old people at home? *British Medical Journal, 282,* 266–282.

Wolfson, L. I., Whipple, R., & Amerman, P. (1985). Gait and balance in the elderly: Two functional capacities that link sensory and motor ability to falls. *Clinics in Geriatric Medicine, 1,* 649–660.

Wolfson, L. I., Whipple, R., Amerman, P., & Tobin, J. N. (1990). Gait assessment in the elderly: A gait abnormality rating scale and its relation to falls. *Journal of Gerontology: Medical Sciences, 45,* M12–19.

Woolacott, M. H., Shumway-Cook, A., & Nashner, L. (1982). Postural reflexes and aging. In J. A. Mortimer, F. J. Pirrozolo, & G. J. Maletta (Eds.), *The Aging Motor System* (pp. 98–119). New York: Praeger.

[6]

The Postural Control Scale

Nancy E. Dayhoff

Postural control is the ability to control the body in space during mobility as a result of the integration of neural and musculoskeletal dynamics (Horak, Shupert, & Mirka, 1989; Woollacott, 1990; Woollacott, Inglin, & Manchester, 1988). Integration results in "the ability to maintain equilibrium in a gravitational field by keeping or returning the center of body mass over its base of support" (Horak, 1987, p. 1881). Translated into clinical terms, integration results in the ability to walk, sit down and stand up, reach for objects, and continue maintaining balance. Loss of balance that is uncorrected results in a fall. Two behavioral components have been identified as reflecting integration: (1) automatic postural adjustments or balance during stance, and (2) voluntary postural adjustments during movement.

Postural dyscontrol has been identified as a risk factor for falls both for persons living in the community and for those in nursing homes. For example, Wilde, Nayak, and Issacs (1981) concluded from a study of older adults living in the community that postural dyscontrol was a significant contributing factor in at least 67% of falls. Other authors have suggested that postural dyscontrol can be implicated in falls in one of several ways: (1) in the presence of postural dyscontrol, environmental disturbances (such as slippery or uneven flooring) may directly contribute to falls; (2) postural dyscontrol jointly with other risk factors (such as age, medications, confusion) may directly influence falls; or (3) postural dyscontrol may contribute directly to falls and/or mediate the influence of other risk factors for falls (Maki, Holliday, & Fernie, 1990; Manchester, Woollacott, Zederbauer-Hylton, & Marin, 1989; Pyyko, Jantti, & Aalto, 1988; Sobel & McCart, 1983).

The studies to date have used technological measures of postural control, with balance, sway, and functional gait as indices of postural dyscontrol. However, technological measures of postural control are expensive, require special training for use, and may stress the patient beyond what an acutely ill older adult can tolerate. Therefore, there is a critical need for an observational measure of postural control that is valid, reliable, and clinically feasible for use with hospitalized patients.

An ideal clinical assessment tool would measure the intensity and magnitude of the factors constituting postural dyscontrol, would be sensitive to small differences, would provide for comparable measurement over time, and would be reliable with minimal training of staff nurses. Such a tool could help identify whether postural dyscontrol contributes to falls, and if so, interventions could be tested to improve postural control in order to decrease falls and improve mobility, and monitor changes in postural control during hospitalization (Corcoran & Fischer, 1987; Tinetti, 1986).

Among the existing valid and reliable observational measures of the behaviors associated with postural control, the balance and gait performance scales developed by Tinetti (1986) have the requisites for clinical behavioral measurement. However, the number of assessments (22 items) and the requirement that the patient walk 100 feet—50 feet at a relatively rapid pace (Tinetti, Williams, & Mayewski, 1986)—make these scales impractical for hospitalized patients, who may have only bathroom privileges or who may be too weak or have other symptoms that would interfere with walking at a rapid pace. Therefore, a briefer, more clinically useful version of the Tinetti scales was developed by the author. The study reported here examined the psychometric properties of the new scale.

METHOD

Development of the Postural Control Scale

Fourteen items from the Tinetti scales were selected as appropriate for hospitalized patients. The 14 items are assumed to be behavioral correlates of three factors in postural control: automatic balance, voluntary control of balance, and gait. Because balance and gait are inexorably intertwined, no one item is linked to a single factor in postural control, but the composite score should reflect control.

Standard conditions were established for assessment. The patient sat in a chair without arms, stood up and maintained the stance for 5 seconds, walked 10 feet, turned around, and returned to sit in the chair. The distance of 10 feet was selected because, in a two-bed hospital room, it is the usual distance from the bed next to the window to the bathroom.

Using the scoring system established by Tinetti, the 14 items were tested in a pilot study with 38 hospitalized persons. The distance of 10 feet was well tolerated, but inter-rater reliability for the scoring of 12 of the 14 items was not as high as desired. The scales were therefore modified to enhance reliability, and the new scale was named the Postural Control Scale (PCS). Figure 6.1 depicts 6 items from the scale.

To test the psychometric properties of the PCS, 123 older patients hospitalized primarily for medical problems such as cardiovascular, endocrine, and pulmonary pathologies were evaluated simultaneously by two research assistants trained in the use of the PCS. Research assistants (RAs) were graduate nursing students and staff nurses. Two RAs observed the patient simultaneously from the same viewpoint and recorded their observations independently.

RESULTS

Seventy-four of the patients were female and 49 male. Their ages ranged from 50 to 90; the average age was 75. Of the total sample, 42 had fallen at least once during the preceding 3 months. The majority (74) walked without an assistive device; 21 used a cane and 17, a walker. During walking, 97 had no therapeutic equipment, 12 were receiving in-

FIGURE 6.1. Examples of items from Postural Control Scale.

Directions	Skill Assessed	Score = 1	Score = 2	Score = 3	Score = 4	Comments	Score
Have client sit in chair for 1 minute and observe. (Chair should be facing wall and three meters from wall.)	1. Sitting balance	Steady and stable without holding onto chair.	Holds onto chair while sitting.	Leans or slides down in chair.	Requires assistance to prevent falling out of chair.		
Ask client to rise from chair and stand still for 5 seconds with eyes open.	2. Rising from chair	Able to rise in a single movement.	Pushes up with arms, legs, or walking aid but successful in one attempt.	Multiple attempts required but successful in rising.	Unable to rise from chair without another person's assistance.		
Observe distance between toe of stance foot and heel of swing foot; observe from side; do not judge first few or last few steps; observe one side at a time.	6. Step length	Approximately 1 to 1-1/2 the length of person's foot between the stance toe and swing heel on both sides.	Approximately less than one length of person's foot equal on both sides.	One foot moves up to other foot and not passed.	Giant steps; length exceeds 1-1/2 length of person's foot.		
Observe from behind.	8. Step continuity	Begins raising heel of one foot (toe on) as heel of other foot touches the floor; no stop or break in stride.	Places entire foot (heel and toe) on floor before begining to raise other foot, but does not stop in stride.	Stops completely between steps.			
Observe from front.	9. Walking stance	Approximately 1-4 inches between feet as they pass.	Feet have space between as one passes other (greater than 4 inches).	Feet almost touch each other (less than 1 inch).	Feet touch each other during step.		
Observe for lateral sway. (Observe from front.)	11. Trunk stability	Trunk does not sway and is not held rigid.	Trunk slightly sways but stays within the width of the hips.	Trunk is held rigid.	Trunk sway exceeds the width of the hips.		

travenous medications, and 3 were using portable oxygen. Data were unavailable for 11 subjects.

Subjects' scores on the PCS were distributed across the possible range (1 to 4) on each behavior, suggesting that the scale provides differential measures of intensities of postural dyscontrol and is sensitive to differences in behaviors. For example, for the behavior "rising from the chair," 14 subjects were able to rise in a single movement; 79 used their arms, legs, or walking aid to push up, but were successful in rising in one attempt; 16 required multiple attempts before a successful rise; and 14 were unable to rise from the chair without another person's help.

Evidence of Validity

To examine criterion-related validity, self-report of a fall or no fall in the 3 months prior to measurement (in the hospital or prior to hospitalization) was used as the criterion variable. Because the criterion variable was dichotomous, logistic regression was used to determine how well the items on the scale distinguished between fallers and non-fallers (Press & Wilson, 1978). This analysis classified patients as fallers or non-fallers based on the scale items. Seventy-two percent of the patients could be correctly classified (Table 6.1). The non-fallers were more accurately classified (91.5%) than the fallers (34%). If a non-faller is misclassified as a faller, that person might be unduly restricted during hospitalization, which could decrease the patient's functional independence. Misclassification of a faller as a non-faller could have more adverse effects: the person might fall because preventive or remedial measures were not instituted.

Of the 14 items on the PCS, 6 significantly contributed to the classification of patients as fallers or non-fallers: sitting balance, rising from the

TABLE 6.1 Criterion-Related Validity: Classification of Subjects as Fallers or Non-Fallers Based on Logistic Regression

	Actual Group			
	Fall		No Fall	
Predicted Group	n	%	n	%
Fall	14	34.0	7	8.5
No Fall	27	66.0	75	91.5
Total	41		82	

chair, trunk stability, walking stance, step length, and step continuity (see Figure 6.1). This suggests that a brief assessment can classify patients at risk for falls because of postural dyscontrol.

Evidence of Reliability

Inter-rater reliability for each item on the scale, using an analysis of variance model for estimating generalizability coefficients, was acceptable, with a range of .46 to .98 (mean = .80). The internal reliability of the scale was also acceptable, with an alpha of .88 for the total sample, and .87 for both faller and non-faller samples examined separately.

DISCUSSION

The findings of this study add to the findings of Tinetti et al. (1986), Morse, Tylko, and Dixon (1987), and Hogue, Studenski, and Duncan (1989). For example, rising from a chair and gait parameters were found to distinguish fallers from non-fallers in all four studies. Also, similarities in sitting balance were found using the PCS and the Mobility Scale (Hogue et al., 1989). Differences in findings among the four studies may be attributed to differences in scaling of items, different tests of validity and reliability, and differences in subjects used for the testing. For example, Tinetti studied residents of nursing homes and Hogue studied persons in their homes, while this study used hospitalized patients.

The six behavioral categories noted above may be used as a brief but sensitive assessment of postural control. In this study, the indicators were more successful in classifying non-fallers than fallers. Classifying persons who do not fall is important since restriction of older adults who are not likely to fall could compromise unnecessarily their functional status. The moderate percentage of fallers classified by the PCS does not negate the importance of the findings. As Tinetti (1986) suggests, falling is a complex phenomenon, and combinations of risk factors must be explored. These findings suggest that additional patient variables need to be examined along with postural dyscontrol, to increase the accuracy of identification of persons at risk for falls. An additional assessment that might be added to the scale is having the patient reach for an object placed on the floor from both a sitting position and a standing position. That would assess the patient's ability to perform the reaching movements of bending over for the object and returning to the sitting and standing positions (Tinetti, 1986). Observations of the patient's ability to reach without assistance or with the assistance of an environmental aid (i.e., a chair arm or wall) or the assistance of another person may provide evidence of the patient's limits of stability. Evidence of limits of stability may not be captured by the items on the Postural Control Scale. Once additional assessment factors are identified, prospective studies should be conducted to establish the individual or joint effects of postural dyscontrol and these other variables as significant risk factors for falls in hospitalized older adults.

The Postural Control Scale also needs to be tested against objective measures of postural control. If the validity of the PCS is confirmed by technical measures of voluntary control and automatic balance adjustments, the scale can be used to identify subjects for testing of nursing interventions to improve postural control.

Clearly, before fall prevention interventions can be developed and tested, risk factors that are amenable to nursing interventions must be identified. Currently used risk factors, such as age, medications, and diagnoses, are not amenable to nursing interventions. It is likely that most currently used variables are indirect indicators of some common etiology, and based on existing research, postural dyscontrol may be one common etiology. Laboratory research suggests that interventions may be successful in improving some aspects of postural control. Testing of nursing interventions to affect postural control, however, is contingent on the use of valid and reliable measures that are sensitive to small changes in control. The Postural Control Scale is a measure that staff nurses can use to begin identifying fallers and non-fallers.

ACKNOWLEDGMENTS

This research was partially supported by the Community Medical Research Institute, Inc., Community Hospitals of Indianapolis, IN. The author acknowledges research assistants Diane Buell, BSN, and Saberina Bishop, BSN; graduate nursing students, Indiana University School of Nursing, and staff nurses of Community Hospital East: Beverly Burns, BSN, RNC; Therese Brandon, BSN; Teresa Golab, BSN; Sheryl Boyer, BSN; and Gloria Mercer, RN, for assistance with data collection.

REFERENCES

Corcoran, K., & Fischer, J. (1987). *Measures for clinical practice*. New York: The Free Press.

Horak, F. B. (1987). Clinical measurement of postural control in adults. *Physical Therapy, 67*, 1881–1885.

Horak, F. B., Shupert, C. L., & Mirka, A. (1989). Components of postural dyscontrol in the elderly: A review. *Neurobiology of Aging, 10*, 727–738.

Hogue, C. C., Studenski, S., & Duncan, P. (1989). Assessing mobility: The first step in preventing falls. In S. G. Funk, E. M. Tornquist, M. T. Champagne, L. A. Copp, & R. A. Wiese (Eds.), *Key aspects of recovery: Improving nutrition, rest and mobility* (pp. 275–280). New York: Springer.

Maki, B. E., Holliday, P. J., & Fernie, G. R. (1990). Aging and postural control: A comparison of spontaneous and induced-sway balance tests. *Journal of the American Geriatrics Society, 38,* 1–9.

Manchester, D., Woollacott, M., Zederbauer-Hylton, N., & Marin, O. (1989). Visual, vestibular and somatosensory contributions to balance control in older adults. *Journal of Gerontology, 44,* 118–127.

Morse, J. M., Tylko, S. J., & Dixon, H. A. (1987). Characteristics of the fall-prone patient. *The Gerontologist, 27,* 516–522.

Press, S. J., & Wilson, S. (1978). Choosing between logistic regression and discriminant analysis. *Journal of the American Statistical Association, 73*(364), 699–705.

Pyykko, I., Jantti, P., & Aalto, H. (1988). Postural control in the oldest olds. *Advances in Oto-Rhino-Larnygology, 41,* 146–151.

Sobel, K., & McCart, G. (1983). Drug use and accidental falls in an intermediate care facility. *Geriatrics and Gerontology, 17,* 539–543.

Tinetti, M. E. (1986). Performance-oriented assessment of mobility problems in elderly patients. *Journal of the American Geriatrics Society, 34,* 119–126.

Tinetti, M. E., Williams, T. F., & Mayewski, R. (1986). Fall risk index for elderly patients based on number of chronic disabilities. *American Journal of Medicine, 80,* 429–434.

Wilde, D., Nayak, L., & Issacs, B. (1981). Prognosis of falls in old people at home. *Journal of Epidemiology and Community Health, 35,* 200–204.

Woollacott, M. H. (1990). Changes in postural control and the integration of postural responses into voluntary movements with aging: Is borderline pathology a contributor? In T. Brandt, W. Paulus, W. Bles, M. Dieterich, S. Krafczyk, & A. Straube (Eds.), *Disorders of posture and gait* (pp. 221–228). New York: Thieme.

Woollacott, M., Inglin, B., & Manchester, D. (1988). Response preparation and postural control: Neuromuscular changes in the older adult. *Annals of New York Academy of Science, 525,* 42–53.

[7]

A Risk Model for Patient Fall Prevention

*Mary E. Soja, Thomas A. Kippenbrock,
Ann L. Hendrich, and Allen Nyhuis*

Patient falls are frequent in health care institutions, and these falls result in injuries. Jones and Smith (1989) report that patient falls account for 40% of all hospital incidents. Tinetti, Speechley, and Ginter (1988) report that 6% of nursing home residents have serious injuries after falling. These include fractures, cerebral contusions, severe sprains, hematomas, and hemothoraces. According to Stehlin (1988), over 200,000 hip fractures occur each year because of falls. Rowe (1982) has noted that the death rate from falls increases significantly with aging.

The literature on falls identifies the following potential risk factors: general weakness, decreased mobility of the lower extremities, sleeplessness, incontinence, confusion, depression, substance abuse, impaired speech, advanced age, decreased vision, vertigo, difficulty regaining balance, proprioceptive problems, history of falls, impaired gait, use of walking aids, intravenous therapy, poor mental state, nocturia, temperature elevation, and admission related to either orthopedics or oncology (Gryfe, Ashley, & Amies, 1977; Hendrich, 1988; Isaacs, 1985; Janken, Reynolds, & Swiech, 1986; Melton & Riggs, 1985; Morse, Tylko, & Dixon, 1985; Peck, 1986; Witte, 1979). This study compared fallers and non-fallers as a basis for identifying and weighting the most significant risk factors for hospitalized patients as a basis for developing a model for risk assessment and fall prevention.

METHOD

In order to compare risk factors of fallers and non-fallers, a retrospective case-control study was conducted at a large Midwestern acute care teaching hospital, using data derived from chart audits. The fall sample consisted of every patient over the age of 3 who fell during one calendar month (March 1989) at the institution. Some patients fell more than once during the study month, but to avoid statistical bias, only one incident per patient was audited for the fall sample ($n = 71$). A matched control sample was selected by randomly examining charts for patients admitted in March 1989 to the same nursing units to which patients in the fall sample were admitted. (Comatose patients were excluded from the control sample.) The control sample included 161 patients.

A risk factor assessment instrument developed by Hendrich (1988) was modified for use in the study. Demographic data such as age, gender, and admitting diagnosis were recorded, along with the occurrence of risk factors identified in the literature or derived from the authors' clinical experiences (see Table 7.1).

Charts for the fall sample were audited for two time periods: within 24 hours of admission and within 24 hours of the fall. Charts of the control sample were reviewed within 24 hours of admission and on the day closest to the midpoint of the patient's stay. Chart reviews were conducted by registered nurses with audit experience. The reviewers noted the presence or absence of each risk factor listed in Table 7.1. Inter-rater reliability was found to be 97.5% in a subset of the charts reviewed.

RESULTS

The sample of 71 fallers had a mean age of 58, and 52% were male; the 161 control patients had a mean age of 54, and 50% were male. The most frequent diagnostic categories in the fall sample were central nervous system (19%), diabetes (15%), cardiovascular (14%), and infections (14%). The most frequent diagnoses in the control sample were cardiovascular (21%), infections (12%), gastrointestinal (11%), and diabetes (11%).

A multivariate risk factor model was developed using logistic regression techniques. The mathematical definition of relative risk (RR) was:

$$RR = \frac{\text{Chances of falling if risk factor present}}{\text{Chances of falling if risk factor absent}}$$

TABLE 7.1   Risk Factors Used in the Falls Assessment Instrument (in addition to demographic data)

Risk factors	
1. Walking aids/devices	12. Depression
2. Intravenous therapy	13. History of falls
3. Impaired speech	14. Admission for syncope or previous admission for syncope
4. Impaired vision	
5. Incontinence	15. Orthopedic diagnosis
6. General weakness	16. Admission related to cancer
7. Decreased mobility of the lower extremities	17. 24 hours post surgical procedure
	18. Cardiovascular diagnosis
8. Sleeplessness	19. 100°F oral temperature elevation
9. Nocturia	20. 101°F rectal temperature elevation
10. Urinary frequency	21. Confusion
11. Foley catheter	

The most significant risk factor was clinical depression (relative risk or RR > 30). That is to say, the chances of falling were more than 30 times greater for patients who were depressed than for patients who were not depressed (see Table 7.2).

Other significant risk factors identified in the fall patient sample were age 70 or over, decreased mobility of the lower extremities, generalized weakness, abnormal elimination needs (i.e., incontinence, nocturia, and/or urinary frequency), and a 24-hour post surgical procedure time factor. The chances of a patient falling were between two and seven times greater if one of these risk factors was present (2 < RR < 7). One negative risk factor (i.e., a factor that reduced the risk of falling) was temperature elevation (≥ 100F oral, ≥ 101F rectal), probably because febrile patients stayed in bed.

Interactions between risk factors were also significant. For example, patients under the age of 70 who had a history of falls were at much higher risk than patients with a history of falls aged 70+ (RR = 53 vs. RR = 1.4). Likewise, confused patients under age 70 were at higher risk than confused patients aged 70+ (RR = 15 vs. RR = 1.4). The patients under age 70 tended to be patients with neurologic deficits.

When a patient's cumulative relative risk was greater than 10, the authors considered this patient at "extremely high risk for falls." Using this criterion, the risk model predicted patient falls with a sensitivity of 90% (i.e., 90% of all fallers were classified by the model as at extremely high risk for falling) and a specificity of 74% (i.e., 74% of non-fallers were classified as not at risk for falling).

DISCUSSION

The relative risk values from the multivariate analysis have been adapted for clinical nursing assessment by mathematically converting them to integer weights, referred to as risk points. For example, a patient with depression is assigned 10 points. A patient with decreased mobility of the lower extremities is assigned 5 points. See Table 7.2 for risk factors and the assignment of points.

If a patient has more than one risk factor, the risk points corresponding to the identified risk factors are summed to determine the final risk score. Thus, a patient over 70 years of age would receive 5 points for age and 1 point for a history of falls. These would be added together for a total of 6 points. For example, a 74-year old patient (5 points) admitted to the hospital complaining of generalized weakness (4 points), who walks with a walker (5 points), would receive 14 points, or a risk score of 14. This risk score then can be used as a reference to determine the level of nursing interventions needed for fall prevention.

Three levels of interventions have been established based on the patient's risk score:

1. Minimum level, a score of less than 4 points, indicates a need for interventions of call light in reach, bed in low position and brakes locked, side rails up, and assessment of gait to determine assistance needed.
2. Moderate level, a score of 4 to 7 points, indicates a need for all the minimal level interventions as well as special room and arm band

TABLE 7.2 Risk Factors and Point Assignments

Risk factor	Relative risk	Confidence interval	Points
Fall history with age < 70	52.61	(7.24, 382.2D)	+12
Depression	33.02	(7.43, 146.78)	+10
Confused patient age < 70	15.11	(3.55, 64.41)	+ 8
Age ≥ 70	5.28	(1.76, 15.80)	+ 5
Decreased mobility of the lower extremities	6.20	(2.38, 16.12)	+ 5
Generalized weakness	3.68	(1.47, 9.22)	+ 4
Abnormal elimination needs	3.37	(1.07, 10.68	+ 4
24 hours post surgical procedure time factor	2.32	(0.87, 6.16)	+ 3
Confused patient age ≥ 70	1.42	(0.29, 6.88)	+ 1
Fall history with age ≥ 70	1.42	(0.24, 8.54)	+ 1
Temperature elevation ≥ 100F oral or ≥ 101F rectal	0.37	(0.12, 1.09)	− 3

identification (e.g., highlighted or using another color of paper such as red), adequate night lighting, frequent assessment of the patient's elimination needs, and assistance as needed.

3. Maximum level, a score of more than 7, indicates a need for interventions at the minimal and moderate levels plus weight-sensitive bed alarming device; a commode, bedpan, or urinal within easy reach of the patient; and reorientation of the confused patient. A safety device may be deemed necessary.

This study verified previous findings in the fall literature but condensed the list of significant risk factors that identify patients with the potential to fall. The use of the three proposed levels of nursing interventions can help prevent patient falls and resulting injuries. Additional benefits of the intervention levels are conservation of resources and nursing time and improved assessment by clinical nurses.

ACKNOWLEDGMENTS

Partial financial support from the Indiana University–Purdue University at Indianapolis Project Development Program Grant is gratefully acknowledged.

REFERENCES

Gryfe, C. I., Ashley, M. I., & Amies, A. (1977). A longitudinal study of falls in an elderly population. I. Incidence and morbidity. *Age and Ageing, 6*, 201.

Hendrich, A. L. (1988). An effective unit-based prevention plan. *Journal of Nursing Quality Assurance, 3*, 28–30.

Isaacs, B. (1985). Clinical and laboratory studies of falls in old people. *Clinics in Geriatric Medicine, 1*, 513–524.

Janken, J. K., Reynolds, B., & Swiech, K. (1986). Patient falls in the acute care setting: Identifying risk factors. *Nursing Research, 35*, 215–219.

Jones, W. J., & Smith, A. (1989). Preventing hospital incidents: What we can do. *Nursing Management, 20*(9), 58–60.

Melton, J. L., & Riggs, L. B. (1985). Risk factors for injury after a fall. *Clinics in Geriatric Medicine, 1*, 525–540.

Morse, J. M., Tylko, S. J., & Dixon, H. A. (1985). The patient who falls and falls again. *Journal of Gerontological Nursing, 11*(11), 15–18.

Peck, W. A. (1986). Falls and hip fractures in elderly. *Hospital Practice, 21*(12), 720–726.

Rowe, J. W. (1982). Falls. In J. W. Rowe (Ed.). *Health and disease in older age* (p. 394). Boston: Little, Brown.

Stehlin, D. (1988). The silent epidemic of hip fractures. *FDA Consumer, 22*(4), 18–23.

Tinetti, M. E., Speechley, M., & Ginter, S. F. (1988). Risk factors for falls among elderly persons living in the community. *New England Journal of Medicine, 319,* 1701–1707.

Witte, N. S. (1979). Why the elderly fall. *American Journal of Nursing, 79,* 1950–1952.

[8]

Managing Falls: Identifying Population-Specific Risk Factors and Prevention Strategies

Kathleen Heslin, Jayne Towers, Colleen Leckie, Heather Thornton-Lawrence, Karen Perkin, Mario Jacques, Joyce Mullin, and Lynn Wick

The majority of patient falls are preventable. Predictors of falls include impaired mobility, weakness, (Morse, Morse, & Tylko, 1989; Morse, Tylko, & Dixon, 1987), diminished lower extremity strength and diminished activities of daily living (Tinetti, 1987), use of a walking aid, multiple secondary diagnoses (Morse et al., 1987; Morse et al., 1989), age (Tinetti, 1987), time of day (Morse, Prouse, Morrow, & Federspell, 1985; Morse et al., 1987; Swartzbeck & Mulligan, 1982), previous history of falls (Tinetti, Williams, & Mayewski, 1986; Morse et al., 1985; Morse et al., 1987; Morse et al., 1989), cognitive changes (Morse et al., 1985; Morse et al., 1987; Morse et al., 1989), sensory deficits (impaired vision) (Jarvinen & Jarvinen, 1968; Cohen & Lasley, 1985; Witte, 1979), impaired elimination patterns, pain, respiratory therapy (Morse et al., 1987), and medications (Hendrick, 1988).

Fall rates differ between acute care and long-term care settings. In the acute care setting 2.5 falls per patient are reported for every 1000 bed days, whereas up to 422 falls per 1000 bed days are reported in long-term care settings. Further, approximately 40% of these falls result in injury, 3% of which are serious (Morse et al., 1985; Morse et al., 1989). The purpose of this study was to identify factors contributing to fall injuries in acute, long-term, and residential health care settings, and to develop appropriate prevention strategies for these settings.

METHOD

Setting and Sample

The study was conducted in a 966-bed teaching hospital located in a residential community of southwestern Ontario. The facility has 581 acute care, 138 long-term care, and 247 residential care beds. The average length of stay is 7.5 days for the acute care service, 142.7 days in the long-term care setting, and 268.5 days for residential care. The occupancy rate is 87% for the acute care center, 95% for long-term care, and 98.9% for residential care. The fall rates at the time of the study were 2.16% for acute care, 1.46% for long-term care, and 9.83% for residential care.

A fall was defined as an event in which the patient came to rest on the floor from a lying, standing, or sitting position. Situations in which professional staff partially prevented the fall were excluded from the study. Falls that occurred on obstetrics, psychiatric, or pediatric units were also excluded. A retrospective review of incident reports and selected charts was done for 1,080 fall incidents; 225 of these data sets were excluded either because of incomplete data or failure to meet inclusion criteria. Thus the sample size for the analysis was 855 fall incidents.

Data Collection

To identify factors contributing to falls, data were collected on age, location of the fall, and seven risk factors: confusion, mobility deficits (impaired mobility or immobility), generalized weakness, assistive devices, safety devices, medical diagnoses , and previous falls. In addition, the type of injury was noted. Points were given for each risk factor, to derive a total risk score.

Location of the fall was recorded as "from bed," "in the bathroom," "ambulating," "wheelchair," "commode," "stretcher," or "chair."

Cognitive status was recorded as either alert or confused. Confusion was defined as impaired memory, inability to follow instructions, and/or impaired thought process. Each of these factors in confusion was scored as 1 point; thus the patient's risk score for confusion could range from 0 to 3.

Impaired mobility was defined as impaired gait or balance, or inability to walk outside the bedroom without support. Normal gait was operationalized as walking with head erect and striding unhesitantly with arms swinging freely at the side; normal gait was scored 0. Impaired gait was considered to be characterized by shuffling, narrow-based small steps, and a decreased walking speed; each of these three factors was scored 1 point. Small steps were indicative of decreased stride length (one foot or less), with variability in the length of successive steps. Patients with impaired gait typically grasped onto furniture, walls, the bed, or a walking aid for support, and were unable to walk without assistance (Wolfson, 1985; Morse et al. , 1989). Impaired balance was defined as unsteady gait with postural instability when standing (sway). Instability when standing results in inability to accommodate to even small destabilizing forces (Wolfson, 1985); it received a score of 1 point.

Immobility was defined as patients' inability to initiate movement on their own, requirement of a wheelchair and placement in the wheelchair by staff (no ambulatory aid was scored as 1; walking aid was scored as 2; and wheelchair aid was scored as 3).

Generalized weakness was defined as deficits in two out of six activities of daily living. If the patient was unable to stand or get out of bed independently, unable to feed himself, unable to turn in bed while fully conscious, unable to sit on the side of the bed without sliding off, or verbalized an experience of weakness (Tinetti, 1987), the patient was categorized as weak and assigned a score of up to 2 points depending on degree of weakness.

Assistive devices were defined as ambulatory aids such as canes, walkers, or wheelchairs, and use of one or more received a score of 1.

Safety devices included call bells, side rails, and restraint use. Patients received a score of 1 if none of the devices were in use, a 2 if side rails and call bells were used, and a 3 if the patient was restrained by posey jacket or waist or wrist restraint or was tied down with a sheet.

Medical diagnoses that were considered risk factors included cancer, neurologic, musculoskeletal, cardiovascular, orthopedic, gynecologic, surgical, and internal medicine. Conditions included within the internal medicine group were pneumonia, HIV, asthma, COPD, weakness, epistaxis, diarrhea, dehydration, diabetes, gastrointestinal disorders, cellulitis, colitis, nephrologic or urologic disorders, herpes zoster, dementia, hyperthyroidism, and pancreatitis.

Injuries resulting from falls were grouped into these categories: none, minor, and major. Minor injuries consisted of contusions, abrasions, and lacerations. Major injuries included fractures, multiple fractures, head injuries, and mortality within 24 hours.

RESULTS

Fall Characteristics: Acute Care

Of the 358 falls that occurred in the acute care center, only 17% were by patients under the age of 60; 49% of fallers were between the ages of 60 and 79, and the remainder of fallers (34%) were 80 or older (see Table 8.1). Marginally more falls (38%) occurred on the night shift (2301–0700 hours) than during the day shift (33%) or evening shift (29%). Overall, however, 54% of falls occurred between 0700 and 1900, and the remaining 46% occurred from 1900 to 0700. Nevertheless, a significantly greater number of falls from bed [$\chi^2(4) = 33.64$, $p < .001$] occurred during the night ($n = 88$). Fifty-nine percent of the patients who fell had a medical diagnosis within the internal medicine category; other diagnoses were relatively equally distributed among musculoskeletal (12%), neurologic (13%), and surgical (16%) categories (see Table 8.1).

One-half of the patients fell from bed (49%), 36% fell while they were ambulating, and the remaining 15% fell from a chair, wheelchair, or commode. At least 12% of those patients who fell while ambulating were attempting to get to or from the bathroom. The majority of the patients (56%) had some form of impaired gait, and 21% were patients requiring total assistance: however, 23% were identified as having no mobility deficits. Approximately one-half (54%) of the patients who fell were considered alert, while 46% were confused. The great majority of patients who fell from bed (98%) had restrictive devices (call bells and side rails), and 2% were using restraints at the time of their fall.

Sixty-three percent of those who fell incurred no injury, while 31% suffered some form of minor injury including contusions and abrasions. Major injuries accounted for 6% of the falls: these included fractures, dislocations, and head injuries (see Table 8.2). Two patients died within 24 hours of incurring the major injury.

The association between risk factors and injury was examined using

TABLE 8.1 Frequency Distribution of Characteristics of Fall Population in Acute, Long-Term, and Residential Care Settings

	Acute care (358 falls)		Long-Term care (55 falls)		Residential care (437 falls)	
	n	%	n	%	n	%
Age						
≤ 59	61	17	25	32	12	3
60–79	175	49	18	22	133	30
≥ 80	122	34	12	46	292	67
Shift						
day (0701-1500)	118	33	22	40	156	36
evening (1501-2300)	104	29	16	29	184	42
night (2301-0700)	136	38	17	31	96	22
Medical Diagnosis Category						
Internal medicine	211	59	27	50	301	69
Musculoskeletal	43	12	2	3	31	7
Neurologic	47	13	26	47	105	24
Surgical	57	16	0	0	0	0
Location						
Ambulation	129	36	1	2	154	35
Bed	175	49	36	65	194	44
Chair/wheelchair	54	15	18	33	89	20
Mobility Deficits						
No deficits	82	23	2	4	105	24
Impaired gait/balance	201	56	25	46	183	42
Total assistance	75	21	28	51	149	34
Cognitive Status						
Alert	193	54	31	56	232	53
Confused	165	46	24	44	205	47

chi square analyses, including the Fisher Yates correction factor for cell sizes less than 5. Patients who injured themselves were most likely to be over the age of 80 ($p < .001$), to have impaired mobility ($p < .01$), to experience generalized weakness ($p < .05$), to have fallen from a chair or wheelchair ($p < .07$), and to be in a restraint ($p < .1$) (see Table 8.3). The best combination of predictors of injury was determined using a stepwise logistic regression model. The greatest predictors of injury in acute care were age ≥ 80 ($p < .001$) and mobility deficits ($p < .01$). There were insufficient data to examine recurrent falls in the acute care population.

TABLE 8.2 Frequency of Injuries Resulting from Falls

	Acute care (358 falls)		Long-Term care (55 falls)		Residential care (437 falls)	
	n	%	n	%	n	%
No injury	226	63	45	82	319	73
Minor injury	111	31	10	18	92	21
Major injury	21	6	0	0	26	6

Fall Characteristics: Long-Term Care/Chronic Care

Of the 55 falls in the long-term care setting, 40% occurred during the day shift, with the remainder equally distributed between the evening and night shifts (see Table 8.1). An unusual age distribution was seen, with 32% of the fallers being under the age of 59. Upon closer examination, it was discovered that three patients who suffered from Huntington's chorea accounted for 45% of the falls in the long-term care setting; the mortality age for this group is typically less than 60 years. The remainder of the falls were distributed as expected—22% within the 60–79 year-old group, and 46% among those 80 and over.

The majority of residents (65%) fell in the bedroom area; 33% of the falls occurred from chairs, whereas only 2% occurred during ambulation. Such figures are consistent with the mobility status of patients in this setting: 51% were considered very dependent and were confined to a wheelchair, while another 46% had very limited mobility, although they were able to ambulate with assistive devices or the assistance of two individuals. Only 4% were categorized as able to walk independently. One-half of the patients had a diagnosis in the internal medicine category, and 47% had some form of neurologic disorder (principally Huntington's chorea); the other 3% were diagnosed as having musculoskeletal disorders. Surprisingly, no major injuries resulted from the falls in the long-term care setting. The majority of residents (82%) suffered no injury at all, while 18% suffered some form of minor injury (see Table 8.2).

Long-term care residents who injured themselves were likely to have a neurologic deficit ($p < .01$), to have fallen from a wheelchair or chair ($p < .04$), and to be age 80 or over ($p < .08$) (Table 8.3). The best combination of predictors of injury in long-term care was neurologic diagnosis ($p < .01$) and age 80 and over ($p < .1$). Falls were most likely to recur if the resident had mobility deficits ($p < .1$), had neurologic defi-

TABLE 8.3 Comparison of Risk Factors for Injury and Recurrent Falls in Acute, Long-Term, and Residential Care Settings

		Chi square coefficient (χ^2)		
			Setting	
Outcome	Risk factor	Acute care ($n = 358$)	Long-Term care ($n = 55$)	Residential care ($n = 437$)
Injury	Age	17.97^a	2.97^d	ns
	Neurologic Dx	ns	6.60^b	ns
	Internal medicine Dx	ns	ns	10.34^c
	During ambulation	ns	ns	9.93^c
	Impaired mobility	15.10^b	ns	9.51^c
	Generalized weakness	10.62^c	ns	ns
	Chair/wheelchair	8.67^d	4.12^c	ns
	Restraint	7.27^d	ns	5.42^d
	Confusion	ns	ns	ns
	Time of day	ns	ns	ns
Recurrent Falls	Confusion	—	ns	6.03^b
	Neurologic Dx	—	2.54^d	6.14^c
	Impaired mobility	—	2.19^d	3.38^d
	Weakness	—	ns	3.82^d
	Restrictive device/ transfer aid	—	2.04^d	ns
	Time of day	—	ns	ns
	Age	—	ns	ns

$^a p < .001$
$^b p < .01$
$^c p < .05$
$^d p < .1$

cits ($p < .1$), or was in restraints ($p < .1$). These associations were relatively weak, however.

Fall Characteristics: Residential Care

Four hundred and thirty-seven falls occurred in the residential care center. Thirty-six percent of these falls occurred during the day shift, 22% occurred during the night shift, and 42% occurred during the evening shift. The age distribution of the fallers in the residential setting was as expected: 3% of those who fell were between the ages of 40 and 59, 30% were between 60 and 79, and 67% were 80 and over (see Table

8.1). Forty-two percent of the residents who fell had some impaired gait, and 34% required total assistance for any kind of transfer movement; however, 24% ambulated without assistance. More residents (44%) fell from bed than while ambulating (35%); a considerable proportion (20%) fell from a wheelchair. Approximately one-quarter (24%) of those who fell in the residential care setting had some form of neurologic diagnosis; 7% had a musculoskeletal disorder. The great majority (69%) of those who fell had internal medicine diagnoses.

The outcomes of falls in the residential care setting were very similar to those in the acute care setting: 73% of the residents did not incur any injury as a result of their fall, whereas 21% suffered some form of minor injury and another 6% suffered a major injury. The number of injuries did not differ significantly on different shifts.

Risk factors found to be associated with injury using chi square included a diagnosis in the internal medicine category ($p < .03$), ambulation ($p < .04$), mobility deficits ($p < .04$), and use of restraints ($p < .1$). The best combination of predictors of injury in residential care was use of a restrictive device ($p < .01$) and falls occurring from chairs and wheelchairs ($p < .05$). Falls were more likely to recur if the resident was confused ($p < .01$), had neurologic deficits ($p < .04$), or had mobility deficits ($p < .1$) and generalized weakness ($p < .1$) (see Table 8.3).

Interventions

Because of the multifaceted nature of the risk factors and the variability of the settings, an intervention model was designed to target specific care settings and types of falls (see Figure 8.1). The acute care area initiated a bed sensor program, followed by a benzodiazepine utilization prevention plan, and assessments of impaired mobility. The long-term care setting began with restraint-free cushions and enhancements to the bed-wheelchair transfer plan, and then initiated a wheelchair preventive maintenance and specialization purchase program. The residential care area developed a trial bed-to-bathroom rest-stop strategy, altered the dinner hour, and recommended gait assessments. Further interventions were identified as part of a long-term, comprehensive fall prevention program.

Acute Care Interventions

Sensor for Bed-Based Falls The initial intervention for the acute care setting was directed toward bed-based falls; this intervention consisted of a fall-risk assessment (see Figure 8.2), nursing care plan, spot-the-dot,

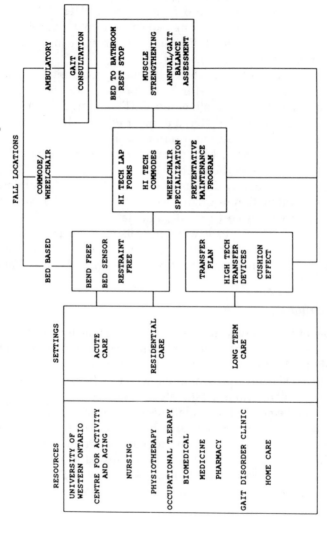

FIGURE 8.1. Collaborative intervention model for fall prevention.

FIGURE 8.2. Fall prevention assessment form.

RISK FACTOR ASSESSMENT	Date:										
	Time:										
Risk Factor	Score:										
Age 65 - 79	.5										
Age 80 >	1										
Confusion (unable to follow instruction to stay in bed)	2										
Attempts to get out of bed/Agitation	5										
Previous fall related to patient condition	1										
Impaired mobility, balance or gait	1										
Generalized weakness	1										
Alterations in elimination (frequency, urgency, nocturia, incontinence, IV Lasix)	1										
Medications within 24 hours (benzo-diazepines, tranquilizers, narcotics, and anesthesia)	1										
Immobile	-5										
Risk Assessment Total Score											

FLOW SHEET

Level I - Score .5 - 2*											
Level II - Score 2.5 - 4**											
Level III - Score ≥ 4.5***											
Patient education delivered to: Patient											
Patient education delivered to: Family or Sitter											
Nurse's initial											

Note: *Implement interventions for Level I (see Table 8.4).
    **Implement interventions for Levels I and II (see Table 8.4).
    ***Implement interventions for Levels I, II, and III (see Table 8.4).

and bed sensor. The assessment was developed from the risk-factor analysis. Each factor found to predict falls was given a score reflecting its importance. Three additional risk factors were added to the assessment form based on the literature. These factors were (1) medications—sedatives, tranquilizers, narcotics, and general anesthetic—within 24 hours (Hendrick, 1988), (2) alterations in elimination—frequency, urgency, and nocturia or incontinence (Morse et al., 1987), and (3) previous falls. Spot-the-dot consisted of color coded markers placed at strategic positions to alert staff of fall risk (central call bell receiver at the nursing station, above the bed, and at the entrance to the patient's room). The bed sensor was a pressure-sensitive magnetic plasticized pad connected to a call bell control unit.

The intervention trial period in the acute care setting was 3 months, for a total of 13,425 patient days, on two large medical and two large surgical units, which accounted for 50% of acute care falls. Each patient was assessed on each shift using the risk assessment form, and was assigned a risk category—Level I (possible risk), II (potential fall risk), or III (actual fall risk), with corresponding interventions (see Figure 8.2). The reverse side of the form provided details to guide the assessment (see Table 8.4). A bed-sensor system was assigned to each patient who was evaluated at Level III and thus received a nursing diagnosis of actual fall risk. The patients were kept on these bed-sensor systems for as long as their assessment indicated that they were at the level of actual fall risk. For patients whose risk-factor scores were below the critical limit and who were at the level of potential fall risk, spot-the-dot was used (Hendrick, 1988).

Post-implementation analyses indicated a dramatic decrease in the number of bed-based falls during the 3-month trial. Pre-implementation, the medical and surgical units accounted for both the majority of acute care bed-based falls ($n = 140$) and the majority of acute care major injuries ($n = 7$). During the implementation period, no bed-based falls or injuries were incurred by patients on the surgical units using the bed-sensor system. On the medical units, four patients using the bed-sensor system had bed-based falls, and one of these suffered a severe injury. One fall, however, occurred as a result of an equipment failure: the sensor failed to ring. (Subsequent evaluation indicated that it was a failure of the call bell system that connected to and activated the sensor alarm.) One fall occurred with a patient who was confused and experiencing urinary urgency, and the other two falls involved patients who were both agitated and confused. The alarm delay times sub-sequently were readjusted from 4 to 2 seconds; since that time, no further falls have occurred. Overall, there was an 85% reduction in bed-based falls using the sensor system (see Figure 8.3).

Six patients on the medical units who were assessed at Level II, potential for fall, and who received the observation intervention of spot-the-dot, fell from bed. A chart audit of these patients revealed that they were all receiving benzodiazepines (Ativan, Oxazepam, Lorazepam); 50% of them suffered from angina or hypoxia up to 12 hours before the fall. Use of benzodiazepines and hypoxia were there-

TABLE 8.4   Guidelines for Completing Fall Risk Assessment and Flow Sheet

---

POLICY:

1. A fall risk assessment will be completed on all newly admitted patients, excluding critical care, pediatrics, obstetrics, and psychiatry.
2. A flow sheet will be initiated for all Level II and Level III patients.
3. The flow sheet will be kept at the patient's bedside with other flow sheets.
4. Fall risk reassessment and documentation on the flow sheet should be completed once per 12-hour tour for all Level II and Level III patients, and maintained (for 3 days) for Level II patients who return to Level I.
5. For those patients scoring Level I on admission, reassessment is not required unless there is a significant change in patient condition related to fall risk factors.
6. If in the nurse's judgment the patient does not require a bed sensor and the risk score is above 4.5, an * must be placed next to the score. A note must be written in the core progress notes identifying the reasons for the decision and a reassessment done every 12 hours.
7. All actual fall episodes must be documented on the Fall Report form.

PROCEDURE:

1. Complete the fall risk assessment by marking the corresponding score in the appropriate column for the risk factors that apply to the patient. It may be necessary to collaborate with the registered nurse when completing the assessment. Consider the following:

   Confusion: inability to follow instructions, impaired short-term memory, impaired thought process (psychosis), and conditions that potentiate agitation such as septicemia and hypoxia.

   Attempts to get out of bed: attempts to get out of bed related to factors such as agitation, alcohol, or poor pain control.

   Previous fall related to risk factors: note previous falls related to patient condition such as weakness, impaired mobility, or confusion. Do not include previous falls related to environmental factors such as faulty equipment.

   Impaired mobility: impaired gait (shuffling, small steps, slow pace, holding onto nurse, bed, walls, chairs, IV poles for support) and/or impaired balance (unsteady when standing or sitting).

   Generalized weakness: absence of 2 out of 6 ADL, unable to feed self, unable to turn self in bed yet is fully conscious, verbalizes is feeling weak, unable to sit on bed for 10 minutes without sliding off.

   Alterations in elimination: medications such as diuretics that may alter elimination patterns including Lasix IV bolus and hs diuretics.

   Immobile: patient who is unable to initiate movement to get out of bed, patient who cannot attempt any self-movement. A *negative* score of 5 is assigned to prevent eligibility for a bed sensor.

2. Add the values for each risk factor indicated, and place the total score in the total score column.

TABLE 8.4 *Continued*

3. Determine the patient's fall risk by referring to the Assessment Key and institute the corresponding intervention. (Refer to Standard Care Plan, Potential for Injury: Falls.)
4. Complete the patient education section ensuring that education is delivered to patient/family or sitter regarding the use of the fall prevention system.
5. Initiate Fall Flow Sheet when a potential or actual fall risk is determined, by placing a check in the appropriate column. Note:

Possible Fall Risk—Level I Intervention:	call bell in reach, bed in low position, side rails up, nonslip footwear.
Potential Fall Risk—Level II Intervention:	spot the dot, assess and assist ambulation, elimination needs checked, nursing care plan, screen medications.
Actual Fall Risk—Level III Intervention:	bed sensor.

fore added to the list of risk factors and assigned a weight of 1; with these additions, no subsequent bed-based falls were experienced.

Changes in the age-related risk categories also were made on the assessment tool based on response from the surgical units. Several surgical patients received assessment scores indicating Level III, actual risk of fall, when there was no active attempt by the patients to get out of bed. It appeared as though their ages were qualifying a number of patients for Level III status who would not necessarily need a bed sensor. Therefore, the weighting for the age category 80 and over was readjusted from 1.3 to 1.

One additional risk was added to the assessment tool following the intervention period: persistent attempts to get out of bed. Nurses on both the medical and surgical units perceived that patients who made persistent attempts to get out of bed were at extreme risk for falling and required a bed sensor. At the same time, immobility was added as a negative factor: the nurse deducted 5 points from the total assessment score for those patients who met the criteria for actual risk of falling but who, because of their pronounced incapacity or feeble state, were unable to initiate the movements needed to get out of bed.

A survey of staff satisfaction with the sensor system was administered following the trial period. Thirty percent of the nurses reported that they now had more time to spend with their patients, while 75% perceived that their care was enhanced, 65% perceived a reduction in use of restraints, 80% felt they had more control in preventing bed-based falls, and 70% believed their fall-risk assessment skills were improved.

FIGURE 8.3. Minor and major injuries from bed-based falls.

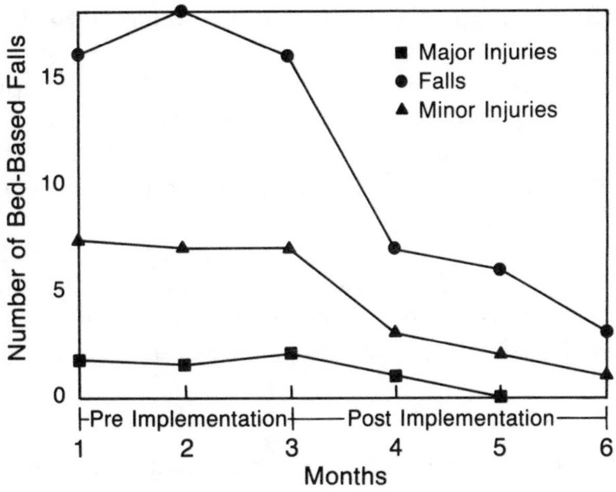

Note: Intervention started at Month 3.

Benzodiazepine-Free Program In a collaborative project of the Departments of Nursing, Pharmacy, and Medicine, the 150 medical consultants within the health center were surveyed in February 1991 to elicit information on trends in prescriptions of benzodiazepines. The survey indicated that at any given time, 50% of all patients had an order for benzodiazepines. The principal reason for prescribing benzodiazepines given by physicians responding to the survey was patient/family request. Canada, unlike the United States, has not signed the International Agreement for Controlled Substances related to the use of benzodiazepines. The Province of Ontario has the highest number of prescriptions per person per annum in the world (13 per patient).

The following strategies have been formulated:

1. A proposal was submitted to the Pharmacy and Therapeutics Committee to reduce the hospital formulary from eight to two forms of benzodiazepines.
2. Benzodiazepine ward stock will be reduced by approximately 50%.
3. A prescription shift to p.r.n. will be promoted.
4. Education regarding the complications with use in the frail elderly and cardiorespiratory-compromised patients will be provided in medical and nursing teaching rounds, followed by a utilization review audit and a comparison of benzodiazepine use with concurrent fall events.

Impaired Mobility Assessments Historically, all physiotherapy consultations in this acute care setting have been initiated with a written physician's order, in an attempt to prioritize referrals based on scarce resources. However, nurses are in an ideal position to screen patients with impaired mobility for direct referral to physiotherapy. Factors associated with impaired gait and balance are standard questions on the nursing admission forms, and it is well documented that patients with impairments in mobility benefit from appropriately assigned mobility aids.

In a collaborative project between nursing and physiotherapy, a referral screening form will be developed for physiotherapy consultation, assessment, assignment, and patient instruction regarding the use of walking aids. Collaborative transfer plans will also be developed.

Long-Term Care Interventions

A sample of residents in the long-term care setting ($n = 40$) was tested for fall risk using the fall assessment form developed for the acute care setting intervention period. This assessment indicated that 100% of the sample required use of the bed sensor, yet 50% of the patients had never fallen from bed at any time during their extended stay in this setting (average = 147 days). Therefore, it was decided that the risk assessment tool used for acute care was not appropriate for long-term care. Closer examination of the fall types in the long-term care setting revealed fall proneness during the bed-to-chair transfer process in addition to falls from wheelchair and bed related to a diagnosis of Huntington's chorea. Thus bed falls, bed transfers, and wheelchairs were targeted for intervention.

Restraint-Free Cushion Effect Patients with Huntington's chorea had significant, repeated involuntary neuromuscular actions that resulted in falls from bed. These actions were rapid, making a sensor intervention inadequate for prevention. Thus a new intervention was designed to protect these patients from injury. Restraints were removed, bed rails were padded with cushions, and the bed was surrounded with mattresses. Since the initiation of this intervention, these patients have remained injury free while having room for in-bed movement.

Bed-to-Chair Transfers Approximately 50% of the bed-based falls in the long-term care setting occurred during the transfer process. Such falls were attributed to problems with the transfer process and equipment failures. Problems occurred when staff had a false sense of resident cooperativeness during the process; in fact, residents often would unpredictably resist and counteract the transfer. The intervention consisted of a transfer plan collaboratively developed by physiotherapy, occupational therapy, and nursing staff, with a commitment to use the plan for all transfers. The transfer plan provided details on the transfer device to be used, staff body mechanics (positioning of hands and feet), the transfer side of the bed, height of the bed, resident alignment, number of staff required, and time of day (frequency and duration). Changes in transfer requirements were reviewed by team members on a p.r.n. basis and at regularly scheduled biannual case review meetings. There was a subsequent 55% reduction in bed-based falls.

In addition, two high-tech transfer devices were purchased for two of the four long-term care units, and a monthly maintenance program was initiated for the remaining transfer equipment. With the combination of a transfer plan and transfer devices, there was a 92% reduction in bed-based falls on Unit 1 and 97% on Unit 2. This result was confounded, however, by the death of the two patients with Huntington's chorea who had had 45% of the falls.

It was noted that in most of the long-term care wheelchair falls, contributing factors were inaccessibility of the wheelchair brakes and wheelchair instability. Wheelchair purchase plans were developed involving product evaluation review with capital costing projections, and two specialized wheelchairs were purchased. Also a monthly wheelchair preventive maintenance program was initiated. The two wheelchairs were customized for individual resident postural control and support needs. No residents have fallen from these specialized chairs.

Residential Care Interventions

Rest Stop   A significant number of injuries occurring in the residential care setting ($p < .05$) were associated with ambulation. A nurse clinician in long-term/residential care worked with nursing staff to create the "rest-stop" concept, a specific plan of care for the frail elderly identified as having potential or actual risk for falling. A personalized, stable chair was positioned midway from bed to bathroom as a "rest stop." Use of this intervention has eliminated bed-to-bathroom falls for patients with whom this intervention was tested over a 3-month period. This intervention has been extended to placing chairs in strategic positions in the corridor with very positive results.

Dinner Hour   Forty-two percent of the falls in the residential setting occurred during the evening (1500-2300) shift. Melton and Riggs (1985) have noted that the frail elderly are particularly sensitive to postprandial hypotension, in which systolic blood pressure drops an average of 25 mmHg up to 60 minutes after a meal. The resident population had their evening meal at 1700–1800 hours, and began preparing for bed at 1900 hours. Because there is possibly an association between mealtime, a delayed hypotensive event, and a fall event, plans are in place to separate the mealtime by an additional hour from the bedtime preparation activity; this intervention was developed in collaboration with nutrition services, and results are pending completion of a pilot test.

Gait Assessments   Because approximately one-third (35.2%) of the residential care falls occurred during ambulation, and injury was associated with impaired mobility ($p = .04$), a gait assessment program was recommended. Currently, residents in residential care are dependent on home care physiotherapy for development of their ambulation plan of care. In Ontario, home care funding for physiotherapy is very limited. However, recent amendments to Long-Term Care Reform legislation will enable p.r.n. physical assessments; as this legislation becomes enacted, gait assessments will be implemented.

Muscle Strengthening   The initial data collected identified the residential care population as frail elderly over the age of 60 (95%), 76% of whom had impaired or severely impaired mobility. A number of researchers (Aniansson & Zethernan, 1984; Isaacs, 1985; Kaufman, 1985; Melton & Riggs, 1985; Rice, 1989; Riffle, 1982; Vandervoort & McCamas, 1986) have proposed muscle strength training programs for the frail elderly in order to improve functions needed for daily living, such as ambulating. Researchers at the Centre for Activity and Aging (Dr. P. Rechnitzer and Dr. A. A. Vandervoort, 1991) and the author have designed a research proposal to test outcomes of a muscle strengthening program for the residential care population. This study will be conducted when funds become available.

DISCUSSION

Clinical Support

Implementation of these interventions in practice requires educational and clinical support for staff. Staff nurses require inservice training that clarifies and reinforces risk-factor assessment, specifically cognitive and mobility status. Because the effectiveness of a bed-sensor system is dependent on risk-factor assessment, clinical nurse specialists are needed as consultants to staff in the assessment process. On-site consultation resources can be created by appointing unit fall resource nurses (one per shift) who can respond to queries from their peers regarding assessment and intervention strategies. It is particularly useful to have unit resources in place for the first 6 months of implementation and to structure an audit component into fall prevention activities.

Of interest in this study was the lack of effectiveness of traditional preventive approaches such as use of call bells in preventing falls.

Considering that 98% of the patients who fell from bed had a call bell in place, their ineffectiveness seems evident. It may be that subclinical confusion is challenged by internal factors such as hypoxia, cardiac ischemia, urinary stress, and mood-altering drugs such as benzodiaze-pines. The patient is initially assessed as alert and able to use a call bell, but the effects of illness stress and/or drugs compel the patient to rapid, independent at-risk activity, which suggests that we need to develop and use methods to assess subclinical confusional states.

Also of interest was the specificity of risk factors based on type of facility. In the acute care setting, the need for bed sensors was based on the patients' propensity to attempt to get out of bed unassisted, whereas in long-term care the patients were less likely to initiate independent bed exit activity (among the non-Huntington's population); rather, falls were more likely to occur in the transfer process. In the residential care population, transient confusion may be less of a risk factor, and mobil-ity, strength, and agility factors more dominant, thus requiring a differ-ent focus in assessment and treatment.

Of critical importance is the impact of interventions on the type of fall. It is clear that factors contributing to the fall event and subsequent injury differ greatly. Effective fall management requires targeting both intrinsic factors, with interventions such as muscle strengthening, gait training, and mood-altering drug reduction, and extrinsic factors, using transfer plans, transfer devices, a safe environment (such as a cushioned floor), alert systems, wheelchair specialization, preventive maintenance, and rest stops. It is the interactive effect of these interventions that con-tributes to effective fall prevention.

Collaboration

Collaboration is critical to effective fall prevention. As these in-terventions illustrate, a number of disciplines and services must interact to address various risk factors. Each discipline should take a leading role when the predominant risk factor is related to their service: clinical pharmacy should handle reductions in benzodiazepine utilization; nurse managers should look after equipment purchases; the physiother-apists should handle transfer plans and mobility assessments; nurse clinicians should tend to nurse alert systems, consultation, and educa-tion; and occupational therapy should implement home prevention and wheelchair positioning and specialization.

Future

A number of variables that were not explored in this study may be contributing factors to falls; these require further study and additional interventions, such as diet, drug, and exercise therapy for the osteoporosis population and examination of the effect of illness-induced stress on patients' ability to manage their hospital environment; and the effects of lighting and pathways; washroom space; height of beds; polypharmacy; transient confusional states; and neurologic phenomena.

REFERENCES

Aniansson, A., & Zethernan, C. (1984). Effect of a training programme for pensioners on condition and muscle strength. *Archives of Gerontology, 3,* 229–241.

Cohen, T. E., & Lasley, D. J. (1985). Visual depth illusion and falls in the elderly. *Clinics in Geriatric Medicine, 1,* 601–620.

Hendrick, A. L. (1988). An effective unit-based fall prevention plan. *Journal of Nursing Quality Assurance, 3,* 28–36.

Isaacs, B. (1985). Clinical and laboratory studies of falls in old people. *Clinics in Geriatric Medicine, 1,* 513–520.

Jarvinen, K. A., & Jarvinen, P. H. (1968). Falling from bed as a complication of hospital treatment. *Journal of Chronic Diseases, 21,* 375–378.

Kaufman, T. L. (1985). Strength training effect in young and aged women. *Archives of Physical and Rehabilitative Medicine, 65,* 223–226.

Melton, L. J., & Riggs, B. L. (1985). Risk factors for injury after a fall. *Clinics in Geriatric Medicine, 1,* 525–533.

Morse, J. M., Morse, R. N., & Tylko, S. J. (1989). Development of a scale to identify the fall prone elderly. *Canadian Journal of Aging, 8,* 366–376.

Morse, J. M., Prouse, M. D., Morrow, N., & Federspell, G. (1985). A retrospective analysis of patient falls. *Canadian Journal of Public Health, 76*(3), 116–118.

Morse, J. M., Tylko, S. J., & Dixon, H. A. (1987). Characteristics of the fall-prone patient. *The Gerontologist, 27,* 516–522.

Rice, C. L. (1989). Strength in an elderly population. *Archives of Physical and Rehabilitative Medicine, 70,* 391–397.

Riffle, K. L. (1982). Falls, kinds, causes, and prevention. *Geriatric Nursing, 35,* 165–169.

Swartzbeck, E. M., & Mulligan, W. L. (1982). A comparative study of hospital incidents. *Nursing Management, 13,* 39–43.

Tinetti, M. E. (1987). Factors associated with serious injury during falls by ambulatory nursing home residents. *Journal of the American Geriatrics Society, 35,* 644–648.

Tinetti, M. E., Williams, T. F., & Mayewski, R. (1986). Fall risk index for elderly patients based on a number of chronic disabilities. *American Journal of Medicine, 80,* 429–434.

Vandervoort, A. A., & McCamas, A. J. (1986). Contractile changes in opposing muscles of the human ankle joint with aging. *Journal of Applied Physiology, 61,* 361–367.

Witte, N. S. (1979). Why elderly fall. *American Journal of Nursing, 79,* 1950–1952.

Wolfson, L. (1985). Falls and the elderly: Gait and balance in the elderly. *Clinics of Geriatric Medicine, 1,* 649–653.

[9]

A Program to Reduce Frailty in the Elderly

Elizabeth McNeely, Sandra D.Clements, and Steven L. Wolf

Though frailty occurs more frequently in the older population, Knight and Walker (1988) firmly state that frailty "is not, however, a consequence of age" (p. 358). Interestingly, the *Encyclopedia of Aging* (Maddox, 1987) does not include the word *frailty* as a term associated with aging. And in fact, frailty remains an ill-defined and elusive concept. Though frailty is not synonymous with aging, age-related changes may cause alterations in the management and outcome of life activities. According to a geriatric assessment text, a frail individual is "a person whose management of day-to-day tasks is tenuous" (Gallo, Reichel, & Anderson, 1988)—this definition implies that most people may be frail at many points in their lives.

The notion that a frail individual is a person whose life activities are tenuous reflects a functional perspective and implies that approaches to intervention need to be broad. Indeed, a noted gerontologist (Neugarten, 1984) suggests that a functional approach should be used in all rehabilitation and health-promotion activities with the older adult population.

One of the challenges for clinicians and researchers alike is to identify which factors influence functional capabilities. With major health problems such as falls in the elderly, many factors and relationships may be important. Indeed, the literature on falls in the elderly clearly indicates that causes of falling and injuries from falls are multifactorial and must be considered from biological, psychological, and sociological perspectives (Tinetti & Speechly, 1989).

   The subtlety and complexity of functional frailty and a need for interventions to reduce frailty and falls in the elderly led to the initiation of a set of 3-year, nationwide clinical trials sponsored by the National Institute on Aging and the National Center for Nursing Research (#U01-AG-09124). This multisite cooperative study focusing on frailty and injuries among the elderly population is entitled "Frailty and Injuries: Cooperative Studies of Intervention Techniques," or FICSIT. FICSIT studies are being conducted at eight sites nationwide and use a variety of clinical protocols to investigate innovative interventions.

   A total of 1500 subjects, ranging from community dwellers to nursing home residents, are participating in the studies. All sites are collecting information for a common data base, which includes demographics, cognition, gait, balance, strength, and function. Each site has an intervention protocol and collects specific data related to that protocol. Falls, near-falls, and fall-related injury data will be examined throughout the 3-year study period. Meta-analysis will be used to examine the different protocols and combine the site results into useful data on common outcomes of falls and fall-related injuries.

SITE DESCRIPTIONS

Site One is located in Portland, OR, at Kaiser Foundation Hospitals. Community-dwelling subjects identified as at high risk for falls participate in walking, generalized physical conditioning, and guided mental imagery. Site Two is at Yale University, New Haven, CT. Researchers at this site are comparing the number of falls and fall injuries in an ambulatory control population who receive "usual health care" to the number in an experimental group who receive a risk-abatement strategy targeted at potentially alterable risk factors for falls (e.g., muscle weakness, visual and hearing impairments, etc.). Site Three is located at the University of Washington in Seattle. Community-dwelling subjects with leg weakness at a level associated with increased risk of impaired health and falls are given strength training, endurance training, or a combination of the two. Site Four is located in San Antonio, TX, at the Audie L. Murphy Memorial Veterans' Hospital Extended Care Therapy Center. Subjects are nursing home residents who do not usually "qualify" for physical therapy under reimbursement guidelines; in this study they receive intensive physical therapy. Site Five is located in Atlanta, GA, at the Emory University Center for Rehabilitation Medicine and Wesley Woods Geriatric Hospital. Researchers at this location are investigating balance training for community-dwelling older adults. Site Six is at Hebrew Rehabilitation Center for the Aged in Boston, MA. The subjects, who are frail, institutionalized "fallers," are receiving vigorous progressive resistance training of the legs and/or multinutrient supplementation. Site Seven is at the University of Iowa in Iowa City. Investigations at this site concentrate on nursing home residents and are examining the use of hip joint protective clothing and assistance to the toilet during elimination rounds. Site Eight is at the University of Connecticut in Farmington, CT. Community-dwelling subjects are exposed to balance training, strength training, or a combination of the two. Thus, in the FICSIT projects the problems of frailty and fall-related injuries are being approached systematically with a variety of subjects and interventions. This chapter briefly describes one of the clinical trials, at Emory University and Wesley Wood Geriatric Hospital, Atlanta, GA.

METHOD

The Emory/Wesley Woods FICSIT research team includes a nurse gerontologist, a physical therapist, a behavioral neurologist, a medical sociologist, an environmental architect, a clinical neuropsychologist, a psychiatrist, a biostatistician, a nutritionist, and a Grand Master of the Chinese exercise Tai Chi Chuan. The study uses a pre–post experimental design with random assignment of subjects to one of three protocols—static exercise, dynamic exercise, and a nonexercise health education group.

All participants are age 70 or older, living in a nonsupervised situation, ambulatory, and free of progressive neurologic conditions or severe cognitive impairment. A screening history and physical are used to ensure that subjects meet these criteria.

Initial recruitment for subjects was begun by chart reviews at the Wesley Wood Geriatric Hospital and outpatient clinic. After the media publicized the FICSIT program nationally and locally, community interest generated further inquiries and interest in participating.

Subjects ($N = 215$) are enrolled in 15-week intervention or control sessions. There are 10–12 subjects in each of the dynamic exercise, static exercise, and health education protocols during each 15-week period.

Protocols

The two intervention protocols used at Emory/Wesley Woods contrast both cultural and technological approaches to balance training. "Static exercise" is a Western, high-technology biofeedback intervention. "Dynamic exercise" is a Far Eastern, low-technology intervention. A third group (the control group) attends a health education seminar but has no exercise protocol.

Static Exercise   Static exercise training is done using a computerized balance machine. The protocol involves biofeedback training for maintaining balance. The subject stands on electronic force plates in front of a CRT screen and, by shifting the center of body mass, moves the cursor on the screen toward specified targets. When the subject shifts body weight on the electrically sensitive foot plates, the cursor traces the pattern on the screen recorded by the computer.

Electronic force sensors simulate proprioceptive reactions of weight transfer balancing by the subject. Balance training takes place as targets are moved and reconfigured and the platform under the foot plates is tilted and turned. The complexity of tasks increases as the sessions progress. For safety, the subjects are placed in a suspension harness during the sessions. The 15-week one-hour sessions are under the direction of a physical therapist skilled in biofeedback training.

In the pilot study that included three sessions of this protocol with 10 older persons, the findings (shown in Table 9.1) indicated that improvement occurred with the biofeedback training. Specifically, all subjects showed ability to shift weight more quickly from pre- to posttest within each session as well as across the three training sessions. At the start of the protocol (Session 1 pretest), subjects took an average of 7.83 seconds to complete the weight shift; by the posttest of Session 3 they could accomplish this task in an average of 2.65 seconds. The improvements from pre- to posttest within sessions and from session to session were both significant [$F(1,7) = 25.9$, $p = .001$ and $F(2,6) = 5.73$, $p = .041$, respectively]. The interaction between session and time (pre- to posttest) was also significant [$F(2,6) = 6.22$, $p = .034$], indicating that subjects showed greater improvement during the first session than they did during Sessions 2 and 3. The long-term effects of trained muscle response in older persons are part of the ongoing investigation.

TABLE 9.1   Number of Seconds to Complete Weight-Shift Movement in Static Exercise Group: Interaction between Session and Time

	Pretest		Posttest	
	Mean	SD	Mean	SD
Session 1	7.83	2.63	4.47	2.11
Session 2	4.41	1.96	3.13	1.13
Session 3	3.74	1.10	2.65	0.48

Dynamic Exercise The second protocol is the practice of Tai Chi Chuan—Yang style (Tai Chi). Tai Chi was once a martial art and has evolved into a dance-like, well controlled set of slow, deliberate, opposing, that is, Yin and Yang, body movements. Approximately 60% of older adults in the People's Republic of China practice Tai Chi daily. Scenes from China reveal hundreds of people of all ages practicing Tai Chi as an energizing and relaxing activity. Tai Chi is mandatory in Chinese schools and the practice is widespread in the Eastern world.

Even though Tai Chi has been practiced for hundreds of years by thousands of people of all ages, very little scientific data on the specific effects of Tai Chi are available. A few reports in Western journals have indicated the potential health benefits of Tai Chi (Koh, 1982; Zhuo, Shephard, David, & Philby, 1984). The Grand Master of Tai Chi Chuan who leads the dynamic exercise groups also searched the Chinese literature for research information on Tai Chi. The search revealed some studies of the physiologic and psychologic benefits of Tai Chi, but the studies are of questionable scientific rigor. Clearly, the benefits of Tai Chi need further scientific investigation (Qu Mianyu, 1986).

Nevertheless, the fact that the practice of Tai Chi is both time honored and popular indicates that regular practice of Tai Chi may indeed be beneficial. Tai Chi's slow deliberative movements and mind/body awareness are congruent with the flexibility and balance exercise needs of the older adult.

Interestingly, the response to publicity about this study in the media indicates that older people in Western cultures are anxious to learn Tai Chi. A number of inquirers said that they would participate in the study only if they could be assured of assignment to the Tai Chi protocol. Though this assurance could not be offered, the inquiries clearly showed that this form of exercise is acceptable to older adults in Western society.

The protocol is a set of 10 selected Tai Chi movements known as "forms." There are over 108 forms in the practice of Tai Chi. However, for this study the Tai Chi leader and principal investigator selected 10 forms that represent components of potentially lost or impaired movement in an older population. The routine is designed to gain a sense of body control and movement mastery. Tai Chi exercises demand concentration and a sense of body awareness.

The sessions are held twice a week. Each session lasts approximately 1 hour. To date, two groups ($n = 20$) have completed the 15-week intervention, and one group ($n = 10$) has completed postintervention testing. Although the quantitative data have not yet been analyzed, the participants have reported anecdotal data. Many individuals attest to increased flexibility and confidence in body balance and freedom of movement. One man said that he could now balance on one foot to get into his trousers, whereas before, he was sitting down to dress. In addition, the social interaction and camaraderie provided the first group with the motivation to continue meeting weekly on their own to practice the forms as a group—as all participants are encouraged to do postintervention.

Health Education Seminars The 1-hour health education seminar is conducted weekly by a nurse. The seminars engage participants in discussions about topics relevant to aging challenges, for example, memory enhancement skills, nutrition, medication use/abuse, legal aspects, dental care, living wills, etc. The protocol prohibits discussions about exercises or injury control, but the group is allowed to change the predetermined topics if other areas of interest evolve. The seminar subjects are requested to keep records of falls and near-falls and injuries, and are measured in the same way as the other study subjects.

Data Collection

Common data base items collected on all subjects in all FICSIT studies include demographic information, height, weight, chronic health conditions, sleep patterns, and medications. In addition, cognitive function and psychosocial data are collected, using the Folstein Mini-Mental State Examination, the Tinetti Falls Efficacy Scale, a Quality of Life Scale by Ware, the Katz IADL, portions of the Sickness Impact Profile, and the Center of Epidemiological Studies—Depression Scale (CES-D).

Additionally, all sites collect a set of physical measurements. These include near-vision acuity, gait, static balance, handgrip dynamometry, and passive knee, hip, and ankle range of motion, and isometric strength.

At Emory/Wesley Woods (Site Five), the investigators also collect information on nutrition intake, blood lipids, body composition, isometric, and cardiovascular endurance. Supplementary psychosocial data at Site Five include the Affect Balance Scale, which measures frequency of positive and negative emotional states. Also, the Wechsler Adult Intelligence Scale-Revised (WAIS-R) vocabulary items provides an IQ estimate. The WAIS-R digit symbol and Reitan Trail marking test (Trails A & B) measure cognitive fluency and effectiveness of information processing. The Choice Control Mastery Scale measures the individual's perceived control of health status and life events. Finally, the investigators ask about recent exercise patterns in a format designed by the Centers for Disease Control. The common data base items and the Emory/Wesley Wood site-specific items are collected pre- and postintervention; measurements are again repeated 4 months after the intervention.

In addition, randomly selected subject homes are surveyed to provide a descriptive inventory of features relevant to activities of daily living, instrumental activities of daily living, and social activities. The survey was developed by the Research & Training Center for Accessible Housing at North Carolina State University to characterize homes of persons with disabilities.

These data are collected under the supervision of the environmental architect on the research team. Data are collected on the plan of the house, measures of elevations, height of shelves, stairs, storage areas, and the path to the mailbox. Comments from the occupants that are relevant to dwelling in the residence are also solicited.

The purpose of the behavior-relevant environmental survey is to determine the interaction of daily activities and intervention conditions (e.g., reaching, bending, rotating, balance, and stamina) with falls and injury control. These data are then related to self-ratings by subjects on the performance of daily tasks.

DISCUSSION

Interventions that improve quality of life are important for older adults. While much of the research to date on the benefits of exercise has focused on cardiovascular outcomes, the multisite FICSIT studies are examining exercise interventions targeted to improving functioning and reducing injury in the elderly.

Though the FICSIT studies are still in the initial intervention phases, they have important implications for nurse clinicians and researchers working with the older adult population. For example, from the preliminary work reported here, it appears as if static exercise that involves biofeedback training for maintaining balance shows promise for improving older adults' ability to shift body weight to more quickly regain a center of balance. While quantitative data are not yet available to evaluate the benefits of Tai Chi Chuan, anecdotal data indicate that the slow, controlled movements of this dynamic exercise appeal to the elderly and may increase flexibility and confidence in body balance and movement. The expected outcome of the Emory/Wesley Woods site is new approaches that will enable older adults to improve balance and reduce the likelihood of falls and delay the onset of frailty.

Clinicians can expect to hear and read about a variety of innovative approaches from the various FICSIT study sites. Collectively, the FICSIT studies will provide a set of critical interventions to reduce injuries among the elderly. We thus anticipate that the findings from FICSIT initiatives will have a positive impact on both quality of life and injury control in the older adult population.

REFERENCES

Gallo, J. J., Reichel, W., & Anderson, L. (1988). *The handbook of geriatric assessment*. Rockville, MD: Aspen.

Knight, B., & Walker, D. L. (1988). Toward a definition of alternatives to institutionalization for the frail elderly. *The Gerontologist, 25,* 358–363.

Koh, T. C. (1982). Tai Chi Chuan and ankylosing spondylitis—a personal experience. *American Journal of Chinese Medicine, 1*(4), 59–61.

Maddox, G. (1987). *The encyclopedia of aging*. New York: Springer.

Neugarten, B. (1984). Psychological aspects of aging and illness. *Psychosomatics, 25,* 123–125.

Qu Mianyu. (1986). Taijiquan: A medical assessment. In *Simplified Taijiquan* (pp. 6–9). Chinese Sports Editorial Board: Beijing: Chinese International Book Trading Corporation.

Tinetti, M. E., & Speechly, M. (1989). Prevention of falls in the elderly. *New England Journal of Medicine, 320,* 1055–1059.

Zhuo, D., Shephard, R. J., David, G. M., & Philby, M. J. (1984). Responses during Tai Chi Chuan exercise. *Canadian Journal of Applied Sport Sciences, 9,* 7–10.

[10]

Evaluation of Two Interventions to Reduce Falls and Fall Injuries: The Challenge of Hip Pads and Individualized Elimination Rounds

Jo Ellen Rude Ross, Meridean L. Maas, Jeffrey C. Huston, Carolyn J. Kundel, Paul J. Woodward, Teresa A. Gyldenvard, Lati Modarressi, Marta Heffner, Jeanette Daly, Marcia Casselman, Michael S. Sellberg, Patricia Tunink, J. Christopher Smith, George Woodworth, and Thomas Kruckeberg

Falls are the leading cause of injury and loss of independence among the elderly and one of the most difficult problems facing caregivers of elderly persons in long-term care institutions. Margulec, Librach, and Schadel (1970) found that 95% of injuries sustained among elderly living in long-term care facilities resulted from falls. Sixty-one percent of those experiencing fractures died shortly after the fall. Femur fractures are among the worst injuries one can sustain in a fall. In a year-long study of persons over 50, Jensen and Tondevold (1979) found a hip fracture mortality rate of 27%. Fisher et al. (1991), who used Medicare records to determine the incidence of hip fractures and resulting fatalities, found a mortality rate of 12.5% during the first 90 days following hip fracture; 24% had died within a year. Magaziner and associates (1989) followed 1814 elderly community dwellers who had sustained hip fractures and were hospitalized: 4.3% died during hospitalization, and a total of 17.4% died during the first year. Eighteen percent were dependent on a caregiver for assistance with daily activities one year after hospitalization.

For many elderly, a particularly high-risk activity is toileting. Rainsville (1984) noted that 54% of falls took place while patients used or attempted to use the commode, urinal, or bathroom. Foerster (1981) found that 45 of 105 falls (43%), and 50% of night falls, were related to bathroom use. Walshe and Rosen (1979) determined that 30% of falls in a community hospital occurred while the patient was going to the bathroom. On an oncology/neurology/neurosurgery unit, one quarter of falls occurred in the bathroom; 47.5% were sustained in ambulation to and from the toilet (Coyle, 1979). Among nocturnal falls, 60% were related to toileting—65% for men and 58% for women. Among day falls, 45% were related to toileting for males and 24% for females.

The pilot studies we have conducted were designed to test the effectiveness of two interventions in reducing the number of falls and the injuries due to falls among institutionalized elderly in intermediate care sites. The first intervention was a hip pad designed to reduce the likelihood and extent of injuries due to falls by redistributing and absorbing the shock load of the hip (greater trochantor) when a fall occurred. The second intervention was designed to prevent falls by providing assistance to and from the toilet during elimination rounds. This chapter reports the findings from the series of pilots of the two interventions. These pilot studies were part of a large cooperative investigation of falls among the frail elderly entitled "Frailty and Injuries: Cooperative Studies of Intervention Techniques" (FICSIT).

HIP PAD INTERVENTION

Generally, evaluations of interventions to prevent injury have found that the more "passive" an intervention, the greater its impact. An example of a "passive" intervention is the passive automobile restraints (automatic seat belt or air bag) now installed because not everyone will actively buckle the seat belt. Haddon (1974) has emphasized the importance of passive interventions in preventing unintentional injury.

Hip joint protective pads are designed to reduce the occurrence and/or severity of hip injuries due to falls. Hip pads are passive in that once they are on, they provide passive protection when a fall occurs. The design consists of a molded piece of plastic curved to fit the curvature of the body. In the center, "stress risers" (elevations in the plastic) provide structural stability and strength. The plastic portion of the hip pad is positioned over a large area of the hip in order to reduce the stress of the shock load in that region. The molded plastic is inserted into a $\frac{5}{8}$–1 inch thick piece of foam, which absorbs the energy of the impact load. The pads are inserted into strategically located pockets in a pantlike garment. The garments are individually tailored to fit snugly enough so that pads remain positioned over the hip.

Because the hip pads are designed for the frail elderly, including persons with impaired mobility and/or incontinence, the crotch of the garment is cut away to facilitate toileting or to allow incontinence pads to be worn. Velcro is placed on the center front and on each leg to allow easy application and removal. The protective clothing is comfortable enough to be worn all the time. Individuals receiving this intervention were asked to wear the hip pad garment 24 hours a day.

The pilot studies of the hip pad intervention were designed to answer several questions: (1) Do elderly who are identified as being at risk to fall believe themselves to be at risk? (2) Will elderly nursing home patients wear hip pads, and to what extent? (3) What factors are associated with compliance in wearing hip pads? (4) When falls occur, do the elderly wearing hip pads have fewer and less severe injuries to the hip than those who are not wearing hip pads?

ELIMINATION ROUNDS

Because many falls appear to be related to the need for elimination, the use of scheduled toileting rounds may reduce the number of falls if assistance is offered during this high-risk activity. Individuals in the elimination-rounds intervention group were placed on individualized rounds based on their elimination patterns. First, the pattern of elimination was documented for a set period of time. After ascertaining elimination times, a schedule for assisting residents was prescribed, and a staff person assisted the resident to and from the bathroom, remaining with the resident during elimination; the staff member provided assistance with clothing as needed.

The pilots of the elimination-rounds intervention were designed to answer the following questions: (1) Are patients compliant in seeking assistance with scheduled toileting? (2) Are staff compliant in carrying out individually scheduled toileting? (3) Can accurate toileting patterns be established? (4) Can toileting schedules be effectively maintained? (5) Does individualized scheduled toileting reduce the number of patient falls?

PILOT STUDIES

Six pilot studies were conducted on the two interventions. Four of the six pilots tested only hip pads; one pilot evaluated both interventions using random assignment of subjects to four groups, one hip pad group, one elimination-rounds group, one group that had both interventions, and a comparison group; and the sixth pilot tested only elimination rounds. Elderly residents (age 65 and older) of four long-term care facilities were recruited as subjects for each of the pilots. Many were cognitively impaired, as determined by the Global Deterioration Scale (Reisberg, Ferris, deLeon, & Crook, 1982). Consent was sought from the individual if cognitively intact, or from a family member.

Data were collected on the "wearability" of hip pads, compliance in wearing the pads, problems with the hip pad garment for Alzheimer's patients, and tissue perfusion when the garment was worn in bed; patients' compliance with elimination rounds; and staff compliance in carrying out the elimination rounds intervention. Data on falls and injury rates were collected for both interventions.

Hip Pad Studies

The pilots on hip pad use indicated that certain elderly will wear hip pads; however, many do not want to be bothered with them. To summarize the results of the studies involving hip pads, we learned that:

1. Compliance was much higher in cognitively intact individuals.
2. Subjects who had had significant injuries or significant fall events in their lives demonstrated greater compliance.
3. Men tended to be more compliant in wearing the hip pads than women.
4. Because many cognitively intact residents felt little fear of either falling or injury, they did not wish to wear hip pads and therefore did not participate.
5. Some subjects with late stages of dementia became agitated while wearing the garment, as well as when wearing the garment and pads.
6. Lying on the hip pads compromised skin perfusion in very thin individuals, although no problems occurred during the pilots.

Because a hip fracture is a rare event, even among the frail elderly, to adequately answer the question of whether hip pads significantly reduce hip injuries and hip fractures would require thousands of subjects.

Moreover, poor compliance in wearing the hip pads by cognitively impaired experimental group subjects reduces the difference between hip pad and control groups, necessitating even more subjects to test the effectiveness of the pads. Therefore, the next phase of study of hip pads will examine compliance rates in cognitively alert individuals and in persons who are in early stages of dementing illnesses. The majority of subjects will come from community groups such as Parkinson's support groups, individuals who have sustained hip fractures, and residents in apartments associated with nursing homes. Results from the next phase of study will indicate whether the hip pads show enough promise to conduct a large clinical trial in which thousands of individuals would wear hip pads, and the rate of hip fractures and hip injuries in experimental and control groups would be compared.

Meanwhile, other hip pads or devices to reduce hip injuries may come onto the market. For such devices, nurses should note what has been done to demonstrate: (1) effectiveness in reducing hip fractures, as determined by a randomized study; (2) wearability of the device (comfort, heat production and dissipation beneath, etc.); (3) acceptance by the elderly (demonstrated compliance); (4) skin perfusion beneath the device; and (5) initial and repeating costs.

Elimination-Rounds Studies

We learned the following from the elimination-round pilots:

1. Intensive efforts by researchers were needed to ensure a reasonable staff compliance rate of 80%.
2. Because subjects were noncompliant in asking for help in toileting, despite an 80% rate of staff compliance, half of the falls reported during the study period occurred during toileting.
3. Nursing home staff viewed incontinence as the outcome endpoint rather than "falls which did not occur."
4. Diagnosis of the type of incontinence is necessary in order to determine which types of patients may be helped in reducing falls due to toileting. Individualized toileting schedules may not be appropriate for persons with overflow and functional incontinence, but may be appropriate for those with stress and urge incontinence.
5. Subject compliance is a very important factor, and it needs to be actively facilitated in patients with sufficient cognitive ability.

Falls in general and falls occurring during efforts to transfer to a commode or move to the bathroom represent "soft" endpoints. The

FICSIT definition of a fall is "unintentionally coming to rest on the ground, floor, or other lower level." This definition specifically excludes coming to rest against the wall or other structural components. Also excluded are events where the person comes to rest on furniture such as a chair or bed (FICSIT Operations Manual, 1990). Because so many patients who fall are cognitively impaired, the ability of subjects to appreciate the nuances of the definition of a fall is questionable; therefore they may not report falls. To further define a fall as one related to elimination requires an assumption of even greater ability to distinguish circumstances. Attempts to accurately determine whether falls are related to elimination or not would require physical evidence such as the infamous "pool of urine," a fall in the bathroom or off of the commode, eye witness accounts, and/or reliable patient report.

DISCUSSION

Although the results of the pilot studies have not yet shown definite trends, both interventions hold promise for the prevention of falls and injuries among the institutionalized elderly. Additional studies are needed to develop and test methods of measuring falls and injuries in the elderly, particularly in those who are cognitively impaired and are thus unable to provide accurate descriptions of their falls.

Studies are also needed to develop reliable and valid measurements of elimination-related falls and to describe the relationship of elimination to falls in this population. Although individualized elimination schedules can be established for many institutionalized elderly, the schedules are not useful if the elderly person has overflow incontinence. Further, assisting patients with elimination is labor intensive, and convincing staff and administrators that it is more beneficial than use of incontinence pads or disposable diapers is difficult. For persons with stress and urge incontinence, however, staff compliance with the intervention may be greater because the intervention is observed to reduce wetness. For studies in which reduction of incontinence with individualized toileting is the primary outcome, measurement of falls as a secondary outcome would be advantageous. Reduction of falls would serve as an additional benefit to patients and staff and would further support the toileting intervention. In addition, the acute care setting may provide a better initial site for individualized scheduled toileting than the long-term care setting.

The next phase of our study will further assess the feasibility of the use of hip pads as a passive intervention to prevent or minimize injuries from falls in the elderly. The purposes of this phase will be to identify populations at high risk of falls and hip fracture who are suitable for compliance studies on wearing hip pads, and to refine and evaluate a multistaged compliance program to maximize wearing of hip pads. If these goals are achieved, a randomized clinical trial will be proposed to determine the hip pad's effectiveness in reducing hip fracture and other hip injuries.

ACKNOWLEDGMENT

This study was supported by Grant #1-U01-NR0638 from the National Center for Nursing Research, NIH.

REFERENCES

Coyle, N. (1979). A problem-focused approach to nursing audit: Patient falls. *Cancer Nursing, 2,* 389–391.

Fisher, E. S., Baron, J. A., Malenka, D. J., Barrett, J. A., Kniffin, W. D., Whalery, F. S., & Bubolz, T. A. (1991). Hip fracture incidence and mortality in New England. *Epidemiology, 2,* 116–122.

Foerster, J. (1981). A study of falls: The elderly nursing home resident. *Journal of the New York State Nurses Association, 12,* 9–17.

Haddon, W. Jr. (1974). Editorial: Strategy in preventive medicine: Passive vs active approaches to reducing human wastage. *Journal of Trauma, 14,* 353–354.

Jensen, J. S., & Tondevold, E. (1979). Mortality after hip fractures. *Acta Orthopaedica Scandanavica, 50,* 161–167.

Magaziner, J., Hyg, M. S., Simonsick, E. M., Kashnor, M., Hebel, J. R., & Kensora, J. E. (1989). Survival experience of aged hip fracture patients. *American Journal of Public Health, 79,* 274–278.

Margulec, I., Librach, G., & Schadel, M. (1970). Epidemiological study of accidents among residents of homes for aged. *Journal of Gerontology, 25,* 342–346.

Rainsville, N. H. (1984). Effect of an implemented prevention program on the frequency of patient falls. *Quarterly Review Bulletin,* 287–291.

Reisberg B., Ferris, S. H., deLeon, M. J., & Crook, T. (1982). The Global Deterioration Scale (GDS): An instrument for the assessment of primary degenerative dementia. *American Journal of Psychiatry, 139,* 1136–1139.

Walshe, A., & Rosen, H. (1979). A study of patient falls from bed. *Journal of Nursing Administration, 9,* 31–35.

[11]

Elderly Exercise: Relationship to Ambulatory Function, Fall Behavior, and Well-being

Betty J. Reynolds and Corre J. Garrett (deceased)

Aging normally is accompanied by a decrease in activity, which can lead to decreased balance and gait changes, as well as psychological effects including decreased well-being. All of these can precipitate falls in the elderly, with a resulting loss of independence and confidence and a premature need for institutionalization.

A major challenge for nursing is to promote independence in the elderly and postpone problems resulting from inactivity. Experts agree that activity in the form of exercise includes benefits related not only to the musculoskeletal system (balance and gait) and mental function (i.e., well-being), but also to cardiovascular and metabolic function.

This study was designed to determine whether a planned exercise program had an effect on balance (altering postural stability), gait (decreasing proneness to trip and stumble), fall behavior, and well-being in a noninstitutionalized elderly sample.

METHOD

Participants for the program were 41 volunteers recruited through an announcement placed in a rural eastern North Carolina countywide mailing of the Council on Aging Newsletter. People aged 60 and above were invited to come for an initial screening.

Screening included a comprehensive history and physical examination, an EKG, hematocrit and hemoglobin determination, and urinalysis. The tests were performed at a Geriatric Ambulatory Center and evaluated by a geriatric medical consultant and cardiologist, to exclude any high-risk subjects. Exclusion was based on cardiac problems such as heart block or evidence of a major past infarct. Three volunteers were screened out because of cardiac problems. The program thus began with 38 participants.

Intervention

A retired registered nurse who operated a local exercise studio was hired to conduct a program of moderate exercise for 1 hour, three times a week, for 3 months. The sessions, held during midmorning, were accompanied by music. The program was designed according to American College of Sports Medicine (1986) guidelines, with exercises specifically planned for the older adult (Biegel, 1984; Parker, 1983; Stempfly, 1984). The program involved a collection of movements exercising all the joints of the body, in addition to a warm-up and cool-down period. Warm-up included exercises in breathing, stretching, and hugging oneself. The first exercise set focused on wrists, fingers, and hands, and the next on ankles, toes, and feet. Then came exercises of the neck, head, face, and eyes, followed by exercises of the shoulders, elbows, and arms. The next set of exercises focused on hips, knees, and legs, and the final group on trunk, back, front, and sides. Some exercises could be performed seated, others while standing with a chair back for support. For example, seated exercises included rounding shoulders forward, then pulling the shoulders back. Exercises performed while standing holding a chair back included stepping back with one foot, bringing feet back together, then repeating with the other foot. The exercises also included dancing and rhythmic movements and exercise-producing games performed to music. (A complete list of the exercises is available from the author.)

Data Collection

Data on balance, gait, and fall behaviors were collected before and after the exercise program. Balance was evaluated by a gerontological nurse practitioner using neurologic tests of cerebellar function for coordination and balance, such as finger to nose, heel to shin, rapid alternating movements, and the Romberg test, which measures the ability to maintain balance standing with feet together and eyes closed. Balance also was measured by the participant's ability to retrieve an article from the floor from a standing position, while retaining balance, and by the ability to stand on one foot at a time for 5 seconds. All participants passed all coordination and balance tests, except for standing on one foot at a time for 5 seconds.

Gait, including right and left stride (distance between two consecutive ipsilateral heel strikes), right and left step length (perpendicular distance between two consecutive contralateral heel strikes), right and left step width (distance between two consecutive contralateral heel strikes), right and left foot angle (angle of the foot as compared to straight ahead), and velocity (amount of time to walk 6 meters), was measured according to the procedure established by Cerny (1983). Paper table covers, produced in rolls, were used to lay out a 6-meter run. The paper was taped to the floor, and the examiner attached small triangles of moleskin saturated with ink to the underside of the toe and heel of the participant's shoe. The subject's walk across the 6-meter length of paper was timed with a stop watch. Two runs were made, and the second run was recorded for the measurement of velocity. The same process was used after the program for post-data.

Falls during the 3 months prior to the program were determined using Rubenstein and Robbins' (1984) Fall History Instrument. This 22-item instrument was created for use with noninstitutionalized elderly fallers to develop a systematic approach to determine the incidence and causes of falls. Falls in the noninstitutionalized elderly often are not recognized as falls because no injury results; therefore such falls may go unreported. To avoid recall bias, the Fall History Instrument was used to jog each participant's memory of actual falls. The instrument asks questions regarding the fall such as, "Were there obstacles causing the fall?" and "Do you have any trouble walking and/or using assistive devices?" Following the exercise program, the instrument was administered again to determine falls during the 3 months of the program.

On completion of the program, an instrument that compared recollected well-being 3 months prior to the program with well-being during the last month of the program was mailed to participants for anonymous return. This instrument was adapted, with permission, from the General Well-Being Schedule (GWBS) designed by Dupuy (McDowell & Newell, 1987); it serves as an indicator of subjective feelings of psychological well-being, and reflects both positive and negative feelings. For the current study, the instrument was shortened from 18 to 10 items, using only three of the six subscales: Anxiety, Positive Well-being, and Vitality. A 6-point scale was used for each item; total scores, therefore, ranged from 1 to 60. In order to compare perceptions of general well-being in the past and present, items asked subjects to report not only current, but also past feelings. To avoid a Hawthorne effect from the exercise program, the instrument was administered a second time 9 months after the completion of the program. Participants were asked to compare current well-being with well-being upon completion of the program. The second mailing also included 10 questions on independent exercise behaviors since the completion of the program.

RESULTS

Twenty-two participants attended more than 50% of the exercise sessions and were in attendance on the last day of the exercise sessions when post-data were collected. The 22 participants who completed all measures included 17 women and 5 men whose ages ranged from 60 to 75 years; one participant was black, and the rest were white.

Participants' ability to balance on the left foot was unchanged after the intervention; however, balance on the right foot increased following the program. Of the 11 participants who could not balance 5 seconds or more on the right foot before the exercise program, 5 (45%) could do so at the program's completion; only 1 (9%) of the 11 who were able to balance for 5 seconds or more before the program was no longer able to do so after the program. This improvement in balance was significant [McNemar's $\chi^2(1) = 2.67$, $p < .09$; an alpha of .10 was used for significance testing because of the small sample size].

Several parameters of gait changed. Increases were noted in stride length, step length, right foot angle, and velocity. The increases in right stride, left stride, right step length, and velocity were all statistically significant. Decreases were noted in step width (see Table 11.1).

The number of falls experienced by participants decreased from five during the 3 months prior to the program to one during the program. While this decrease was not significant [$\chi^2(1) = 2.67$, $p < .20$], it does indicate that the program has some potential to reduce falls.

We can report by simple observation that as time progressed, conversations became livelier, and we saw more smiling faces. The general attitude of the participants appeared to be happier, and bodies were carried taller and straighter.

Participants reported that their well-being was greater at program completion (a mean improvement of 7.55 points on the Well-being Scale) than at 3 months before the program. Statistically significant increases occurred in the total score for well-being [$t(21) = 3.49$, $p < .001$] as well as for seven of the items when the instrument was administered immediately following program completion. When participants were asked 9 months later to recall well-being on program completion, recalled scores were even higher (mean increase = 1.94 points).

TABLE 11.1 Gait Measurements Pre- and Post-Exercise Program

Variable	Pre-program N = 22		Post-program N = 22		Paired t-test
	mean	SD	mean	SD	t value
Stride right (cm)	121.49	18.33	126.26	18.69	2.39[a]
Stride left (cm)	122.19	18.75	126.26	18.69	2.02[a]
Step length R (cm)	59.64	10.08	63.69	9.22	2.71[b]
Step length L (cm)	61.54	9.11	62.51	9.99	.56
Step width R (cm)	6.20	3.11	6.16	3.66	−.09
Step width L (cm)	6.56	3.37	6.16	3.66	−.73
Foot angle R (cm)	0.87	0.59	0.92	0.58	.52
Foot angle L (cm)	0.62	0.62	0.62	0.42	.00
Velocity (cm/sec)	10.81	2.37	11.46	2.06	1.89[a]

[a] $p < .05$, 1 tailed
[b] $p < .01$, 1 tailed

As noted above, 10 additional items were added to the last mailing of the well-being questionnaire. These items concerned independent exercise behavior since the end of the program and whether or not the participant would join a subsequent organized exercise program. The responses revealed that none of the participants had continued to exercise at home alone after the class was disbanded. All, however, said that they would gladly join another class for exercise when another one was started.

DISCUSSION

It is reasonable to expect that similar exercise programs would be beneficial for the elderly in many settings. Nurses employed in public health, home care, or mental health settings might enlist participants from their clients. Various other community settings such as churches, meal sites, or YWCAs probably have populations who would profit from exercises. Participants also might be found in retirement villages, day-care centers, and skilled care facilities. Exercises can be carried out with almost every elderly person. There are standing, sitting, and lying down exercises for nearly all elderly.

Since none of the participants in this study continued to exercise independently, obviously organized programs should be ongoing. Any benefits accrued from the exercises are probably lost if the exercises are not continued. The increased socialization experienced by the participants in organized programs is also important. Indeed, the "together" time of the exercise classes may have been as important to the participants' increased well-being as the exercises themselves.

Exercise interventions for the elderly are not only vital to reduce the number of falls experienced by the elderly, but are also cost effective. The program described here cost approximately $40.00 per participant. This amount reflects primarily the fees for the EKGs and laboratory work. A small portion of the price per person was spent to pay the exercise instructor and her travel expenses and supplies. Compared to the cost of falls and their sequelae, $40.00 is negligible. Of equal importance, but without dollar value, is the fact that patient well-being increased during the program, which may have increased productive activity in some of the participants.

ACKNOWLEDGMENT

This research was partially supported by an East Carolina University Research/Creative Activity Award.

REFERENCES

American College of Sports Medicine. (1986). *Guidelines for exercise testing and prescription* (3rd ed.). Philadelphia: Lea and Febiger.

Biegel, L. (Ed.). (1984). *Physical fitness and the older person.* Rockville, MD: Aspen Press.

Cerny, K. (1983). A clinical method of quantitative gait analysis. *Physical Therapist, 63,* 1125–1126.

McDowell, I., & Newell, C. (1987). *Measuring health: A guide to rating scales and questionnaires.* New York: Oxford University Press.

Rubenstein, L. Z., & Robbins, A. S. (1984). Falls in the elderly: A clinical perspective. *Geriatrics, 39(4),* 67–78.

Parker, B. (1983). *Sit down and shape up: A handbook of fitness and exercise for older adults.* New York: Leisure Press.

Stempfly, P. P. (1984). *Keep movin': Get fit, stay fit, pass it along.* Springfield, OH: Wonderhorse Press.

[12]

A Falls Prevention Program for the Acute Care Setting

Linda M. Hollinger and Patricia A. Patterson

It has been suggested that approximately 25% of falls in acute care settings result in some degree of injury (Morse, Tylks, & Dixon, 1987). Falls may be fatal, especially among the elderly. Even if falls do not result in injury, fear and anxiety about future incidents may decrease the patient's independence and mobility.

Falls are most often examined retrospectively, resulting in underestimation of rates. Many falls are also self-reported or unwitnessed, leading to inaccuracies in the reports. Few studies have taken a prospective approach, assessing patients at risk for falls upon admission to an acute care setting, implementing a falls precaution program, and evaluating the program's effectiveness at regular intervals (Whedon & Shedd, 1989).

Data collected in the Department of Medical Nursing at Rush–Presbyterian–St. Luke's Medical Center over a 6-month period in 1989 revealed a total of 86 patient falls. The Quality Assurance Committee of the department therefore identified patient falls as a critical variable to be studied. The majority of the patients who fell were elderly or experiencing neurologic disorders.

The purpose of this study was to develop and implement a falls precaution assessment and prevention program in this acute care setting. The effectiveness of the program was evaluated by examining changes in the rate of falls after program implementation. Factors associated with falls that occurred after the program was implemented were identified, and nursing staff were surveyed regarding their perceptions of the effectiveness of the assessment tool and falls prevention measures.

METHOD

A task force made up of interested staff and leadership personnel from the Department of Medical Nursing reviewed the literature and analyzed the data collected on patient falls in the department as a basis for developing a falls prevention program. Goals included identifying patients at risk for falls, instituting appropriate precautions to ensure patient safety, and evaluating the effectiveness of the program.

The Fall Assessment Tool was developed to be completed by registered nurses as part of the admission assessment and every 7 days thereafter or whenever the patient's status changed, as determined by nursing judgment. The tool assesses patient factors (e.g., history of falls, confusion, and age) and environmental factors (e.g., first week on the unit and attached equipment) identified in the literature as risk factors for falling (see Table 12.1). The nurse circles the numerical score for all factors that apply to the patient and/or environment. The circled scores are tallied and fall precautions are initiated for all patients with scores of 15 or greater.

Based on information obtained from the Fall Assessment Tool, fall prevention measures were individualized, using the Fall Prevention Measures Tool, to reflect the needs of each patient at risk to fall (see Table 12.2). Prevention measures included putting the bed in low position and half/full siderail use, limitations on activity, a bedside commode, nonskid footwear, frequent toileting, a restraint order, personal items and call light within reach, frequent visual checks of the patient, a night light, assistive devices, frequent environmental orientation, and reminders of attached equipment and safety precautions. Stickers indicating "Fall Precautions" were placed on the patient's medical record and nursing care plan, and on a patient arm band.

Before the program was implemented, volunteer representatives from each of the medical units received in-service education on the new instruments, the stickers available to identify patients at risk, and the new policy. The issues covered in the new policy included its purposes, the way in which the tools were to be used, and the responsibilities of registered nurses and unit clerks. Under this new policy, the volunteer representatives were responsible for training staff on their individual units, serving as unit resource persons during the pilot, and acting as liaison between the units and the program task force.

The Unit Clerk Supervisor informed the departmental clerks about their responsibility for placing "Fall Precautions" stickers on the medical record and the nursing care plan, and on the patient's arm band. Memos explaining the Fall Precautions Program were distributed to the various support services that had direct contact with patients.

TABLE 12.1   Fall Assessment Tool

Please circle all factor scores that apply to the patient and/or environment.

	Initial score	Reassessed score
Patient factors		
History of falls	15	15
Confusion	15	15
Age (over 65)	5	5
Impaired judgment	5	5
Sensory deficit	5	5
Unable to ambulate independently	5	5
Decreased level of cooperation	5	5
Increased anxiety/emotional lability	5	5
Incontinence/urgency	5	5
CV/respiratory disease affecting perfusion and oxygenation	5	5
Medications affecting BP or level of consciousness	5	5
Postural hypotension with dizziness	5	5
Environmental factors		
First week on unit	5	5
Attached equipment (e.g., IV pole, chest tubes, appliances, O₂ tubing, etc.)	5	5
TOTAL POINTS	__	__

Implement fall precautions for score of 15 or greater.
Fall precautions may not be indicated for patients with chronic problems that are compensated for.

Assessed for Fall Risk

Date _____   Signature _____
Date _____   Signature _____
Date _____   Signature _____
Date _____   Signature _____
Date _____   Signature _____

TABLE 12.2 Fall Prevention Measures

Check off applicable measures. Add "fall precautions" to clinical record and care plan. Date, initial, and sign when fall precautions are implemented and when reassessed. These fall precautions are in addition to general safety measures for all patients.

_____ Place green ID bracelet indicating "Fall Precautions" on patient's wrist.

_____ Bed in low position

_____ Bed in locked position

_____ Siderails

Siderail up   1 _____   2 _____

Siderail noc only   1 _____   2 _____

_____ Activity order

Bedrest   _____

Up ad lib   _____

Up w/asst.   _____

_____ Bedside commode

_____ Nonskid footwear

_____ Toileting schedule   Frequency _____

_____ Slow position changes

_____ Restraint order (check patient hourly w/restraints)

Posey belt   _____

Posey vest   _____

Wrist (soft)   1 _____   2 _____

Leathers   _____

_____ Personal items within reach

_____ Call light within reach

_____ Visual checks of patient   Frequency _____

_____ Night light P.R.N.

_____ Assistive devices

W/C   _____

Walker   _____

Cane   _____

Other   _____

_____ Orient patient to environment   Frequency _____

_____ Alert patient to attached equipment/safety precautions

_____ Other measures   _____

Precautions Implemented/Reassessed

Date _____   Signature _____

Date _____   Signature _____

Date _____   Signature _____

Date _____   Signature _____

This program was implemented for a 6-month period. Data on patient falls were reported on patient incident forms. The fall rate was calculated as follows:

$$\frac{\text{Number of patient falls}}{\text{Number of patient bed days}} \times 1000$$

As part of the program evaluation, the nursing staff were surveyed to determine their perceptions of the program's effectiveness.

RESULTS

During the 6-month program there was a significant decrease in the rate of falls from the 6 months preceding implementation of the program $[t(7) = 2.60, p < .05, \text{1-tailed}]$. Prior to the program, the mean fall rate was 4.06; after the program, the rate had decreased to 2.63 (see Table 12.3). Interestingly, the two units that showed the greatest decrease in falls (Units #6 and #7) both had structured fall programs in place before the program began; the new program clearly enhanced the effectiveness of the programs that had already been instituted.

Seventy-four percent of the patients who fell were 65 years of age or older; 70% of fallers aged 65 or older had some reported neurologic problem, while only 14% of fallers under the age of 65 had some form of neurologic disorder (see Table 12.4). Seventy-one percent of fallers were

TABLE 12.3 Patient Fall Rates Pre- and Postprogram by Unit[a]

| Unit | Fall rate | |
	Preprogram	Postprogram
1	4.76	2.18
2	4.46	5.05
3	1.28	2.13
4	5.71	3.81
5	3.04	2.64
6	5.00	2.18
7	5.31	2.25
8	2.89	0.80
Mean	4.06	2.63

[a]Corrected for multiple fallers: $t(7) = 2.60, p < .05$, one-tailed test.

TABLE 12.4 Comparison of Selected Characteristics of Fallers and Nonfallers

Characteristic	Percentage of fallers[a]	Percentage of nonfallers[b]
Age $\geq$ 65 years	74	54
Neurologic Problems[c]		
$\geq$ 65 years of age	70	39
< 65 years of age	14	6
Female	71	64
Activity Level		
Up ad lib	14	20
Up with assistance	78	76
Bedrest	8	4
Taking Narcotics	38	49
Diagnosis of Hypertension	42	44
Level of Consciousness		
Alert, oriented $\times$ 3[d]	62	78
Oriented $\times$ 1–2[e]	26	20
Confused	12	2

[a] n = 81 (total of 90 falls)
[b] n = 50 (random sample of 5–6 patients per unit drawn as comparison group during period of the study)
[c] Percentage of fallers $\geq$ 65 and < 65 who had neurologic problems.
[d] oriented to the 3 indices of person, place, and time
[e] oriented to 1 or 2 of the indices of person, place, and time

female. There was no significant difference in the number of narcotics administered to fallers and non-fallers, or in other patient characteristics except for age and diagnosis of neurologic disorders.

Ninety-four percent of all reported falls occurred in patient rooms. Seventy-four percent occurred while the patient was attempting to get to the bathroom, and 92% of those falls were unwitnessed; 78% of patients who fell were classified as able to be up only with assistance.

Falls were significantly related to patient acuity on three units (r = .621 to .736, p < .01); to the number of hours of supplemental agency nursing care used on two units (r = .782 to .961, p < .01); and to the difference between recommended and actual hours of staffing on three units (r = −.659 to .494, p < .05). That is, significantly more falls occurred when patient acuity was high, when more supplemental staff were used, and when actual hours of staffing were less than the hours recommended, based on patient acuity and census information. One unit was an exception to this pattern. On that unit falls were not less frequent when actual staffing hours were below recommended; this appeared to be due to the large number of orientees on the unit, which resulted in increased staffing hours by inexperienced staff.

Patient factors related to falls included having a history of falls, unsteady gait, a longer hospital stay, poor vision or hearing, confusion or disorientation, emotional lability, incontinence, multiple medications, and postural hypotension.

Environmental and other extrinsic factors associated with falls included poor room design; inadequate room lighting; environmental hazards such as IV poles, unlocked bed wheels, or overbed trays; inadequate staffing patterns; a high level of patient acuity; and increased reliance on agency or temporary nursing personnel.

Nursing staff were asked to complete a Fall Precautions Survey 6 months after implementation of the program, using a Likert-type scale ranging from "strongly agree" to "strongly disagree." The scale included items about the fall assessment and fall prevention measures tools, consistency of usage of the new tools on various units, ability to appropriately identify patients at risk of falling, in-service education, and responsibilities of the health care team.

The surveys revealed an overall positive response to the fall precaution program. Staff perceived that the Fall Assessment Tool and the Fall Prevention Measures Tool were clear, easy to complete, and patient specific. Nearly three-fourths of the staff felt they had received adequate in-service education. Seventy-nine percent agreed that fall risk could readily be assessed as part of the patient admission process. Sixty-nine percent agreed that the fall precaution policy clearly indicated work responsibilities for the nursing staff and unit clerk to complete during the patient's admission process.

Although 48% of the staff agreed that the fall assessment tool appropriately identified patients at risk for falls, 41% felt the tool was "overly sensitive" in placing a patient on fall precautions; the criteria of age, being a new admission, and having an IV were considered particular problems. In some cases, staff felt they would not have placed newly admitted elderly patients on fall precautions. Although greater age was significantly related to increased falls, the staff nurses did not appear aware of the relationship between falls and age-related changes that predispose the elderly to potential injury. Thus, their view of the tool as oversensitive may reflect the nurses' lack of understanding of aging processes, both normal and abnormal. According to the policy, all patients were to be reassessed for fall precautions after one week. Sixty percent of the staff perceived that reassessment for fall precautions was done inconsistently. Policy revision might incorporate nurses' judgment as to the need for reassessment based on patient status rather than using a set time frame.

Implementation of our fall precautions program also decreased the use of restraints in the clinical setting, as reported by nurses during the post-implementation survey. No pre-implementation data are available for comparison, however.

DISCUSSION

The "Fall Precautions Program" enabled our department to assess a clinical issue, devise and implement a plan of action, and measure patient outcomes. We concluded that a "Fall Precautions Program" that is successfully utilized by nursing staff can identify patients at risk for falls and guide implementation of prevention measures. A confounding factor in this study, however, is that the strategies used served to increase staff awareness of patients at risk for falls. Thus, it may not have been the fall precautions program that decreased patient falls, but simply the fact that staff nurses' awareness of fall preventions was heightened.

The tools developed for our program have enabled our staff to maintain better reporting of patients at risk for falls. Nurses are constantly reminded of patients at risk and are able to share this information in reports, care plans, and documentation of patient care progress. Future recommendations include periodic assessments of patient fall rates and resulting injuries.

REFERENCES

Morse, J., Tylks, S., & Dixon, H. (1987). Characteristics of the fall-prone patient. *The Gerontologist, 27*, 516–522.

Whedon, M., & Shedd, P. (1989). Prediction and prevention of patient falls. *Image: Journal of Nursing Scholarship, 21*, 108–114.

[13]

Reducing Restraints: One Nursing Home's Story

Lois K. Evans and Neville E. Strumpf

In the United States, the use of physical restraints escalated after the mid-1960s (Evans & Strumpf, 1989). Data from a 1988 national survey conducted by the Health Care Financing Administration (HCFA, 1988) indicated that an average of 41% of nursing home residents were restrained on a regular basis. At the same time, regional studies estimated that about 60% of nursing home residents received psychotropic medications.

However, in recent years, physical restraints have been increasingly called into question as an intervention to prevent older adults from falling. Now physical restraints are viewed as, at best, an unvalidated technique to be used cautiously and only with informed consent (Miles, 1990); at worst, they are seen as an archaic and unacceptable practice symbolizing poor-quality care. The research literature suggests that restraints do not guarantee safety—the ostensible reason for their use. Falls by nursing home residents are not decreased by restraints; and restrained elders are more likely to receive serious injuries when they fall (Tinetti, Liu, Marottoli, & Ginter, 1991). Injuries resulting directly from restraints have also been documented, and 200 deaths per year may occur from strangulation and accidental burning as elders attempt to escape from their restraints (Rigert & Lerner, 1990). In addition, serious physical changes can result from the prolonged immobilization imposed by restraints—for example, pressure sores, nosocomial infections, and incontinence; restrained patients also have a higher risk of mortality than nonrestrained patients (Lofgren, MacPherson, Granieri, Myllenbeck, & Spratka, 1989). Problems in appetite and elimination occur, and functional status and mobility decline from muscle wasting and loss of balance (Evans & Strumpf, 1989). Finally, patients in restraints are often socially isolated, and they may experience periods of disorganization, confusion, panic, fear of abandonment, anger, agitation, loss of self-esteem, withdrawal, and depression (Evans, Strumpf, & Williams, 1991). While many American nurses hold strong beliefs about the efficacy of restraints in the care of older people and have a minimal repertoire of alternative interventions for problematic behavior (Evans & Strumpf, 1990), staff too may suffer when working in an environment characterized by routine restraint use. The dehumanizing effects of these practices may well contribute to the high burnout and turnover among caregivers; some now even refer to routine restraint as neglectful care (Capezuti, Strumpf, & Evans, 1991; Evans, 1991). The increasing public and professional awareness in recent years of the iatrogenic effects of physical restraint on frail elders, a changing ethical and legal climate, and growing efforts to do away with restraints culminated in 1987 in the Nursing Home Reform Act (PL 100-203, 1987), which requires reduction in the routine use of physical restraint.

Since the new regulations went into effect in October 1990, nursing homes across the nation have been struggling to provide a reasonably safe environment while attempting to comply with guidelines stressing individualized, less restrictive care. Missing from the guidelines, however, is a clear method for changing practice. Thus, the purpose of this pilot study was to develop and test the effects of a structured staff education program on the prevalence of restraint use and on resident and staff outcomes on one unit in a nursing home.

Models of planned change provided the conceptual framework for the study (Brooten, Hayman, & Naylor, 1988; Lewin, 1951). One way to "unfreeze" or produce disequilibrium in social systems, a condition necessary for change, is to alter the belief system through education. During pre-intervention data collection and throughout the educational program, staff were expected to become more aware of the problems surrounding restraint use. Education provided the opportunity for staff to "move"—that is, to change their paradigm for viewing patient behavior and patient care, and to examine, accept, and try out innovations. "Refreezing" was expected to occur when staff accepted new ways of caring and established the regimens as part of the system, as indicated by post-intervention policy change, improved resident care plans, decreased restraint use, and improved resident and staff outcomes.

METHOD

It was expected that a program of 10 restraint education sessions for nursing staff on one unit of a nursing home would result in:

1. improvements in staff outcomes (burnout, beliefs about restraint efficacy and knowledge of alternatives);
2. reduction of restraint use;
3. improvements in resident outcomes (function, cognition, and affect); and
4. no increase in the number of serious resident injuries.

The study used a pretest–posttest design; that is, patients and staff were evaluated before and after the intervention. Limitations of this design were monitored by keeping a careful record of all events that could affect the outcomes. For example, from prior experience, we were aware that restraint use can drop initially when a study of the practice is announced. Thus, resident and staff data were collected in one preliminary observation (P1), but these data were not used to examine changes following the intervention. Data were collected again 1 month later (T1), followed immediately by a 4-month educational intervention, and then data were collected 1 month after completion of the intervention (T2). Because restraint use appeared to continue dropping in the weeks following the posttest observation (T2), further data on restraint use were collected 3 months following the intervention (T3).

Sample and Setting

The study site was a 120-bed not-for-profit nursing home adjacent to the University of Pennsylvania. A 62-bed skilled care unit was selected for the study because of its higher prevalence of restraint use.

Resident subjects were noncomatose patients, age 60 and above, who verbally agreed to be interviewed and/or to have their records reviewed. No one refused to participate. Over the course of the study, 79 residents, ranging in age from 63 to 100 (mean = 82) were enrolled. Average length of nursing home stay was 1.3 years, and level of education was approximately the tenth grade. More than 75% of subjects were female, and 60% were widowed; just over half were recipients of Medicaid. Subjects had an average of 6.7 medical diagnoses or problems, with cardiovascular disease (71%), musculoskeletal problems (56%), and mental status changes (56%) most prevalent.

Staff subjects were all full- or part-time clinical nursing staff who agreed to participate. A total of 33 were enrolled over the course of the study. The average subject was aged 38, had 13 years of education, and was female. Slightly under half were licensed nurses (5 RNs, 9 LPNs), and 44% had had continuing education in gerontology.

Loss of subjects occurred between P1 and T1 and between T1 and T2 due to death, discharge, transfer, or resignation. Thus, the sample available for the pre–post analysis differed from the total sample enrolled.

Instruments and Procedures

At each data collection point, restraint prevalence was determined through 18 observation rounds, conducted twice each shift over a 72-hour period by teams of nurses who recorded the restraint status of every resident. Restraint was defined as "any device placed on or near the body which limits freedom of voluntary movement" (Evans et al., 1991, p. 82). In this definition, restraints include vest, belt, mitt, and limb restraints and the geriatric chair with fixed tray table.

Cognitive function of residents was measured using the Mini Mental State Examination (MMSE) (Folstein, Folstein, & McHugh, 1975). Affective state was determined using the Cornell Scale, a 19-item depression inventory which relies on information from interviews with both the resident's caregiver and the resident and which has been shown to have high reliability, sensitivity, and validity with demented subjects (Alexopoulos, Abrams, Young, & Shamoian, 1988). Functional status was determined by a staff-completed Psychogeriatric Dependency Rating Scale (PGDRS), which measures function in three areas: orientation, behavior, and physical function (Wilkinson & Graham-White, 1980). Items to estimate risk of falls and risk of treatment interference and to describe the pattern of restraint use were added to this questionnaire. Data on medical problems, use of medications, significant negative health events, and plan of care for the 30 days prior to and including the days of restraint observation were obtained from health care records.

Staff subjects completed two instruments: (1) the Maslach Burnout Inventory (Maslach & Jackson, 1981), a 22-item tool that measures burnout in three areas (emotional exhaustion, depersonalization, and reduced personal accomplishment) and that has moderate to high internal consistency, test–retest reliability, and correlations with independent behavioral ratings; and (2) the Perceptions of Restraint Use Questionnaire (PRUQ) (Strumpf & Evans, 1988), a 17-item Likert scale that measures beliefs about the efficacy of physical restraint with the elderly. This instrument has face and content validity and high internal consistency. In addition, staff subjects were asked to list alternatives for managing fall risk, treatment interference, and disruptive behaviors. Finally, institutional records of incidents, injuries, and restraint policies were examined.

Intervention

The experimental intervention was a program of ten 45-minute restraint education sessions conducted by a gerontologic clinical nurse specialist. The program modules were developed by the investigators in consultation with an educational consultant and two gerontologic nurse clinicians. The program focussed on developing awareness of myths, effects of restraint, and legal and ethical issues, and emphasized a systematic way to assess behavior and develop interventions for three problematic behaviors: fall risk, treatment interference, and disruptive behavior. Module titles included, for example, "Making Sense of Behavior," "Feelings and Beliefs about Restraints," "Working with Residents Who Fall," "Managing Wandering Behavior," and "Making Decisions about Restraints." Each module contained an overview, main objectives and key points, a structured content outline, and background materials, including references for the educator.

To capitalize on adult education principles, an interactive teaching method was used. A balance between theoretical and clinically relevant information was sought by alternating role playing, experiential exercises, homework assignments such as keeping a behavioral monitoring log, slides, video clips, lecture, and discussion. Each of the 10 sessions was presented for day, evening, and night shift nursing staff. Refreshments provided a modest motivation to attend, and University of Pennsylvania Certificates of Participation were awarded in a special ceremony and reception at the conclusion of the program. Although 38 staff (33 study participants and 5 other staff) attended from 1 to 10 sessions, not all of them completed pre- and post-testing.

RESULTS

Staff Outcomes

Among the 33 staff who participated in the study, only 13 completed both pre- and post-test instruments; thus, summary data are reported only for these 13 staff members. These staff attended an average of 4.8 sessions of the Restraint Education Program.

At Time 1, staff scores on the three composite subscales in the burnout inventory demonstrated a low level of burnout as compared to national norms for health care workers. No statistically significant change occurred in these scores from pre- to post-test, although there was improvement on the personal accomplishment subscale, indicating that staff felt better about their work. The 8 staff who completed pre- and post-PRUQ instruments showed a significant change in their beliefs about restraint efficacy, with average scores dropping from 4.25 to 3.88 on a 5-point scale, $[t(7) = 2.41, p = .047]$, where higher scores indicated greater belief in the efficacy of restraints (see Figure 13.1). The post-test score (3.88) closely resembles our findings in a 1987 study in which

FIGURE 13.1. Pre- (T1) and post- (T2) Restraint Education Program scores for the Perceptions of Restraint Use Questionnaire (PRUQ) (*n* = 8) and identification of alternatives to restraint use (Alt) (*n* = 13).

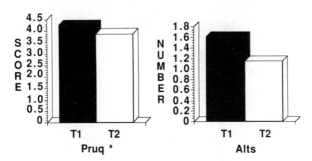

Note. * $p < .05$

American nursing home staff scores averaged 3.65, but this score still represents a much greater willingness to restrain older adults than among Scottish nurses, who averaged 2.77 in a cross-cultural study (Evans & Strumpf, 1990). The mean number of alternative interventions named by the 13 subjects was low compared to those named by Scottish nurses (Evans & Strumpf, 1990), and the number actually declined pre- to post-test, from 1.62 to 1.15. However, the range of types of alternatives identified expanded, especially in psychosocial and activity interventions. Thus there was improvement in some staff outcomes but not in others.

Restraint Prevalence

True to prediction, restraint use was lower initially (preliminary observation = 46.6%) but returned to "baseline" at T1 (prevalence = 52.6%). A slight increase to 53.6% was noted at 1-month posteducation (T2), but the prevalence declined over the next 2 months to 47.3% at T3 (see Figure 13.2). This figure, however, is higher than the national average of 41% reported by HCFA in 1988. Thus, while reduced restraint use was predicted, this was not found to be the case. However, one important change in the type and pattern of restraint was noted: At T1, vests (72%), geriatric chairs (34%), and mitts (3%) were in use, whereas at T2, restraining devices consisted mainly of geriatric chairs or recliners with tray tables (71%) with few vests (29%) and no mitt restraints. Further, the pattern of restraint use changed from round-the-clock use to use only when residents were out of bed.

FIGURE 13.2. Restraint use prevalence pre- (P1 & T1) and post- (T2 & T3) Restraint Education Program (n = 43).

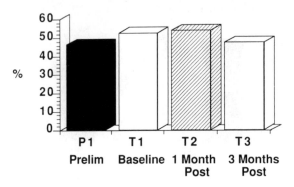

Resident Outcomes

Forty-three subjects were present at both T1 and T2; subjects missing data on any instrument were excluded from these analyses; thus the n differs in different analyses. Resident subject MMSE scores at T1 averaged 10.29 (severely impaired). The decline to 9.35 at T2 was not significant [$t(33)$ = .96, p = .342]. Likewise, the mean T1 score on the Cornell Scale was 12.85 (probable depression), and this score remained stable at T2 [12.62; $t(33)$ = .13, p = .895].

In general, resident function scores (Figure 13.3) indicated a greater level of impairment than that reported in the literature for psychogeriatric and rehabilitation patients (Wilkinson & Graham-White, 1980). Between T1 and T2, there was no difference in overall functional status [PGDRS means of 34.17 vs. 34.21, $t(41)$ = –.03, p = .977] or in two of the composite subscales—behavior [7.69 vs. 5.93, $t(41)$ = 1.55, p = .129] and physical function [22.98 vs. 23.60, $t(42)$ = –1.06, p = .293]. There was a significant change on the third subscale, orientation [from 3.60 to 4.74, $t(42)$ = –3.47, p < .001] indicating that staff viewed the residents as less oriented at T2. Although functional test scores did not significantly alter from T1 to T2, subjects were rated by staff as less behaviorally disturbed at T2. Perhaps, following restraint education, staff were more aware of cognitive dysfunction as a reason for residents' behaviors and viewed them as less troubling.

Interestingly, significant changes in most of the resident functional scores were found between preliminary observations done 1 month before the program began and at T1 observations, just before the educational program. Specifically, residents were more depressed and had greater disorientation, more behavioral problems, and higher overall dependency scores at T1, 1 month following the preliminary observation

FIGURE 13.3. Resident functional status pre- (T1) and post- (T2) Restraint Education Program.

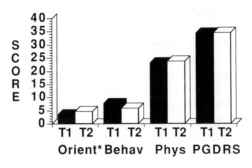

Note. * *p* < .001.

and just before the program. This was the period during which restraint prevalence increased by 6%. The fact that these levels remained consistent during the course of the 4-month educational intervention and into the T2 observation may indicate a retardation in functional decline beyond what might reasonably be expected in institutionalized, frail elders. While improvement in resident function was predicted, this did not occur.

Serious Injuries

It is important to note that no serious injuries occurred in the 30-day period preceding either T1 or T2; thus, as predicted, there was no increase in serious injuries during the study.

DISCUSSION

The major conclusion to be drawn from this analysis is that a systematic educational program for staff in a nursing home can make a difference in attitudes, beliefs, and knowledge, but it is insufficient by itself to produce change in restraint practice over a short time period. Factors that were outside the researchers' control, but that probably influenced the outcomes, included a number of system issues. Just prior to the study, the nursing home had defeated unionization efforts, indicating serious management–staff tensions. During the 8 months of the study, the facility had four different directors of nursing, two different administrators, and two different assistant administrators. During the 4 months of restraint education, the gerontologic nurse specialist was the most consistent leader in the facility. By T2 there had been a 52% turnover of nursing staff on the study unit, and 27% of the residents present at T1 had died or been discharged. Although verbal support for the project and educational program was given by administrative personnel, staff were neither required nor assigned to attend the in-service sessions.

Given these influences, the facts that restraint use did not significantly increase, that functional status did not further decline, that staff came to believe less in restraint efficacy, and that the patterns and types of restraints used over this period became less restrictive demonstrate modest success of the program. We believe that restraint education prepared the staff to begin changing practice once a stable leadership team was in place. And indeed, staff gave anecdotal evidence of a change in practice at the concluding certificate ceremony. One nursing assistant, who had declined to attend any educational sessions, proudly told us about one agitated male resident who had consistently been observed strapped by vest and belt restraints into a geriatric chair with locked tray table; often the chair itself was tied to a railing. Following the educational sessions, this resident's restraints were removed; he was assisted to walk on a scheduled basis and was placed in a regular chair with a wedge cushion to prevent sliding forward. He had had no falls or injuries and was now dressed neatly in slacks, sweater, and shirt. He fed himself, smiled, and was no longer agitated. In another anecdote several months following the study conclusion, the Director of Nursing (DON) described a male resident who walked out of the facility into a heavily trafficked street, was struck by a car, and suffered a fractured hip. Following readmission to the facility, the DON insisted that the resident be restrained "for his safety," but the nursing staff refused, saying they knew his wandering pattern and that he could be appropriately observed and distracted or redirected to the unit before exiting, thus eliminating the need for restraint.

Changing Institutionalized Practice

Reducing restraints in nursing homes will require solid administrative commitment from the Board of Directors, passed on to nursing and departmental supervisory staff in a stable environment supportive of new approaches to care. Furthermore, such a change in practice requires a major shift from a medical to a psychosocial model, from paternalistic approaches to those in which risk taking is accepted as part of the human condition. Dehumanizing, task-oriented approaches must be replaced by individualized, person-centered care, including a focus on rehabilitation.

Policies evolving from this shift in philosophy will sound very different from those in place in most nursing homes today. An interdisciplinary approach, which broadly includes everybody involved with the nursing home, will be essential if a more homelike, less restrictive environment is to be created. And finally, staff training will be essential to facilitate new ways of viewing behavior and efforts to adopt alternative methods of care. Change may come slowly, but change away from routine use of restraint with frail older people remains an important goal, one which can be achieved.

ACKNOWLEDGMENTS

This research was supported by the Alzheimer's Disease and Related Disorders Association, Inc., Grant #PRG-89-155. The authors wish to acknowledge the contributions of the following associates on this project: Lynne Taylor, Karen Knibbe, Cathy Stevenson, Christine Wanich, Joan Wagner, Marianne Johnston, and Carolyn Rohr-Martinek.

REFERENCES

Alexopoulos, G. S., Abrams, R. C., Young, R. C., & Shamoian, C. A. (1988). Cornell scale for depression in dementia. *Biological Psychiatry, 23*, 271–284.

Brooten, D., Hayman, L., & Naylor, M. (1988). *Leadership for change.* Philadelphia: Lippincott.

Capezuti, L., Strumpf, N. E., & Evans, L. (1991). *Reconceptualizing physical restraint as elder neglect.* Unpublished paper. University of Pennsylvania, Philadelphia.

Evans, L. K. (1991, March). Ethical regulation of physical restraints: Is it possible? Paper presented at U. S. Senate Special Committee on Aging and Hastings Center, *Responsible Caring: New Directions in Nursing Home Ethics* hearing. Washington, DC.

Evans, L. K., & Strumpf, N. E. (1989). Tying down the elderly: A review of the literature on physical restraint. *Journal of the American Geriatrics Society, 37*, 65–74.

Evans, L. K., & Strumpf, N. E. (1990). Myths about elder restraint. *Image: Journal of Nursing Scholarship, 22*, 124–128.

Evans, L. K., Strumpf, N. E., & Williams, C. (1991). Redefining a standard of care for frail older people: Alternatives to routine physical restraint. In P. Katz, R. Kane, & M. Mezey (Eds.), *Advances in long term care, 1* (pp. 81–108). New York: Springer.

Folstein, M. F., Folstein, S., & McHugh, P. R. (1975). "Mini-mental state:" A practical guide for grading the cognitive state of patients for clinicians. *Journal of Psychiatric Research, 12*, 189–198.

Health Care Financing Administration. (1988). *Medicare/Medicaid nursing home information: 1987–1988.* Washington, DC: U.S. Government Printing Office.

Lewin, K. (1951). *Field theory in social science.* New York: Harper & Row.

Lofgren, R. P., MacPherson, D. S., Granieri, R., Myllenbeck, S., & Spratka, J. M. (1989). Mechanical restraints on the medical wards: Are protective devices safe? *American Journal of Public Health, 79,* 735–738.

Maslach, C., & Jackson, S. E. (1981). *Maslach burnout inventory manual.* Palo Alto: Consulting Psychologists Press.

Miles, S. (1990, April). *Restraints: Controlling a symptom or a symptom of control.* Paper presented at the Annual Meeting of the American Geriatrics Society, Atlanta, GA.

PL 100-203 (1987). Omnibus Budget Reconciliation Act, Subtitle C, Nursing Home Reform, Washington, DC: U.S. Government Printing Office.

Rigert, J., & Lerner, M. (1990, December 2, 3, 4, 5, & 8). Safeguards that kill. *Minneapolis Star Tribune,* pp. 1A, 18A–22A; 1A, 10A–12A; 1A, 18A–21A; 1A, 18A–20A; 15A.

Strumpf, N. E., & Evans, L. K. (1988). Physical restraint of the hospitalized elderly: Perceptions of patients and nurses. *Nursing Research, 37,* 132–137.

Tinetti, M. E., Liu, W., Marottoli, R. A., & Ginter, S. F. (1991). Mechanical restraint use among residents of skilled nursing facilities. *Journal of the American Medical Association, 265*(4), 468–471.

Wilkinson, I. M., & Graham-White, J. (1980). Dependency rating scales for use in psychogeriatric nursing. *Health Bulletin, 38,* 36–42.

[14]

Research on Falls: Implications for Practice

Lois K. Evans

Over the past 20–30 years, we have simply assumed that certain practices represented good standards of care, and we have allowed these practices to become rituals. The chapters in this book critically examine some of these rituals, including catheter and diaper use as a way of managing incontinence, and the things we do with the cognitively impaired elderly, from use of restraints, to neuroleptic drugs, to not doing anything at all because we assume that these elderly cannot do more. The studies reported here also examined other basic issues—like mobility and elimination. What we begin to see from the research is that some of the old things that we thought were true are not, and we now have the knowledge to address those issues in a new way.

One of the myths we began to tackle several years ago at the University of Pennsylvania was the myth that safety for older people must be provided at all costs. Doris Schwartz, an older colleague of ours, called one day and said, "There's something I need to talk to you about. There's a problem in nursing homes and in hospitals; they're restraining all of my friends and my friends don't like it. I think it's going on too much, and I think you should do something about it." When Doris Schwartz says you should "do something about it," you do something about it! My research partner, Neville Strumpf, and I are convinced that we now have our life's work cut out for us in working on this issue of restraints. The work is very exciting, because it's so multifaceted. It is related not only to falls and mobility; it is also related to continence and to behavioral disturbances in the cognitively impaired. It has ethical and legal dimensions, as well as psychological, sociological, and physiologic aspects.

One thing that seems to be very clear from the research on falls presented in this book is that falls are not accidents. Falls are not random events. They can be predicted to some extent, and once one can predict something, preventive intervention can be developed. Hogue gives a comprehensive overview of what is currently known about falls and the associated risk of injury in older people. The research reported in the chapters on falls focuses primarily on two areas: assessment and intervention. One problem is how to assess who is at risk of falling in various institutions; Soja and Kippenbrock, for example, described an instrument that seems to effectively identify persons at high risk for falls. A particular concern is identifying people who are not only at risk of falling, but at risk of injury from a fall; this, I think, is an even more finely tuned approach to the problem. One of the concerns raised in this book is that while we can identify people who are at risk of falling because of age, medical diagnosis, mobility problems, and the like, we are placing an excessive number of people on "fall-risk precautions" and restricting their mobility unduly. Thus, it is crucial to identify not just *fall-risk* people, but people who are at most risk of receiving *injuries* from their falls. Such people should then be targeted for interventions. The chapter by Heslin and colleagues is particularly interesting in this regard because the authors view risk of injury as the problem, and they have been able to identify specific patient-relevant characteristics that are amenable to change; as a result, interventions can be prescribed to help prevent injuries from falls. The administration in Heslin's facility has taken a new, forward-looking stance in that they have said, "We are not really interested in keeping track of falls as incidents; we are interested in knowing about falls as clinically relevant data for the patient." So the nurses no longer fill out incident reports as though a fall were a "bad thing"; the falls data are put into the patient's chart to help the nurses assess what particular problems the patient has that place him or her at risk for injury and what interventions can resolve those particular problems.

A final group of assessment studies report ways of assessing the mobility status and ambulatory status of patients, not just epidemiologically, but by employing observational means. One good tool is the Postural Control Scale, which is based on Tinnetti's (1986) work and has been finely tuned by Dayhoff from Indiana University.

Intervention studies are focusing on falls prevention in two areas. One emphasizes teaching nurses how to be more aware of people who are at risk of falling and how to make observations and use various techniques to help prevent falls, especially among hospitalized people. (See the studies reported by Hollinger & Patterson and Evans & Strumpf.) There is also some work reported on injury prevention using special technologies; for example, the hip pads study by Ross and colleagues from the University of Iowa is an exciting new development for older adults who would like to continue walking but cannot avoid falling.

Other interventions are aimed at the person. Old persons need to motivate themselves to strengthen their balance, gait, endurance, muscle strength, and muscle tone, so that they are more empowered, personally and physically, to ambulate safely. Some of the interventions that are coming from the FICSIT project—for example, the Tai Chi Chaun and biofeedback exercises, described in the chapter by McNeely et al.—as well as the exercise program described in the chapter by Reynolds and Garrett are good examples of things that nurses can do to empower older people to remain safely mobile through their elder years.

All of the studies reported here are aimed at empowering either nurses or patients. We empower nurses by giving them information about the risk factors for falls in older people and instruments that can be used for early detection of those factors, as well as interventions that can help prevent falls and injuries from falls. The exercise programs and similar interventions are aimed at empowering older people to have safe ambulation and mobility.

We still need to know more clearly *who* is most likely to be injured from a fall, so that we can fine tune our assessments and aim interventions at the people most likely to benefit from them. An underlying theme in all these chapters is that we still believe that falls are bad. I think we have to begin to change our thinking about that—to realize that not all falls are bad, and that, on the continuum of risk taking and quality of life, people want to have some choice about how much to restrict their activity and mobility in order to be protected.

Finally, there is still an underlying attitude problem that has to do with controlling the behavior of older people. For example, in some of the falls intervention chapters, physical restraints still appear on the lists of appropriate nursing interventions to prevent falls in older people. We must look even more deeply at the essence of nursing, which is really caring, using a person-centered approach, to enable the older adult to meet self-defined needs and desires.

REFERENCE

Tinetti, M. E. (1986). Performance-oriented assessment of mobility problems in elderly patients. *Journal of the American Geriatrics Society, 34,* 119–126.

Part III

MANAGING INCONTINENCE

[15]

Managing Incontinence: The Current Bases for Practice

Jean F. Wyman

Urinary incontinence is a significant health problem with potentially serious physical, psychological, and social consequences. Many older adults suffer from incontinence, and it can affect individuals of other age groups as well. Until recently, however, surprisingly little was known about the assessment and management of urinary incontinence. In the early 1980s, work on incontinence began appearing in the health care literature, and the National Institute on Aging (NIA) made urinary incontinence a research priority. From 1984 to 1989, the National Institute of Aging and the Division of Nursing (now the National Center for Nursing Research) sponsored a multisite clinical trial on the behavioral management of urinary incontinence.

The increasing attention paid to incontinence led to an NIH Consensus Development Conference on Urinary Incontinence in October 1988. The outcome of the conference was a summary of current knowledge of the prevalence, costs, consequences, etiology, pathophysiology, diagnostic evaluation, and therapeutic modalities of urinary incontinence, and strategies for increasing public and professional knowledge of incontinence (NIH, 1988).

In 1991, the Agency for Health Care Policy and Research (AHCPR) initiated the development of practice guidelines to assist health care practitioners in the prevention, diagnosis, and management of urinary incontinence. The practice guidelines have been developed by a multidisciplinary panel of nurses, urologists, a gynecologist, a geriatrician, a psychologist, an occupational therapist, and a consumer member. The AHCPR guidelines define a strong role for nurses in the detection, diagnosis, and management of incontinent patients.

This chapter presents a critical review of the research that has been conducted on urinary incontinence, focusing on research applicable to nursing practice. Areas for additional research are also discussed, with recommendations for the direction of research over the next five years.

THE CONDITION OF URINARY INCONTINENCE

The literature on urinary incontinence is vast and often contradictory. The problems with the research are compounded by lack of agreement on the labels for different types of incontinence. Although the International Continence Society (ICS) has attempted to standardize the terminology of lower urinary tract function and ICS definitions are widely used, they are not uniformly accepted.

Urinary incontinence is defined by the ICS as a "condition in which involuntary urine loss is a social or hygienic problem and is objectively demonstrable" (Abrams, Blaivas, Stanton, & Jensen, 1988). Incontinence is rarely determined solely by physiologic factors and is often the result of a complex interaction of physiologic, psychological, social, behavioral, and environmental factors. Two types of incontinence are generally recognized: transient (acute) and established (chronic). Transient incontinence has a sudden onset, usually in association with an acute medical or surgical condition, and often resolves itself with resolution of the precipitating condition. Established incontinence may have either a sudden onset with an acute condition or a gradual onset with no known precipitating cause; it often increases in severity over time (see Table 15.1 for definitions of terms).

Several different classification schemes for established incontinence are currently used. For example, one scheme is based on presenting symptomatology (e.g., incontinence is classified as stress, urge, overflow, or functional [see Table 15.1]). Although these classifications are similar to the North American Nursing Diagnosis Association (NANDA) nursing diagnoses for incontinence, important conceptual differences exist. For example, this classification scheme does not usually include incontinence conditions that require urodynamic evaluation to document their presence. Other classification schemes include the underlying pathophysiologic abnormality (e.g., detrusor instability, incompetent urethral sphincteric mechanism), or functional impairment (e.g., storage/filling phase versus emptying phase problem, or changes in detrusor or outlet resistance activity). Different types of urinary incontinence are not necessarily mutually exclusive. Thus, several types of incontinence may coexist within an individual, each having several possible causes.

TABLE 15.1 Definition of Terms Used for Urinary Incontinence

Term	Definition
Transient incontinence	Sudden onset usually associated with an acute medical or surgical condition; often will resolve itself with resolution of the precipitating condition.
Established incontinence	May have sudden onset with acute condition or gradual onset with no known precipitating cause, and often increases in severity over time.

Types of Established Urinary Incontinence

Functional incontinence	Urine leakage associated with inability or unwillingness to toilet appropriately because of cognitive or physical impairments, psychological factors, or environmental barriers. Bladder and urethral function are normal.
Overflow incontinence	Periodic or continuous dribbling of urine resulting from obstruction and/or overdistension of bladder. Associated with outlet obstruction such as prostatic hypertrophy, bladder neck obstruction, or urethral stricture, or with an underactive detrusor secondary to neurogenic factors or anticholinergic/antispasmodic drugs.
Stress incontinence	Urine leakage associated with sudden increase in intra-abdominal pressure (e.g., cough, sneeze, laugh, exercise). Associated with sphincter incompetence and urethral instability.
Urge incontinence	Urine leakage preceded by strong desire to void. Associated with detrusor (bladder) overactivity.

Behavioral Therapies

Biofeedback	Client receives visual or auditory feedback on own physiologic responses. Used to teach pelvic muscle contraction and to inhibit bladder contractions. Variety of approaches have been used, including pressure and EMG feedback.
Bladder training	(Also termed bladder drill, bladder retraining, bladder discipline.) Scheduled voidings with gradual increases in the voiding interval.
Contingency management	Procedures that involve the systematic and consistent application of rewards and punishments to improve continence. For example, use of social approval and disapproval.
Habit training	Scheduled toiletings with adjustments in schedule based upon patient's voiding pattern. Specific voiding intervals may be increased or decreased.

TABLE 15.1 *(Continued)*

Term	Definition
Patterned urge response toileting	Patient's voiding pattern is determined using special electronic device in undergarment to detect incontinent episodes and then a toileting schedule is tailored to observed pattern.
Pelvic muscle exercise (Kegel exercises)	Set of voluntary muscle contractions designed to strengthen the levator ani muscle complex (pelvic floor muscles).
Prompted voiding	Patients are contacted on a fixed schedule and prompted to void. Assistance provided only if patient requests to void.
Timed voiding	Fixed voiding schedule that remains unchanged during training.

In addition to the complex etiology of the condition, incontinence varies in the frequency, severity, and duration of its symptoms, as well as in the temporal and situational circumstances of episodes. Thus it is important to recognize the heterogeneity of individuals' responses to urinary incontinence as a condition, as well as the social and environmental contexts in which incontinence occurs.

OVERVIEW OF URINARY INCONTINENCE RESEARCH

Research on urinary incontinence has been conducted in several areas: (1) the mechanisms of continence and incontinence; (2) the epidemiology of urinary incontinence, including risk factor identification and physiologic sequelae; (3) psychosocial factors and consequences for incontinent individuals and their caregivers; (4) diagnostic evaluation, including characterization of the type of incontinence, assessment techniques, and outcome measurement; (5) intervention studies, including behavioral, drug, electrical stimulation, surgical, and palliative/ supportive treatments; and (6) economic studies, including the cost of incontinence and the cost effectiveness of different treatment modalities.

Mechanisms of Continence and Incontinence

Basic research on urinary incontinence has focused on the embryology, histology, morphology, anatomy, neuroanatomy, and physiology of micturition in animals and humans. Pharmacologic and neuro-pharmacologic influences on lower urinary tract function also have been studied. The role of pharmacologic influences such as estrogen and other drugs (e.g., diuretics) is still poorly understood.

Micturition and continence are complex functions requiring central and peripheral nervous system coordination. Although we have a basic understanding of these functions, there are still significant areas of disagreement and lack of clarity regarding the components involved in each. Research on the physiology of the lower urinary tract has been limited by lack of instruments that can measure various physiologic parameters, and little is understood about the effects of aging on lower urinary tract function and age's contributions to the development of urinary incontinence. It is believed that age alone is not a risk factor for the development of incontinence; however, many age-related changes, along with drug or disease precipitants that are often outside the urinary tract, may predispose an older individual to incontinence. There also may be cross-cultural differences in the development of urinary in-continence, although such differences are not clearly documented.

Epidemiology of Urinary Incontinence

Most epidemiologic research on urinary incontinence has been con-ducted in older white populations that are predominantly female. Little is known about the prevalence of incontinence in nonwhite, male, and younger populations. The majority of prevalence studies were con-ducted in the 1970s in European countries. The population group sam-pled was usually older adults (most frequently defined as 60 or 65 years and over) drawn from medical practice registries. More recent studies conducted in the United States have included large-scale community-based surveys of older adults (Diokno, Brock, & Herzog, 1986).

The exact prevalence of urinary incontinence is unknown. Prevalence rates vary from 8 to 51% in community-dwelling populations, and from 38 to 55% in long-term care institutionalized populations (Herzog & Fultz, 1990; Mohide, 1986). The estimated rate of incontinence in the elderly admitted to an acute care hospital is approximately 19% (Sullivan & Lindsay, 1984). These varying prevalence rates reflect differences in the definitions of incontinence, the populations studied, and the survey methodologies. In several of the large-scale health surveys, an un-derreporting bias may have been a factor since questions on in-continence were mixed with other types of questions (Herzog & Fultz, 1990).

In general, the prevalence in women is twice as high as in men. Although the prevalence of incontinence tends to increase with advancing age, the findings on this are not consistent. Most studies indicate a relationship between incontinence and impaired cognitive or mobility function. The most frequent type of urinary incontinence involves mixed symptomatology with both stress and urge symptoms present; this is followed by stress symptoms alone; the least common incontinence type is urge symptoms alone (Herzog & Fultz, 1990). (Prevalence studies do not generally include overflow or functional incontinence.)

Information is lacking on risk factors for the development of incontinence and on the progression of pathophysiology, severity, and remission of symptoms. The natural history of incontinence in community, acute, and chronic institutionalized populations is unknown. There are few established risk factors for urinary incontinence. The findings on the most frequently studied risk factors—age, gender, parity, and body weight—are inconsistent. Other risk factors such as menopause, medication use, co-morbidity of chronic illness, and urinary tract infection have not been explored systematically in continent and incontinent populations

Psychosocial Factors and Consequences of Urinary Incontinence

Urinary incontinence can be a devastating experience with extreme psychosocial consequences for both the affected individual (Wyman, Harkins, & Fantl, 1990; Yu, 1987) and his or her caregiver (Noelker, 1987; Sanford, 1975; Yu & Kaltreider, 1987). A useful framework for examining the psychosocial factors associated with urinary incontinence has four components: (1) perception of and response to urinary incontinence; (2) development or exacerbation of incontinence symptoms; (3) psychosocial consequences for individuals, families, and caregivers; and (4) the role of psychosocial factors in treatment (Ory, Wyman, & Yu, 1986). Unfortunately, few well-designed studies have been done in any of these areas. Previous research has been limited by methodological problems including small and nonrepresentative samples, poorly defined diagnostic criteria, and inattention to specification of relevant symptom characteristics. Another major limitation is the lack of standardized instruments for assessing the psychosocial effects of incontinence.

Several areas of incontinence warrant further research. For example, little is known about the large percentage of incontinent individuals (approximately 50%) who do not seek help. The reasons for not seeking evaluation and treatment are poorly understood, and may vary by cultural and ethnic group. The most commonly cited reasons include the view that incontinence is a normal and inevitable consequence of aging, the fear of surgery, and low expectations regarding treatment (Holst & Wilson, 1988).

Research on incontinent women suggests that the effects of urinary incontinence on daily activities and social life may depend on the type of incontinence but may be independent of the severity of the incontinence, that is, not directly tied to the frequency or amount of urine loss. Little is known about the influence of age, gender, or ethnic differences on the perceived impact of urinary incontinence. There have also been no studies comparing the psychosocial effects of urinary incontinence to those of other chronic health conditions. Further research and treatment programs also must address whether intervention can improve the quality of life for affected individuals and their caregivers (Wyman et al., 1990); this is an important area for study because, although incontinent symptoms can improve, they often are not totally eliminated. Thus patient satisfaction and quality of life may be better indicators of treatment outcomes than objective physiologic measurements.

Diagnostic Evaluation of Urinary Incontinence

Most of the research on urinary incontinence has focused on diagnostic evaluation. Studies of the diagnostic evaluation of incontinence have concentrated on the description, classification, and techniques for studying lower urinary tract dysfunction. The International Continence Society has made significant progress in standardizing the terminology and assessment methods related to urinary incontinence. However, because of increasing knowledge and new technology, wide variations exist between investigatory protocols, and there is continued controversy about description, classification, and assessment techniques.

Although several studies have focused on objective quantification of the severity of urinary incontinence, standardized measurements of incontinence that are accurate, reliable, and valid have not been established. Frequency of incontinent episodes is used as a primary outcome in most intervention studies, yet surprisingly few studies have evaluated the reliability of different methods (e.g., self-report diary and electronic monitoring) of assessing frequency (O'Donnell, Sutton, Beck, & Finkbeiner, 1987; Wyman, Choi, Harkins, Wilson, & Fantl, 1988). Several studies, however, have investigated the reliability of a variety of pad-testing techniques in quantifying the amount of urine lost (Fantl, Harkins, Wyman, Choi, & Taylor, 1987; Kromann-Anderson, Jakobsen, & Andersen, 1989).

In addition to research on objective quantification of urinary incontinence, several studies have attempted to standardize instruments that assess variables associated with continence status, such as (1) pelvic muscle strength, assessed through clinical rating scales (Brink, Sampselle, Wells, Diokno, & Gillis, 1989; Worth, Dougherty, & McKey, 1986), or pressure devices (Dougherty, Abrams, & McKey, 1986) and (2) pelvic muscle activity, assessed through electromyography readings (Perry & Whipple, 1982). Such studies are of particular importance in establishing the reliable and valid outcome measures needed for intervention studies. Work in this area is still preliminary, however.

Several researchers have identified clinical algorithms in the assessment of incontinence (Hilton & Stanton, 1981; Ouslander et al., 1989). These algorithms warrant larger scale clinical testing. However, a potential difficulty in applying an algorithm approach to incontinence assessment and management is the large number of patients with mixed symptomatology. With complex symptomatology, symptoms can be misleading and may not match the underlying etiology. Thus, treatment based on an algorithm may not always be the most appropriate choice or yield the best therapeutic outcome.

The NIH Consensus Statement on Urinary Incontinence (1988) and the new AHCPR practice guidelines delineate procedures that should be included in the core or basic evaluation of all incontinent patients, as well as those referred for specialized evaluation. The core evaluation cited in the NIH Consensus Statement includes history, physical examination, functional and environmental assessment, a voiding diary, and selected laboratory tests. Specialized tests included urodynamic evaluation (e.g., cystometry, uroflowmetry, urethral pressure profilometry), videourodynamic evaluation, ultrasound evaluation, cystourethroscopy, and electromyography studies (see Table 15.2). These specialized tests should be used selectively and are usually reserved for patients in whom simple drug or behavioral trials have failed, those with complex symptomatology, those with failed operations, or those anticipating surgical correction of their problem. Evaluation of incontinent individuals with severe cognitive and mobility impairments is more complex and may require a different strategy. Newer noninvasive techniques such as ultrasound need development and refinement to aid in the evaluation of lower urinary tract function in these patients.

Subjects participating in research protocols may need to follow extensive assessment protocols in order to characterize accurately their type of incontinence. Such characterization is critical in the determination of mechanisms of action for various interventions, as well as in the prediction of response.

TABLE 15.2   Specialized Tests for Incontinence

Test	Definition
Cystometry	Determines pressure–volume relationships in the bladder. Assesses detrusor activity, sensation, bladder capacity, and compliance.
Uroflowmetry	Evaluates micturition to determine evidence of obstruction. Assesses voided volume, flow rates, flow times, and characteristics of the flow pattern.
Urethral pressure profilometry	Evaluates the ability of the urethra to prevent leakage. Assesses both static (at rest) and dynamic (coughing or other straining) urethral closure pressure profiles.
Videourodynamic evaluation	Provides simultaneous video recordings of pressure and flow data with radiographic images of the bladder and urethra during bladder filling and emptying.
Ultrasound evaluation	Noninvasive technique used to determine static and dynamic anatomic relationships of the urethra and bladder. Also used to determine bladder volume.
Cystourethroscopy	Direct visualization of the urinary tract by means of a cystoscope inserted through the urethra.
Electromyography studies	Determines the electrical activity of the striated muscles involved in micturition. May also include nerve condition studies.

Intervention Studies

Treatment for urinary incontinence can be grouped into five categories: (1) behavioral, (2) drug, (3) electrical stimulation, (4) surgery, and (5) supportive. Treatment should begin with the lowest risk, least invasive therapies first—such as the behavioral therapies—and proceed to drug and surgical interventions if necessary. Each of the five categories, with the exception of supportive treatment, has demonstrated effectiveness, ranging in cure rates from 6 to 100%. However, the cure or improvement rates are quite variable. Nevertheless, in a large majority of cases, behavioral, drug, and electrical stimulation therapies provide significant improvement to those individuals with mild to moderate incontinence.

Several studies have indicated that behavioral therapy may be as beneficial as drug therapy in improving incontinence symptoms (Fantl, Hurt, & Dunn, 1981; Ouslander, Blaustein, Connor, & Pitt, 1988; Wells, Brink, Diokno, Wolfe, & Gillis, 1991). Drug therapy can be effective in the management of stress, urge, and mixed incontinence. Generally, surgery is particularly effective in the treatment of genuine stress incontinence and urge and overflow incontinence secondary to an enlarged prostate. Drug and surgical therapies are discussed briefly in the NIH Consensus Statement and will not be elaborated on further here.

Intervention studies reported in the literature often have methodological problems that make it difficult to apply their findings to clinical practice. These problems include the use of small samples, poorly defined diagnostic criteria, the lack of appropriate control groups, the use of multiple interventions within the same protocol, unclear definition of outcome variables, failure to use reliable instruments to measure treatment outcomes, lack of explicit criteria for judging cure or improvement, and different follow-up periods after onset of treatment. The efficacy of concomitant interventions is unclear because empirical evidence on the basic intervention is lacking. Also, long-term follow-up data (i.e., past 3–6 months) are generally missing. Research is needed to develop and test management algorithms using a "stepped-approach" to incontinence care similar to that used in hypertension therapy. Large-scale testing in multiple sites of the most promising interventions is also needed. In addition, further research on how to target treatment to patients with particular characteristics to achieve the best outcomes is important.

Behavioral Interventions Studies of behavioral interventions can be grouped into two categories: (1) self-management strategies for cognitively intact, ambulatory adults, who usually reside independently; and (2) external or environmental management strategies for cognitively or physically impaired adults, who usually reside in institutional settings. Behavioral interventions are of several basic types that can be used singly or in combination: scheduling regimens, pelvic muscle exercises, and biofeedback approaches. Self-management strategies include all three types of interventions. Environmental management strategies are predominantly scheduling regimens, with or without the use of contingency management. Five types of scheduling regimens have been identified: bladder training, habit retraining, timed voiding, prompted voiding, and patterned urge response toileting. Although these regimens share some elements, they contain different elements based on adjustment to the voiding schedule during the training period. In addition to a scheduling pattern, these regimens may include specific techniques taught to help patients control urgency, reinforcements for successful responses to training, and therapeutic interactions between the patient and the health care provider.

Bladder training involves a schedule of voidings with progressive increases in intervoiding intervals. Success rates are reported at 44% to 97% in community-dwelling populations (Fantl, Wyman, Harkins, &

Hadley, 1990). Bladder training is used predominantly in urge incontinence, but recently was found equally effective in the management of stress incontinence (Fantl et al., 1991).

Habit retraining also involves the assignment of a toileting schedule, but differs from bladder training in that the voiding interval may be increased or decreased based on the individual's voiding pattern. Improvement rates have ranged from 28% to 85% in community and nursing home populations (Clay, 1978; King, 1980; Rooney, 1982).

Timed voiding consists of the fixed assignment of a voiding schedule that remains unchanged during the course of the training program. This is the most commonly used technique in acute care hospitals and nursing homes. A success rate of 85% was reported in hospitalized geriatric patients (Sogbein & Awad, 1982).

Prompted voiding, similar to timed voiding, involves asking patients at regular intervals whether or not they need to void, and then assisting them to the toilet if the response is positive. Contingency management techniques, including social approval and disapproval, are used based on whether the person is found wet at the time of prompting, and whether successful toileting is achieved. In one study, 42% of nursing home patients responded to prompted voiding with a reduction in wet episodes to less than once in a 12-hour period (Schnelle, 1990).

A relatively new intervention, patterned urge response toileting, is similar to habit retraining. It involves determining the individual's voiding pattern based on a special electronic device, and then tailoring a toileting schedule based on that pattern. Using this method, Colling and colleagues found improvements in continence in 86% of 51 nursing home patients (Colling, Hadley, Ouslander, Campbell, & Eisch, 1989).

Pelvic muscle exercises have been used primarily in the management of mild to moderate stress incontinence in women, but also may be beneficial for male stress incontinence secondary to prostatectomy. Improvement rates vary from 31 to 91% (Wells, 1990). Pelvic exercises are aimed at restoring the tone and function of the perineal muscles, thus presumably increasing the urethral closure pressure. However, the mechanism by which these exercises improve continence status is poorly understood. Studies examining the mechanism of improvement have shown conflicting findings (Benvenuti et al., 1987; Burns, 1988; Tchou, Adams, Varner, & Denton, 1988). There is no common agreement on the best training regimen to achieve improvement in continence status—that is on the number and type of pelvic muscle contractions, frequency and duration of practice, and whether biofeedback and passive resistive devices increase the benefit of exercise. Also, not all individuals can learn a pelvic muscle contraction despite the best teaching efforts.

Biofeedback is a learning technique to help the individual exert better voluntary control over urine storage. Biofeedback approaches incorporate visual or auditory instrumentation to give continuous information to the individual on her or his physiologic responses. Physiologic responses used in biofeedback include sphincter, detrusor, vaginal, and abdominal pressures; or vaginal, anal, and abdominal electromyography readings. Generally biofeedback is used in conjunction with one of the other behavioral interventions. For example, it is used for stress incontinence to help patients correctly isolate and contract the pelvic muscles (Kegel, 1948). It also is used for urge incontinence to help individuals learn to inhibit bladder contractions (Cardozo, Abrams, Stanton, & Feneley, 1978; O'Donnell, Doyle, & Beck, 1988). Few studies, however, have investigated the increased efficacy of behavioral training when biofeedback approaches are incorporated.

A recent technique developed in Eastern Europe incorporates both pelvic muscle exercise and biofeedback through the use of weighted vaginal cones. The cones, which gradually increase in weight over time, are worn during daily activities for a specified period of time. A success rate of 70% was noted in a 4-week trial period (Peattie, Plevnik, & Stanton, 1988).

Behavioral interventions are poorly understood in terms of their mechanism of action; they improve symptoms but do not appear to change underlying pathophysiology. It is unclear, moreover, which individual characteristics predict success or failure with a particular intervention, and application of the results of a majority of the behavioral intervention studies are limited by the unique population who volunteer to participate in research studies. In addition, most studies have been conducted with women, reflecting the higher prevalence rate of incontinence in females. Behavioral interventions must be tested in more heterogeneous populations that include men. However, the lower prevalence rate of incontinence in men, along with the difference in underlying pathophysiology, makes it difficult to recruit an adequate sample for controlled clinical trials with a male population.

Research on behavioral interventions such as prompted voiding and patterned urge response toileting indicates that they are beneficial to nursing home patients. However, such interventions require a high degree of staff motivation, commitment, and compliance to be effective. Future studies are needed to evaluate various strategies for promoting optimal staff compliance with incontinence management. Further, several studies indicate that there are some patients who do not benefit from traditional behavioral therapies (Fantl et al., 1991; Hu et al., 1989; Schnelle, 1990). Novel treatment strategies must be developed and tested for those patients whose incontinence is intractable to traditional therapies.

Electrical Stimulation   Electrical stimulation of the pelvic floor has been tested as a treatment for urinary incontinence over the past 25 years in Europe. It has been introduced in the United States only recently. Electrical stimulation has been found beneficial in treating incontinence caused by sphincteric incompetence (Eriksen & Eik-Nes, 1989; Fall, 1984) and detrusor instability (Eriksen, Bergmann, & Eik-Nes, 1989; Merrill, 1979), and also may reestablish detrusor contractions in patients with atonic bladders (Sotiropoulos, 1975). Current treatment with electrical stimulation involves the use of external devices consisting of either an anal or a vaginal electrode that delivers an intermittent tetanizing current, which can be adjusted to the individual's tolerance. Success rates of chronic electrical stimulation in stress incontinence vary from 6% to 92% (Eriksen & Eik-Nes, 1989; Leach & Bavendam, 1989). It has been suggested, although not proven, that electrical stimulation may be particularly beneficial in stress incontinence therapy when teaching the technique of pelvic muscle contraction to patients who have weak muscles or are unable to contract their perineum voluntarily. Carefully controlled studies comparing electrical stimulation with traditional forms of therapy are needed.

Supportive Interventions   Supportive interventions are implemented when other therapies fail to control urine loss adequately. These interventions include catheterization, both indwelling and intermittent; external collection devices; prostheses such as penile clamps (generally not recommended) and vaginal pessaries; environmental and fluid manipulations; and incontinence pads and garments.

Catheters and External Collection Devices   Indwelling catheter use is not recommended as a strategy for long-term management of the incontinent patient except in selected cases; virtually all catheterized patients will develop bacteriuria despite every effort at optimal hygiene (Warren, 1986). Other long-term management strategies include condom catheters for men, and intermittent catheterization for those with overflow incontinence. Research is needed in several areas: the natural history of intermittent and condom catheterization, bladder retraining techniques after long-term indwelling catheterization, and the development of an external device capable of collecting urine effectively in incontinent women.

Incontinence Pads and Garments   A variety of incontinence pads and garments are commercially available. Approximately 30 studies have appeared in the literature evaluating the advantages and disadvantages of these products for predominantly institutionalized populations. The majority of the studies, however, were conducted in Europe using products that are not available in the United States. Further, few studies have examined the types of absorbent pads and garments used and their benefits in community-dwelling populations (Brink, 1990). Randomized controlled clinical trials are needed to study pads and garments and their effects on cost, quality of life, and care in both institutionalized and community populations.

Environmental and Fluid Manipulations   Although both environmental and fluid manipulations have been suggested as beneficial in the management of urinary incontinence, no studies have evaluated the effectiveness of such manipulations in reducing incontinence severity. Several studies report voluntary fluid restrictions by individuals to control their incontinence (Brink, Wells, & Diokno, 1987; Herzog, Fultz, Normolle, Brock, & Diokno, 1989; Mitteness, 1987). However, a recent study found that fluid intake in community-dwelling incontinent women had little or no relationship to the frequency of incontinent episodes (Wyman, Elswick, Wilson, & Fantl, in press). Future research should explore the type, timing, and volume of fluid intake in incontinence management.

Studies of the Costs of Incontinence and Incontinence Interventions

Hu (1990) estimated the economic cost of urinary incontinence at $10.3 billion in 1987: $3.3 billion for nursing home patients and $7 billion for elderly persons in the community. Few studies have examined the cost of incontinence in specific settings and the cost-benefits associated with specific interventions. Several studies have examined the cost of incontinence care in nursing homes (Cella, 1988; Ouslander & Kane, 1984), but none has investigated the costs associated with incontinence in acute hospitals and in the community. Several clinical trials on behavioral management of nursing home patients have included a cost-benefit analysis of their interventions (Hu et al., 1989; Schnelle, Sowell, Hu, & Traughber, 1988). No studies to date have examined the costs associated with behavioral therapy in the treatment of hospital inpatients or outpatients or the costs associated with other forms of interventions for these groups.

RECOMMENDATIONS FOR FUTURE NURSING RESEARCH

Urinary incontinence is a complex disorder arising from multiple factors: physical, psychological, social, behavioral, and environmental. Thus, incontinence research needs to be multidisciplinary, incorporating the unique perspectives of several disciplines into collaborative projects. These recommendations for nursing research priorities to improve the scientific base of practice build upon those outlined in the NIH Consensus Conference Statement. They include:

1. basic research on the mechanisms underlying the etiology, exacerbation, and response to treatment of specific forms of urinary incontinence;
2. epidemiologic studies, with emphasis on the identification of risk factors for development of urinary incontinence, its occurrence in specific populations (particularly men, nonwhites, individuals under age 65, acute hospitalized patients, and homebound adults), and the natural history of the various clinical and physiologic subtypes;
3. longitudinal studies on the prevention of incontinence in high-risk populations;
4. development and refinement of instruments to measure physiologic and psychosocial variables (including quality of life) associated with incontinence status, and development of noninvasive techniques to assess lower urinary tract function, particularly for cognitively impaired adults;
5. studies on the psychosocial impact of urinary incontinence on affected individuals and caregivers, including examination of factors involved in help-seeking behavior;
6. development and testing of new strategies using innovative techniques for the treatment of urinary incontinence, particularly in nursing home patients, frail or homebound adults, and patients whose incontinence is intractable to traditional forms of therapy;
7. development and testing of nursing care delivery systems in acute and long-term care settings that foster staff participation in and compliance with incontinence management programs;
8. randomized clinical trials on interventions, including longitudinal follow-up evaluation, algorithms for the systematic assessment and management of incontinent patients, and specific behavioral or pharmacologic interventions, either alone or in combination;
9. identification of factors that predict treatment success in order to target specific treatments to particular client characteristics, and investigation into adherence to interventions and strategies that promote optimal compliance;
10. comparative clinical trials of products and equipment involved in the management of refractory incontinence;
11. studies of the natural history of bacteriuria in the use of condoms and intermittent catheters;

12. investigations into indwelling catheter–related problems such as leakage around catheters and bladder retraining post-catheterization;
13. economic studies that examine the costs and benefits associated with incontinence treatment, with attention to the level of improvement experienced by incontinent individuals;
14. development of strategies to disseminate research innovations into clinical practice, with emphasis on nurses' involvement in the assessment and management of urinary incontinence.

RECOMMENDATIONS FOR NURSING PRACTICE

Although urinary incontinence is a common condition of older adults, it should never be considered a normal part of aging. Nurse clinicians should be sensitive to the reasons for underreporting of incontinence, its burden on affected individuals and their caregivers, and the likelihood that urinary incontinence is a symptom of an underlying problem. Once the underlying problem is identified and treated, most cases of incontinence can either be cured or significantly improved. Those patients who do not receive improvement can certainly be better managed.

Nurses can play a key role in the detection, evaluation, and management of urinary incontinence in the community, acute care hospital, and nursing home settings. They are ideally positioned to become experts in the behavioral management of incontinence, and this is often the only form of intervention needed. While much is still unknown about urinary incontinence, nurses have important contributions to make in improving the care of incontinent patients.

ACKNOWLEDGMENTS

This chapter was adapted from a paper prepared for the Priority Expert Panel for Long-Term Care for Older Adults, National Center for Nursing Research, National Institutes of Health, Bethesda, MD. The author gratefully acknowledges the contributions of Drs. Patricia Burns, Joyce Colling, Kathleen McCormick, and Thelma Wells in the development of the paper.

REFERENCES

Abrams, P., Blaivas, J. G., Stanton, S. L., & Jensen, J. T. (1988). The standardization of terminology of lower urinary tract function. *Scandinavian Journal of Urology and Nephrology, 114*(Suppl), 5–19.

Benvenuti, F., Caputo, G. M., Bandinelli, S., Mayer, F., Biagini, C., & Somma-villa, A. (1987). Re-educative treatment of female genuine stress incontinence. *American Journal of Physical Therapy, 66,* 155–168.

Brink, C. A. (1990). Absorbent pads, garments, and management strategies. *Journal of the American Geriatrics Society, 38,* 368–373.

Brink, C. A., Sampselle, C. M., Wells, T. J., Diokno, A. C., & Gillis, G. L. (1989). A digital test for pelvic muscle strength in older women with urinary incontinence. *Nursing Research, 38,* 196–199.

Brink, C. A., Wells, T. J., & Diokno, A. C. (1987). Urinary incontinence in women. *Public Health Nursing, 4,* 114–119.

Burns, P. A. (1988). Combined pelvic floor exercises and biofeedback. *Proceedings of the NIH Consensus Development Conference on Urinary Incontinence* (pp. 98–102), Bethesda, MD.

Cardozo, L., Abrams, P. D., Stanton, S. L., & Feneley, R. C. L. (1978). Idiopathic bladder instability treated by biofeedback. *British Journal of Urology, 50,* 27–30.

Cella, M. (1988). The nursing costs of urinary incontinence in a nursing home population. *Nursing Clinics of North America, 23,* 159–165.

Clay, E. (1978). Incontinence of urine: A regimen for retraining. *Nursing Mirror, 146,* 23–24.

Colling, J., Hadley, B. J., Ouslander, J. G., Campbell, E. B., & Eisch, J. S. (1989). An individualized behavioral approach to treat urinary incontinence among nursing home residents. *The Gerontologist, 29,* 281A.

Diokno, A. C., Brock, B. M., & Herzog, A. R. (1986). Prevalence of urinary incontinence and other urological symptoms in the noninstitutionalized elderly. *Journal of Urology, 136,* 1022–1025.

Dougherty, M. C., Abrams, R., & McKey, P. L. (1986). An instrument to assess the dynamic characteristics of the circumvaginal musculature. *Nursing Research, 35,* 202–206.

Eriksen, B., Bergmann, S., & Eik-Nes, S. (1989). Maximal electricostimulation of the pelvic floor in female idiopathic detrusor instability and urge incontinence. *Neurology and Urodynamics, 8,* 219–230.

Eriksen, B. C., & Eik-Nes, S. H. (1989). Long-term electrical stimulation of the pelvic floor: Primary therapy in female stress incontinence. *Urologia Internationalis, 44,* 90–95.

Fall, M. (1984). Does electrostimulation cure urinary incontinence? *Journal of Urology, 131,* 664–667.

Fantl, J. A., Harkins, S. W., Wyman, J. F., Choi, S. C., & Taylor, J. R. (1987). Fluid loss quantitation test in women with urinary incontinence: A test-retest analysis. *Obstetrics and Gynecology, 70,* 739–743.

Fantl, J. A., Hurt, W. G., & Dunn, L. J. (1981). Detrusor instability syndrome: The use of bladder retraining drills with and without anticholinergics. *American Journal of Obstetrics and Gynecology, 140,* 885–890.

Fantl, J. A., Wyman, J. F., Harkins, S. W., & Hadley, E. C. (1990). Bladder training in the management of lower urinary tract dysfunction in women. *Journal of the American Geriatrics Society, 38,* 329–332.

Fantl, J. A., Wyman, J. F., McClish, D. K., Harkins, S. W., Elswick, R. K., Taylor, J. R., & Hadley, E. C. (1991). Efficacy of bladder training in older women with urinary incontinence. *Journal of the American Medical Association, 265,* 609–613.

Herzog, A. R., & Fultz, N. H. (1990). Prevalence and incidence of urinary incontinence in the community-dwelling population. *Journal of the American Geriatrics Society, 38,* 273–281.

Herzog, A. G., Fultz, N. H., Normolle, D. P., Brock, B. M., & Diokno, A. C. (1989). Methods used to manage urinary incontinence by older adults in the community. *Journal of the American Geriatrics Society, 37,* 339–347.

Hilton, P. V., & Stanton, S. L. (1981). Algorithmic method for assessing urinary incontinence in elderly women. *British Medical Journal, 282,* 940–942.

Holst, K., & Wilson, P. D. (1988). The prevalence of female urinary incontinence and reasons for not seeking treatment. *New Zealand Medical Journal, 101,* 756–758.

Hu, T. (1990). Impact of urinary incontinence on health care costs. *Journal of the American Geriatrics Society, 38,* 292–295.

Hu, T. W., Igou, J. F., Kaltreider, D. L., Yu, L. C., Rohner, T. J., Dennis, P. J., Craighead, W. E., Hadley, E. C., & Ory, M. G. (1989). A clinical trial of a behavioral therapy to reduce urinary incontinence in nursing homes: Outcomes and implications. *Journal of the American Medical Association, 251,* 2656–2662.

Kegel, A. H. (1948). Progressive resistance exercise in the functional restoration of the perineal muscles. *American Journal of Obstetrics and Gynecology, 56,* 238–248.

King, M. R. (1980). Treatment of incontinence. *Nursing Mirror, 76,* 1006–1010.

Kromann-Anderson, B., Jakobsen, H., & Andersen, J. T. (1989). Pad-weighing test: A literature survey on test accuracy and reproducibility. *Neurourology and Urodynamics, 8,* 237–242.

Leach, G. E., & Bavendam, T. G. (1989). Prospective evaluation of the Incontan transrectal stimulator in women with urinary incontinence. *Neurourology and Urodynamics, 8,* 231–236.

Merrill, D. (1979). The treatment of detrusor instability by electrical stimulation. *Journal of Urology, 122,* 515–517.

Mitteness, L. S. (1987). The management of urinary incontinence by community-living elderly. *The Gerontologist, 27,* 185–193.

Mohide, A. (1986). The prevalence and scope of urinary incontinence. *Clinics in Geriatric Medicine, 2,* 639–656.

National Institutes of Health Consensus Development Conference Statement. (1988). *Urinary incontinence in adults.* Bethesda, MD: Office of Medical Applications of Research, National Institutes of Health.

Noelker, L. S. (1987). Incontinence in elderly cared for by family. *The Gerontologist, 27,* 194–200.

O'Donnell, P. D., Doyle, R., & Beck, C. (1988). Biofeedback therapy of urinary incontinence in older inpatient men. *Proceedings of the NIH Consensus Development Conference on Urinary Incontinence* (pp. 91–93). Bethesda, MD.

O'Donnell, P. D., Sutton, L., Beck, C., & Finkbeiner, A. E. (1987). Urinary incontinence detection in elderly inpatient men. *Neurourology and Urodynamics, 6,* 101–108.

Ouslander, J. G., Blaustein, J., Connor, A., & Pitt, A. (1988). Habit training and oxybutynin for incontinence in nursing home patients: A placebo-controlled trial. *Journal of the American Geriatrics Society, 36,* 40–46.

Ouslander, J. G., & Kane, R. (1984). The costs of urinary incontinence in nursing homes. *Medical Care, 22,* 69–79.

Ouslander, J., Leach, G., Staskin, D., Abelsen, S., Blaustein, J., Morishita, L., & Raz, S. (1989). Prospective evaluation of an assessment strategy for geriatric urinary incontinence. *Journal of the American Geriatrics Society, 37,* 715–724.

Ory, M. G., Wyman, J. F., & Yu, L. (1986). Psychosocial factors in urinary incontinence. *Clinics in Geriatric Medicine, 2,* 657–671.

Peattie, A. B., Plevnik, S., & Stanton, S. L. (1988). Vaginal cones: A conservative method of treating genuine stress incontinence. *British Journal of Obstetrics and Gynaecology, 95,* 1049–1053.

Perry, J. D., & Whipple, B. (1982). Vaginal myography. In B. Garber (Ed.), *Circumvaginal musculature and sexual function* (pp. 61–73). New York: S. Karger.

Rooney, V. (1982). A question of habit. *Nursing Mirror, 154,* 2–6.

Sanford, J. R. A. (1975). Tolerance of debility in elderly dependents by supporters at home: Its significance for hospital practice. *British Medical Journal, 3,* 471–473.

Schnelle, J. D. (1990). Treatment of urinary incontinence in nursing home patients by prompted voiding. *Journal of the American Geriatrics Society, 36,* 34–39.

Schnelle, J. F., Sowell, V. A., Hu, T., & Traughber, B. (1988). Reduction of urinary incontinence in nursing homes: Does it reduce or increase costs? *Journal of the American Geriatrics Society, 36,* 34–39.

Sogbein, S. K., & Awad, S. A. (1982). Behavioral treatment of urinary incontinence in geriatric patients. *Canadian Medical Journal, 127,* 863–864.

Sotiropoulos, A. (1975). Urinary incontinence management with electrical stimulation of the pelvic floor. *Urology, 6,* 312–315.

Sullivan, D. H., & Lindsay, R. W. (1984). Urinary incontinence in the geriatric population of an acute care hospital. *Journal of the American Geriatrics Society, 32,* 646–650.

Tchou, D. C. H., Adams, C., Varner, R. E., & Denton, B. (1988). Pelvic-floor musculature exercises in treatment of anatomical urinary stress incontinence. *Physiotherapy, 5,* 652–655.

Warren, J. W. (1986). Catheters and catheter care. *Clinics in Geriatric Medicine, 2,* 857–872.

Wells, T. J. (1990). Pelvic (floor) muscle exercise. *Journal of the American Geriatrics Society, 38,* 333–337.

Wells, T. J., Brink, C., Diokno, A. C., Wolfe, R., & Gillis, G. L. (1991). Pelvic muscle exercise for stress urinary incontinence in elderly women. *Journal of the American Geriatrics Society, 39,* 785–791.

Worth, A. M., Dougherty, M. C., McKey, P. L. (1986). Development and testing of the circumvaginal muscles rating scale. *Nursing Research, 35,* 166–168.

Wyman, J. F., Choi, S. C., Harkins, S. W., Wilson, M., & Fantl, J. A. (1988). The urinary diary in evaluation of incontinent women: A test-retest analysis. *Obstetrics and Gynecology, 71,* 812–817.

Wyman, J. F., Elswick, R. K., Wilson, M. S., & Fantl, J. A. (in press). Relationship of fluid intake to micturition frequency and urinary incontinence in women. *Neurourology and Urodynamics.*

Wyman, J. F., Harkins, S. W., & Fantl, J. A. (1990). Psychosocial impact of urinary incontinence in the community-dwelling population. *Journal of the American Geriatrics Society, 38,* 282–288.

Yu, L. (1987). Incontinence stress index: Measuring psychological impact. *Journal of Gerontological Nursing, 13*(7), 18–25.

Yu, L. C., & Kaltreider, D. L. (1987). Stressed nurses: Dealing with incontinent patients. *Journal of Gerontological Nursing, 13*, 27–30.

[16]

Urine Control by Elders: Noninvasive Strategies

Betty D. Pearson and Janice M. Larson

Age alone does not cause incontinence. Resnick (1990) concluded that many factors are involved in incontinence, and small improvements in multiple factors appear sufficient to restore continence.

To date, however, practicing nurses have had to rely on general measures of risk for incontinence because information gained from assessments was not appropriately linked to either diagnosis or treatment. Based on an extensive literature review, the authors adapted Brink's (1980) assessment method to evaluate 12 risk factors: inadequate liquid intake, inability to delay urination 10 minutes or more, no sensation of a full bladder, no sensation when urine flows, frequency of urination less than 5 times a day, frequency more than 8 times a day, nocturia more than once a night, dribbling a few drops of urine, inability to stop/restart urine flow, burning on urination, bowel constipation, and dry vagina. These risk factors were matched or linked with strategies that elderly, community-dwelling women could do to achieve normal continence (increases in liquid intake, regular toileting, pelvic floor muscle exercise, and dietary changes). Table 16.1 gives the linkages between criteria for normal continence, risk factors, and treatments.

TABLE 16.1 Linkage of Risk Factors: Criteria for Continence, Risk for In-continence, and Treatments

Criteria for continence	Risk for incontinence	Treatments
$\frac{1}{2}$ oz./lb. body weight liquid intake	$<\frac{1}{2}$ oz./lb. body weight liquid intake	Increase liquids
Able to wait 10 minutes or more after urge	Unable to wait 10 minutes after urge	Regular toileting
Recognition of fullness of bladder	No sense of full bladder	Pelvic floor muscle exercises
Recognition of when urination begins	No sense of when urination begins	Pelvic floor muscle exercises
Urination 5 to 8 times/day	Daytime frequency of urination < 5 or > 8	Regular toileting
Nocturia ≤ 1 time/night	Nocturia > 1 time/night	Regular toileting
No dribbling	Dribbling (a few drops, not noticeably wet clothing)	Pelvic floor muscle exercises
Able to stop/start urine flow	Inability to stop/start urine flow	Pelvic floor muscle exercises
No burning on urination	Burning on urination	Check liquid intake, proper perineal care, & urinalysis
No bowel constipation	Bowel constipation	Increase intake of liquids, bran, and prunes; establish post-meal defecation schedule
Moist vagina	Dry vagina	Vitamins B & E

The study reported here was designed to determine whether the 12 risk factors were associated with incontinence and what the effects of self-treatments were.

METHOD

Of 29 women who volunteered to be assessed for continence status, 5 women were classified as *continent* because they neither lost urine involuntarily more than once a month (Brocklehurst, 1986) nor experienced any of the risk factors. These 5 continent women were dropped from the study. Sixteen women were deemed *at-risk* for loss of continence because they experienced one or more of the 12 risk factors; 8

women were labeled *incontinent* because, regardless of whether or not they were experiencing any of the risk factors, they were losing urine involuntarily more than once a month.

These 24 women, whose average age was 67 years, completed six monthly assessment and instruction sessions. All the women were mobile and free of urinary catheters and environmental problems that confound urine control. No physician-prescribed regimens for incontinence were implemented during the 6 months of data collection. The 8 incontinent women took an average of 2.8 (SD = 2.3) prescription and an average of 1.6 (SD = 1.1) over-the-counter drugs. The 16 women determined at baseline to be at-risk took an average of 2.3 (SD = 1.7) prescription and an average of 1.8 (SD = 1.1) over-the-counter drugs. The incontinent women had an average of 4.7 (SD = 7.8) medical diagnoses and the at-risk women had an average of 4.4 (SD = 2.5). All the subjects understood their medications and managed these without assistance.

Instruments

At the baseline interview, the continence history was recorded in private for each subject. During this interview, and subsequently at monthly assessments, the women were asked about the 12 risk factors, and information was also gathered on demographics, mental status, environmental impediments to reaching the toilet, mobility, medical diagnoses, and current medication usage and management. A pilot test–retest of the data collection instrument using 6 elders resulted in 100% reliability (see Figure 16.1 for instrument).

Ability to follow directions was assessed during the Set Test, in which subjects are asked to name 10 cities, colors, fruits, and animals; scoring is 0–40. Isaacs and Akhter (1972) tested the validity and reliability of this instrument and found them satisfactory. A score of 25 or better was required for this study. All 24 women scored above 35.

Treatments

When risk factors were uncovered during the monthly assessments, treatment information was provided, both verbally and in writing—to ensure that the information was standard. Questions were answered and explanations provided. Instructions and explanations were at no more than an eighth grade level, regardless of the subject's educational level (Doak, Doak, & Root, 1985). All the women did their own treatments.

FIGURE 16.1. Continence history (condensed form).

Date: **Name:**   **Birthdate:**

               Address: **Telephone:**

Medical diagnosis(s):

Medications: Prescription and nonprescription

Ability to follow directions:

Environmental: Properly fitted requisite devices (walking, chair, toilet), suitable
    clothing (for finger dexterity, etc.), adequate lighting

Mobility: Ambulatory, walking aid, chair, bed

Remedial Risk-factors
1. Average 24 hour fluid intake: _____ounces

2. Once you are aware you need to urinate, how long can you wait?

3. Can you tell when your bladder is full?

4. Can you tell when your urine begins to come?

5. & 6. How often do you urinate during the day? & 7. During the night?

8. Do you ever dribble urine when you cough, sneeze, or change position?

9. Can you stop your urine and start it again once you have begun to urinate?

10. Do you ever have burning when you pass urine?

11. Do you have a problem with a decrease in the frequency of your bowel move-
    ments accompanied by difficulty in emptying your bowels?   How often?

12. (Females only). Are you experiencing a "dry" vagina, poor lubrication of the
    vagina?

Diagnostic: Do you ever lose your urine at times or places you do not want to?
    How often? (once per month?, once per day?, etc.)

Other
1. Do you do anything that makes it easier for you to control your urine?
    Your bowels?

2. Is there anything that makes it harder for you to control your urine?
    Your bowels?

Each woman was taught noninvasive strategies appropriate for the
risk factors she experienced and was instructed to continue these treatments for the entire study.

Women drinking less than ½ ounce of liquid per pound of body
weight were instructed to gradually increase daily liquid intake by 4
ounces every 7 days until they reached this amount (Weisburg, 1962).

Adequacy of liquid intake was reassessed, however, if the person reported multiple trips to the toilet at night, burning on urination, or bowel constipation.

Regular toileting was taught as either extending or shortening the time period between bladder emptyings. Both those urinating more than 8 times in 24 hours and less than 5 times in 24 hours learned to set regularly scheduled times to urinate. Women unable to wait 10 minutes after perceiving an urge to urinate were instructed to urinate about every 2 to 3 hours while awake.

Pelvic floor muscle exercises were taught to women experiencing inability to stop and restart the flow of urine, dribbling, inability to sense when urine flowed, and dry vagina. Hand positions rather than anatomic models and diagrams were used for instruction. A cupped left hand representing the bladder and the right index finger depicting the urethra (outlet tube) were used to demonstrate the proper position for prevention of urine loss. This position requires that the urethra be "kinked onto itself," thus allowing the pelvic floor muscles to hold the bladder up; when the muscles are relaxed, the urethra is straightened, and urine flows freely.

Pelvic floor muscle exercises were taught using the principle that opposing muscles need to be recognized and relaxed. Each woman first learned to insert her own moistened finger into her vagina and tighten the abdominal muscles, feeling the vaginal changes. (Men learn to do these using the rectum.) Next, the woman relaxed her abdominal muscles and then tightened the pelvic floor muscles as if trying to stop diarrhea, noting the difference she felt with her finger. This checking procedure was adapted from the process developed and validated for clinicians by researchers (Sampselle, Brink, & Wells, 1989).

During the second monthly visit, most women reported that they had successfully recognized the correct muscles, were doing the exercises the recommended 60 times daily, and were tightening these muscles before and during lifting, rising from a bed or a chair, climbing stairs, and when possible, before sneezing and coughing. Once a week these women did a vaginal check to ensure that they were exercising the correct muscles.

Two dietary treatments were taught. Women experiencing dry vagina purchased vitamin B complex and vitamin E 400 units, with no ingredient exceeding 100% of recommended daily requirements (Cutick, 1984; London et al., 1984; McLaren, 1949). These women also learned pelvic floor muscle exercises, since these increase vaginal moistness.

Constipation was defined as a decrease in usual frequency of bowel movements accompanied by difficult passage of feces (Derezin, 1987). A diagram portraying various types of stools was used by each woman to indicate her usual and current stool type (see Figure 16.2) (Walike-Hansen, 1978). Constipation was treated by having the women eat a serving of bran cereal or two slices of bran bread, and eat three or four prunes or drink 4 ounces of prune juice daily. These women also established a post-meal defecation schedule (Iseminger & Hardy, 1982). The women were encouraged to maintain an adequate level of liquid intake (see Tables 16.2–16.7 for the various treatment instructions).

FIGURE 16.2.   Stool descriptions.

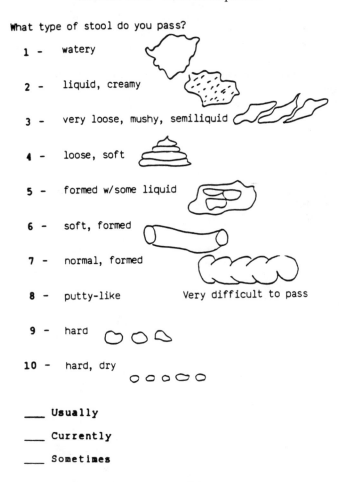

What type of stool do you pass?

1 - watery

2 - liquid, creamy

3 - very loose, mushy, semiliquid

4 - loose, soft

5 - formed w/some liquid

6 - soft, formed

7 - normal, formed

8 - putty-like   Very difficult to pass

9 - hard

10 - hard, dry

____ Usually

____ Currently

____ Sometimes

Note: Adapted from B. Walike Hansen (1978), Stool consistency diagrams. Developed for the tube feeding project, University of Washington, Seattle, WA, and the University of Michigan, Ann Arbor, MI. Used with permission.

TABLE 16.2   Instructions for Increase of Liquid Intake

---

1.   Drink a minimum of $\frac{1}{2}$ ounce of liquid for each pound of body weight each day (24 hours). Your requirement is _____ ounces.
2.   Drink a glass of water, a cup of some juice or other liquid of your choice about every 2 hours.
3.   If you are not drinking this much, increase the amount you drink gradually. Drink an additional $\frac{1}{2}$ cup, about 4 ounces a day, then in 4 days increase another 4 ounces for 4 days and so on until you reach your required amount.
4.   One easy method to keep track of the amount you are drinking each day is to place two containers of the amount of liquid you require in your refrigerator in the morning. These should be empty at bedtime. Another method is to mark down on a pad of paper each time you drink something.

You should gradually increase to the amount you require and continue to drink that amount.
This is a typical day and amount of liquid taken:

Rising	7 ounces or more of water (1 glass)
Breakfast	7 ounces or more of coffee (1 cup)
	4 ounces water ($\frac{1}{2}$ glass)
	4 ounces juice
	4 ounces milk
10:00 A.M.	7 ounces water or juice or other beverage
Noon meal	7 ounces water
	7 ounces beverage
	4 ounces milk
	$3\frac{1}{2}$ ounces soup
3:00 P.M.	7 ounces beverage
Evening Meal	7 ounces beverage
	4 ounces water
Bed Time	$3\frac{1}{2}$ ounces water

In addition, you may take on your own any of these items:

extra juice = 4 ounces	martini = $3\frac{1}{2}$ ounces
can of beverage = 12 ounces ($1\frac{1}{2}$ cups)	ice cream = $3\frac{1}{2}$ ounces
jello = $3\frac{1}{2}$ ounces	wine = $3\frac{1}{2}$ ounces
broth = $3\frac{1}{2}$ ounces	sherbet = $3\frac{1}{2}$ ounces
beer = 7 ounces	and others.

RESULTS

Eight of the 24 women in the study were classified as incontinent at baseline, and 16 at-risk. All 24 women could sense their full bladder and all but 1 could sense when urine began flowing; 4 experienced burning when urinating.

TABLE 16.3 Regular Toileting: Instructions for Persons Emptying Their Bladders Less than 5 Times a Day

---

Emptying your bladder regularly, 5 to 8 times a day, increases your control of urine and decreases the likelihood you will urinate involuntarily. To do so, you must have drunk adequate amounts of liquids ($\frac{1}{2}$ ounce of liquid per pound of body weight).

1. Empty your bladder immediately on arising from bed.
2. Empty your bladder before each meal.
3. Empty your bladder immediately before retiring to bed.
4. Empty your bladder one time each night, if necessary.

Each time you do so, celebrate the fact that you have control of your urine. Drink $\frac{1}{2}$ cup of water each time you go to the bathroom at night.

5. Urinate at least every 2–3 hours during the day.

Example	6:00 A.M.	1:00 P.M.
	7:00 A.M.	4.00 P.M.
	9:00 A.M.	7:00 P.M.
	11:00 A.M.	9:00 P.M. (bedtime)

TABLE 16.4 Regular Toileting: Instructions for Persons Emptying Their Bladders More Than 8 Times a Day

---

Emptying your bladder more than 8 times a day increases your chances of losing control of urine. To urinate only 8 times a day, you must have drunk adequate amounts of liquids ($\frac{1}{2}$ ounce per pound of body weight).

1. Empty your bladder immediately on arising from bed.
2. Empty your bladder after each meal.
3. Follow the instructions for pelvic floor muscle exercises. Do these a total of 60 times a day.
4. Instead of rushing to the toilet in response to need to empty your bladder, pause, sit or stand quietly, relax your abdominal muscles, tighten your pelvic floor muscles; then walk at a normal pace to the toilet.
5. During the day, try to extend the length of time between emptying your bladder. You will probably find you can increase the length of time gradually.
6. Your goal is to empty your bladder ONLY every 2 to 3 hours during the day.

Do not be discouraged; changes take time. It may take you several months to achieve a frequency of only every 2 to 3 hours.

TABLE 16.5 Instructions for Pelvic Floor Muscle Exercises

Recognizing the Correct Muscles

Before you begin exercising the muscles supporting the abdominal contents from below (called the floor of the pelvis or pelvic floor), you must be certain that you are exercising the correct muscles. The following instructions labeled A, B, and C will teach you to recognize the correct muscles. You will want to lie on your back while you learn to identify the correct muscles.

A. Lubricate one finger (water works well) and place it in your vagina or your rectum. Now tighten your abdominal muscles and notice how this changes what you are feeling. THIS IS NOT WHAT YOU WILL FEEL WHEN TIGHTENING THE CORRECT MUSCLES.
B. Now with your abdominal muscles relaxed and while you are blowing air through your mouth, pull in around your lubricated finger as if you were trying to stop a bowel movement. THESE ARE THE MUSCLES YOU DO WANT TO TIGHTEN. Do not tighten your leg muscles.
C. Next time you need to urinate, sit on the toilet with your knees spread apart. Start to urinate, then stop; then start, then stop; then finish. When your muscles are strengthened, this can be done easily.

Pelvic Floor Muscle Exercises

Do these exercises THREE TIMES A DAY, one set while sitting, standing, and lying down. You may do these anytime—any place that is convenient for you.

1. Tighten your pelvic floor muscles; hold for 1 second; relax for 1 second; repeat about 10 times. Next, tighten your pelvic floor muscles; hold for about 10 seconds; relax for about 10 seconds; and repeat about 10 times. (You should tighten these muscles about 60 times a day.)
2. While practicing and using this exercise, make certain that you are keeping your abdominal muscles relaxed. If you also tighten the abdominal muscles, you will put pressure on the urinary bladder and it may empty. It is easier to keep the abdominal muscles relaxed if you breathe out while tightening the pelvic floor muscles. As you tighten your pelvic floor muscles, think about moving these muscles up an elevator, one floor at a time.
3. You should tighten these muscles:
    a. immediately upon getting the urge to urinate, and before moving any other muscles in your body, walking, or changing your position;
    b. before you start to get up from a chair;
    c. before you move to get out of bed;
    d. before and during lifting heavy objects.

DO NOT expect immediate results. Some women and men have done the exercises as directed for 2 to 6 months before they could laugh, cough, sneeze, or lift without leaking urine.

TABLE 16.6 Instructions for Prevention of Constipation

1. Drink a minimum of $\frac{1}{2}$ an ounce of liquid per pound of body weight each day (24 hours).
2. Once a day eat 3 or 4 dried prunes, or drink 4 ounces of prune juice.
3. Eat a serving of bran cereal each day, or eat 2 slices of bran bread (you may toast it if you prefer).
4. Set a regular time each day to have a bowel movement.
5. Do some type of physical exercise for at least 20 minutes. Walk if you can; if not, try tightening and relaxing your abdominal muscles 25 times after you go to bed.

TABLE 16.7 Guidelines for Purchasing and Taking Vitamin B complex and Vitamin E

NOT RECOMMENDED IF YOU HAVE ENDOMETRIOSIS OR ARE TAKING ESTROGEN.

1. Read the label of vitamin B complex available at your usual drugstore, or show these guidelines to your pharmacist.
2. Purchase vitamin B complex whose label lists B1, B2, and so forth, or thiamine, riboflavin, niacin, and so forth, as no more than 100% of daily requirements. Vitamins are effective regardless of whether they are labeled natural or not. Take one each day after breakfast. Note that you may find your urine bright yellow the next time you pass urine. This is okay; it is not harmful.
3. Purchase vitamin E that is labeled 400 IU or 400 units. Take one tablet each day after breakfast. If you have diabetes, request aqua vitamin E from your pharmacist. (It is made by Armour and available from Nature Made or Valu-Rite.)
4. If you forget to take your vitamins after breakfast, they may be taken after lunch. DO NOT take 2 of each if you have missed a day.

DO NOT expect immediate results. Some women need several months before these vitamins are helpful.

Seven of the 8 women who were incontinent at baseline improved to at-risk status at 6 months. Five women were drinking less than the recommended amount of liquids at baseline, and 3 continued low liquid intakes at 6 months. At baseline, 6 women could not wait 10 minutes after the urge to urinate, but 1 of them could do so by the 6-month mark. Three women had a daytime frequency of urination of more than 8 times; 1 continued this and 1 developed this risk. Two of the women initially experienced a daytime frequency less than 5 times but no longer had this risk at 6 months. Four women experienced nocturia more than once a night at baseline, and 1 continued to do so after 6 months. Four women who were incontinent at baseline dribbled a few drops of urine in addition to losing large amounts several times a week; but by the sixth month, these 4 women no longer dribbled urine, though another woman had begun to dribble. Two women were unable at baseline to stop and restart urine flow but could do so before 6 months. Another woman was constipated at baseline but this ceased by 6 months. Five women experienced dry vagina at baseline, but only 1 continued this after 6 months. Figure 16.3 gives a visual representation of these changes, shown as a percentage of those who were incontinent.

A case example may make the changes clearer. Anna (not her real name), who was incontinent at the beginning of the study, experienced 6 risk factors at baseline; by the sixth month she had moved to at-risk status and experienced only 2 risk factors. At baseline, Anna consumed only 40% of the recommended daily liquids and experienced a burning

FIGURE 16.3.   Percentage of 8 incontinent women who experienced a risk at baseline and at Month 6.

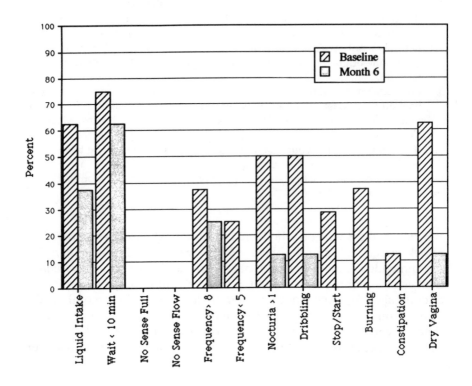

sensation upon urination. She increased her liquid intake to nearly 80% of the recommended amount and was able to eliminate the burning sensation without other treatment. At baseline, Anna was unable to wait longer than 7 minutes after urge to urinate; this urgency persisted despite the fact that she increased her toileting from 5 times a day to 6 or 7 irregularly spaced times each day. Anna also dribbled urine at baseline, in addition to involuntarily losing large amounts several times a week; but she stopped both of these before the sixth month. She was unable at baseline to stop and restart urine flow but could do so at 6 months; she also had a dry vagina at baseline, which became moist by Month 3. Anna learned to perform pelvic floor muscle exercises correctly and also took vitamin B complex and vitamin E 400 units daily. She moved to at-risk status because she no longer lost urine involuntarily though she continued to experience 2 risk factors (inability to wait 10 minutes or more and inadequate liquid intake).

The total number of risk factors for the women who were incontinent at baseline ranged from 3 to 6 (average = 4.88, SD = 1.64); 6 months later they ranged from 2 to 3 (average = 2.13, SD = .99). This decrease in the number of risk factors experienced was significant [$t(7) = 3.67, p = .008$]. The one woman who remained incontinent at 6 months had improved on 3 of 5 risk factors. Another woman who was incontinent at baseline improved on 1 risk factor but developed a new risk factor; all others reduced the number of their risk factors.

At 6 months, 10 of the 16 women who were classified as at-risk at baseline remained at risk, 4 had become risk free, and 2 had become incontinent. Of the 5 at-risk women drinking inadequate liquids, 4 were drinking adequate amounts before Month 6. Another woman, however, had ceased to drink adequate liquids by Month 5. Of the 6 women unable at baseline to wait a minimum of 10 minutes to urinate, 3 improved but another developed this problem. The 1 woman unable at baseline to sense when urine began flowing continued to be unable to do so. Of the 4 women urinating more than 8 times a day at baseline, 3 ceased to do so, but 2 others developed this risk factor. Of the 4 urinating fewer than 5 times daily, 3 met continence criteria before Month 6; of the 5 women urinating more than once a night, 2 no longer did so, but 2 others developed this risk. Of the 5 women who at baseline experienced dribbling, 3 had ceased to do so by Month 6 but 2 others developed this risk. Of the 5 women unable to stop then restart urine flow, all 5 became able to do so by the sixth month; the 1 woman experiencing burning on urination ceased to experience burning. Finally, of the 6 women who were constipated at baseline, 5 no longer were by Month 6; and of the 7 women experiencing dry vagina, 4 had moist vaginas by Month 6. Figure 16.4 gives a visual representation of these findings (shown in percentages).

FIGURE 16.4.   Percentage of 16 at-risk women who experienced a risk at
baseline and at Month 6.

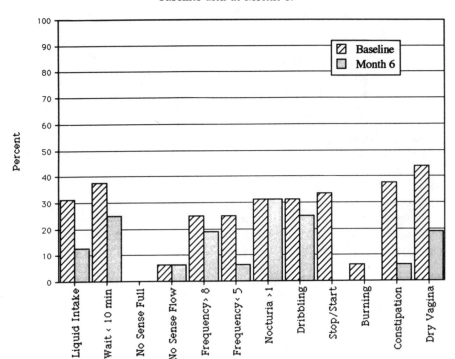

The total number of risk factors at baseline for the at-risk women ranged from 1 to 7 (average = 3.31, SD = 1.62), and, 6 months later, from 0 to 5 (average = 1.88, SD = 1.46). The difference between these averages was significant [$t(15)$ = 1.07, p= .003]. The woman who had most risk factors at both times (7 and 5, respectively) had become incontinent, but another woman had moved from 6 risk factors to none. A second woman who became incontinent experienced 2 risk factors at both times, but not the same 2. Six women developed 1 or 2 new risk factors during the 6 months, but no one increased the total number of risk factors.

The women who were incontinent at baseline experienced a significantly greater number of risk factors at baseline than did the at-risk women [$t(22)$ = 2.22, p = .04], but the difference between the groups in the number of risk factors was not significant at Month 6 [$t(22)$ = .44, p = .67].

The major risk factor changes among the 24 women were a new ability to stop and restart urine flow (7 of 7 or 100% of those with the problem showed improvement) and disappearance of burning on urination (4 of 4 or 100%). Urinating too frequently or infrequently was no longer experienced by 6 of 13 women (a 46% reduction). Constipation was no longer experienced by 6 of 7 women (an 86% reduction), and dry vagina was no longer experienced by 8 of 12 women (a 67% reduction).

DISCUSSION

Nurses in any clinical setting, including long-term care facilities, could use these assessment and treatment strategies to provide positive information to elders about what they can do to care for themselves. When elders are actively involved in their own assessment and treatment, their integrity and functioning are also enhanced. The women in this study reported that they felt more competent and less burdened as a result of the treatments.

The risk factors used here are associated with the state of incontinence. None of the incontinent women were free of risk factors. This is an important confirmation because to be classified as incontinent, women in this study needed only to lose urine involuntarily more than once a month—they did not have to experience any of the risk factors. At baseline, however, each of the incontinent women experienced from 3 to 6 risk factors. It is noteworthy that 7 incontinent women moved from incontinent to at-risk status before the end of the study. Four of the at-risk women became risk free by Month 6. However, two women who were at risk at baseline became incontinent. It should also be noted that some women did develop new risk factors during the 6-month period.

Decidedly longer studies are needed before reaching firm conclusions about prevention of urinary incontinence. The treatment strategies used here are not harmful, however, and thus, as Resnick (1990) suggests, it is possible to offer women recommendations and hope. These strategies cannot work unless used, however. Clearly, nursing practice needs to shift to prevention and treatment using low-cost self-managed or assisted noninvasive strategies. An ounce of prevention continues to be worth a pound of cure.

REFERENCES

Brink, C. (1980). Assessing the problem. *Geriatric Nursing, 1*, 241–247, 275.
Brocklehurst, J. C. (1986). The aging bladder. *British Journal of Hospital Medicine, 35*, 8–10.

Cutick, R. (1984). Special needs of perimenopausal women and menopausal women. *Journal of Obstetric, Gynecologic, and Neonatal Nursing, 13*(2) (suppl.), 68s–73s.

Derezin, M. (1987). Laxatives and fecal modifiers. *American Family Physician, 10,* 126–128.

Doak, D. G., Doak, L. G., & Root, J. H. (1985). *Teaching patients with low literacy skills.* New York: Lippincott.

Iseminger, M., & Hardy, P. (1982). Bran works! *Geriatric Nursing, 2,* 402–404.

Isaacs, B., & Akhtar, A. J. (1972). The set test: A rapid test of mental function in old people. *Age and Ageing, 1,* 222.

London, R. S., Sundaram, G., Manimekalai, S., Murphy, L., Reynolds, M., & Goldstein, P. (1984). Effect of alpha-tocopherol on premenstrual symptomatology: A double blind study. II. Endocrine correlates. *Journal of the American College of Nutrition, 3,* 351–356.

McLaren, H. C. (1949). Vitamin E in the menopause. *British Medical Journal, 1,* 1378–1382.

Resnick, N. M. (1990). Initial evaluation of the incontinent patient. *Journal of the American Geriatrics Society, 38,* 311–316.

Sampselle, C. M., Brink, C. A., & Wells, T. J. (1989). Digital measurement of pelvic muscle strength in childbearing women. *Nursing Research, 38,* 134–138.

Walike-Hansen, B. (1978). Stool-consistency diagrams. In J. Horsley, J. Crane, & K. Haller, *Reducing diarrhea in tube-fed patients: CURN project* (p. 23) (1981). New York: Grune & Stratton.

Weisburg, H. F. (1962). Daily water treatment requirements. In H. F. Weisburg, (Ed.) *Water, electrolyte, and acid-base balance* (2nd ed.) (pp. 63–64). Baltimore, MD: Williams & Wilkins.

[17]

Patterned Urge Response Toileting for Urinary Incontinence: A Clinical Trial

Joyce Colling, Betty Jo Hadley, Joan Eisch,
Emily Campbell, and Joseph G. Ouslander

Behavioral techniques for treating urinary incontinence (UI) involve analysis and alteration of the relationship between the person's symptoms and the maladaptive voiding behavior. These techniques include bladder retraining, habit training, prompted voiding, vaginal cones, electrical stimulation, and pelvic muscle exercises using a variety of techniques including biofeedback. Behavioral interventions are designed somewhat differently for people who are not capable of independent toileting because of physical and/or cognitive impairment, but most behavioral interventions include three primary components: an educational program, scheduled voiding, and positive reinforcement for successful toileting. Prompted voiding and habit training are most often used among debilitated nursing home residents.

Scattered reports of small-scale behavioral intervention studies in nursing homes have appeared in the literature since the mid 1960s (Azrin & Foxx, 1971; Clay, 1980; Collins & Plaska, 1975; Grosicki, 1968; Pollock & Liberman, 1974; Spiro, 1978; Wagner & Paul, 1970). Large-scale clinical trials, however, have been conducted only in recent years (Creason et al. 1989; Engel et al., 1990; Hu et al., 1989; Schnelle et al., 1989). These trials used a 1–3 hour fixed time interval for toileting residents in conjunction with a variety of more subtle behavioral techniques. In contrast, the study reported here individualized the toileting times for residents. Furthermore, the other studies used specially trained research staff to carry out the interventions only during subjects' usual waking hours, while the toileting program in this study was carried out on a 24-hour basis by regular nursing home staff.

The study tested the effects of a noninvasive behavioral treatment called *Patterned Urge Response Toileting* (PURT)[1] on urge/functional urinary incontinence among nursing home residents. Specifically, the study tested the effect of PURT on the:

1. frequency of urinary incontinent episodes and associated volume of urine among incontinent nursing home patients;
2. incidence of complications, e.g., skin irritations and urinary tract infections, among incontinent nursing home patients;
3. psychosocial well-being of incontinent nursing home patients;
4. behavioral capabilities of incontinent nursing home patients;
5. knowledge about urinary incontinence and attitudes of nursing personnel toward caring for incontinent patients; and
6. facility costs for incontinence care.

METHOD

The study used a quasi-experimental design and consisted of a 12-week baseline period, 12 weeks of intervention, and a 12-week post-intervention period. Four nursing homes that had been part of the Robert Wood Johnson Teaching Nursing Home Program participated in the study. These institutions varied in size from 120 to 340 beds and differed in organizational structure, but all were nonprofit facilities. They were located in the West, Midwest, and East Coast. A total of 12 units from these four nursing homes participated in the study. From each nursing home, one or two units were selected to receive the experimental intervention and one or two units (which were as removed from the first units as possible) were selected as control units.

Subjects

Entry into the study occurred in three phases, as shown in Figure 17.1. Of the 763 residents in the units selected for study from the four nursing homes, 218 met the initial eligibility criteria for the study (see Table

[1]We have chosen this acronym to reflect our method of determining and implementing an individualized toileting regimen and to clearly distinguish this method from others reported in the literature.

FIGURE 17.1.   Selection of subjects.

Entry into the study is divided into 3 parts: Initial Screening, Clinical Assessment of Subjects, and Final Exclusion and Inclusion of Subjects. The flow of subjects into the study is shown in the diagram below.

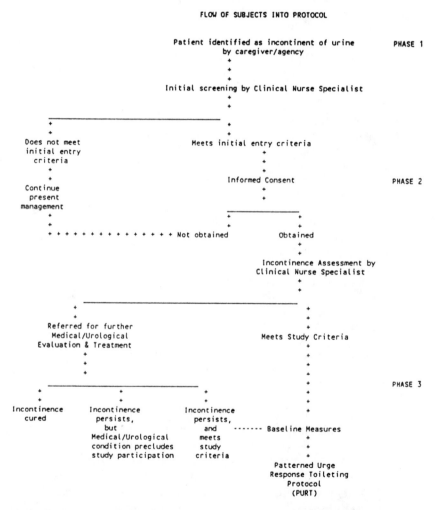

17.1). Consent was obtained from 154 subjects, or 71% of those eligible for the study. Next, a series of assessments was performed by clinical nurse specialists to eliminate residents who were not suitable for the study, such as those who had other medical problems or conditions that required further evaluation.

TABLE 17.1 Initial Entry Criteria and Secondary Exclusion Criteria for Participation in the Study

---

Initial Entry Criteria

    age 65 or older

    incontinent of urine—3 or more episodes of involuntary loss of urine per week for the last two weeks

    no indwelling catheter

    answers correctly either name or place

    toilets without assistance or with assistance of one person

    capable and willing to sign informed consent or has responsible party available to do so for him or her

    approved for entry into the study by the physician

Secondary Exclusion Criteria

    fecal impaction (treat and reexamine for inclusion)

    rectal or pelvic mass

    markedly enlarged prostate and/or prostatic nodule

    severe cystourethrocele/uterine prolapse

    severe atrophic vaginitis (friable, bleeding mucosa)

    new or known duration focal neurologic finding in lumbosacral area

    post-void residual greater than 200 ml

    urinary tract infection—greater than 10 ml colony forming units (treat and reexamine for inclusion)

    hematuria

    uncooperative with diagnostic evaluation

    UI cured by identification and treatment of reversible medical cause (i.e., drug modification)

    genitourinary pathology requiring surgery (i.e., stone, urethral stricture)

    genuine stress incontinence

    voiding frequency—an average of less than 2 hours

The assessments included (1) a detailed medical record review; (2) an assessment of mental, functional, and behavioral status; (3) a focused physical examination; (4) a urinalysis and urine culture and sensitivity; and (5) a simplified urodynamic evaluation. Mental function was assessed using the 10-point Short Portable Mental Status Questionnaire (SPMSQ) (Pfeiffer, 1975). Activities of daily living were assessed using the Katz ADL index (Katz, Ford, Moskowitz, Jackson, & Jaffe, 1963). Behavioral status was assessed using the Hadley, Wood, McCracken (HWM) Behavioral Capabilities Rating Scale for Older Adults (Hadley, Wood, McCracken, & Warshaw, 1988), which was also used as an outcome measure in the study. The physical included a screening neurologic examination as well as pelvic and rectal examinations.

All subjects who had growth of 10^5 or greater of a urinary pathogen from a urine culture were treated with an appropriate antimicrobial, and the bacteriuria was eradicated before the simplified urodynamic evaluation and baseline data collection. The simplified urodynamic evaluation included a post-void residual determination, a stress test (forceful coughing) to detect stress incontinence, and simple cystometry to determine bladder capacity and the presence or absence of involuntary bladder contractions. Procedures for these tests have been described in detail elsewhere (Kane, Ouslander, & Abrass, 1989). The conditions and problems used as secondary exclusion criteria are shown in Table 17.1.

From these assessments an additional 41 people were excluded, which left 113 who entered the study. Eighty-eight of the 113 subjects completed the 9-month study, 51 in the experimental group and 37 in the control group. Of the 25 subjects who did not complete the study, 20 left because of acute illness or death, 2 withdrew consent, and 3 were discharged.

Treatment

The scheduled toileting program was a refinement of habit training. Rather than impose a fixed toileting schedule on patients, an ambulatory electronic monitoring device was used to obtain the exact timing of voiding occurrences for three consecutive 24-hour days for each experimental subject. The voiding pattern of each subject was then precisely identified and translated into an individualized toileting prescription that reinforced the natural voiding pattern of the subject.

The data logger we used in the study to obtain the voiding information weighs about 10 ounces and was connected to a 1-cm temperature-sensitive probe. The small cord attached to the probe was inserted into the subject's absorbent pad or brief so that the temperature sensor was in the most optimal position when the subject voided. Urine is at core body temperature when expelled, which is higher than ambient temperature. The changes in temperature were recorded and stored in the monitor, which recorded the temperature every minute according to real clock time. Data were then printed out in graph form as seen in Figure 17.2. The large spikes of the line show rapid temperature changes and indicate voiding times.

The incontinent times, along with continent voiding times, were plotted on a graph and examined for patterns. A pattern was defined as three or more voids within a similar 1-hour block of time over the 3 days of monitoring. The sample graphs in Figure 17.3 show the distribution of voiding patterns of two subjects.

FIGURE 17.2. Sample of electronic monitor data depicting incontinent episodes. Key: A = incontinent voiding events (note sharp temperature peak and gradual decline); B = monitor off for morning bath; C = monitor off to change wet briefs/bedding.

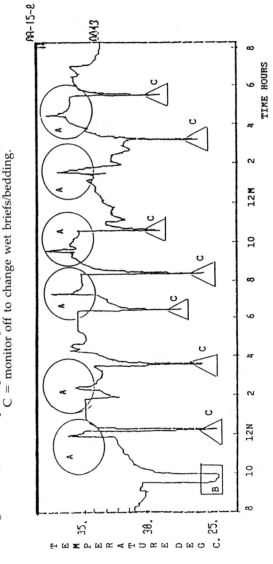

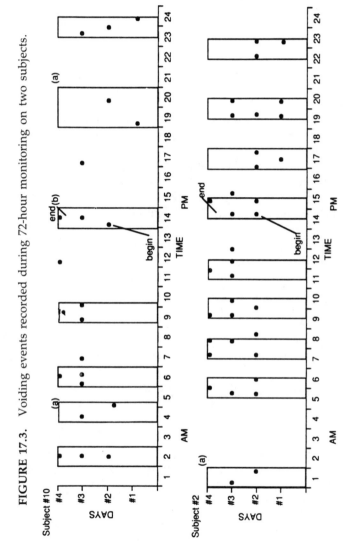

FIGURE 17.3. Voiding events recorded during 72-hour monitoring on two subjects.

Note: (a) Probable pattern. (b) Beginning of monitoring period = 1 P.M. on Day 1; end of monitoring period = 1 P.M. on Day 4.

175

The PURT prescription was then written, directing nursing staff to toilet the resident within 30 minutes of the mean time of the three voids that occurred within any given hour. As would be expected, patterns were different for different subjects , and subjects also differed in the frequency of toileting during a 24-hour period. For instance, 7 probable voiding times were identified for subject 10 (see Figure 17.3). Staff were instructed to toilet this resident as follows: 1:30–2:00 A.M.; 3:40–4:10 A.M.; 5:20–5:50 A.M.; 8:35–9:05 A.M.; 1:20–1:50 P.M.; 7:30–8:00 P.M.; 11:00–11:30 P.M.

An educational program on urinary incontinence (UI) and PURT was developed for the nursing aide staff because almost all of the subjects were either partially or totally dependent on staff to assist them with toileting. The educational program, which was pretested and then videotaped, was given only to staff on the experimental units. It included causes and consequences of UI, and detailed instructions on how to implement the PURT program. Pre- and posttests were given to determine staff's level of knowledge of UI and the PURT program and to assess their attitudes toward caring for incontinent residents. Each staff member who provided care for a resident in the PURT study was given a Daily PURT Prescription Record on which the times for toileting that resident were highlighted. Staff members were also given a written instruction sheet, shown in Table 17.2, that provided step-by-step guidelines for administering PURT.

The program included positive reinforcement to both staff and residents. Reinforcement was constantly provided to the nursing home staff by project staff, who were present on all shifts and on all days of the week to coach, provide corrective feedback, and reinforce correct staff behavior, especially during the first 3 weeks of the program. Positive feedback was also provided to staff on a weekly basis by graphing the

TABLE 17.2 Instructions for Toileting Residents in PURT Program

---

1. At times shown on your toileting sheet, approach resident. State: "Mr./ Mrs., it is time to go to the bathroom/use the commode."
2. Assist resident to toilet even if found wet.
3. Provide privacy for resident, allow 15 min. for toileting.
4. If resident voided correctly, state: "Good, Mr./Mrs., you were able to use the toilet." Or make some other positive comment.
5. Engage briefly in social conversation while making resident comfortable.
6. If resident DID NOT VOID CORRECTLY, remove from toilet after 15 min. DO NOT COMMENT NEGATIVELY OR POSITIVELY OR ENGAGE IN SOCIAL CONVERSATION. Make resident comfortable and leave resident's room.

---

change in continence status of each PURT subject and comparing baseline with current status and with other weeks in the program (see Figure 17.4). These graphs were posted at the nursing station with positive comments from the project staff. Positive reinforcement was also given to PURT subjects, who received praise and attention from nursing staff when they voided at their expected times.

Data Collection

Eight instruments were used to collect data. Urinary incontinence frequency and volume data were collected for one 24-hour period every 3 weeks using the Incontinence Monitoring Record developed by Ouslander (Ouslander, Urman, & Urman, 1986). Urinary tract status was evaluated every 3 weeks using the dipstick and Bacturcult methods to determine the presence or absence of bacteriuria. The color and integrity of the skin were evaluated every 3 weeks using the Oregon Health Sciences University Skin Evaluation Tool. For subjects who were cognitively intact, the Profile of Mood States instrument (McNair, Lorr, & Droppleman, 1971) was administered to collect data on their mood and well-being at 6-week intervals. For all subjects, the Hadley, Wood, McCracken Behavioral Capabilities Rating Scale, based on Dorothy Johnson's model of behavioral systems (Johnson, 1980), was used to determine changes in behavioral capabilities resulting from the intervention. These data were collected every 6 weeks throughout the study. Nursing staff's attitudes toward UI and their knowledge of UI were assessed before the educational program on UI management, after the educational program, at the conclusion of the intervention period, and at the end of the study. Finally, the institutional UI and toileting costs of labor, supplies, and linen were evaluated at baseline, at the end of the intervention period, and again at the conclusion of the study, using direct observation of toileting and changing of subjects who were incontinent.

RESULTS

As seen in Table 17.3, subjects' average age was 85, and both the experimental and control groups were predominantly female, white, and widowed, with high school diplomas. In most cases, they had been admitted to the nursing home from a hospital, and they had resided in the nursing home an average of more than 2 years. The majority of this sample were moderately to severely cognitively impaired, and they were also functionally impaired. Almost three quarters (72%) of the subjects had leakage after requesting to void, 53% leaked large volumes

FIGURE 17.4. An example of a graph comparing a PURT subject's baseline continence status with current status and with other weeks in the program.

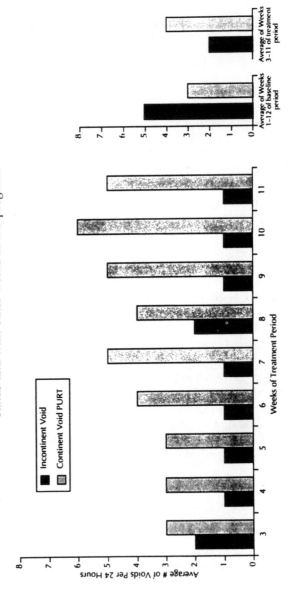

TABLE 17.3 Characteristics of Subjects Who Completed the Study

Characteristic	Experimental group (n = 51)		Control group (n = 37)	
	%	mean ± SD	%	mean ± SD
Age		84.5 ± 6.7		85.4 ± 5.9
Number of months in facility		24.1 ± 21.9		41.2 ± 30.5
Sex				
female	74		92	
male	26		8	
Ethnicity				
white	94		95	
black	6		5	
Admitted from				
own home	23		22	
relative's home	8		5	
hospital	39		27	
other nursing home	24		16	
unknown	6		30	
Functional status[a]		2.6 ± .6		2.6 ± .7
Dependent in:				
bathing	84		78	
dressing	92		81	
toileting	65		62	
transfer	51		39	
feeding	16		24	
Mental status[b]		7.1 ± 2.9		6.5 ± 2.9
Urodynamic status				
residual volume (cc's)		89 ± 87		86 ± 94
volume at strong urge to void (cc's)		243 ± 129		235 ± 133
Incontinence type[c]				
urge	75		70	
mixed stress/urge	25		30	

[a]Katz: 1 = independent; 2 = needs assistance; 3 = dependent
[b]SPMSQ: 0 = high; 10 = low
[c]Determined by clinical history and simple urodynamic evaluation. All subjects had functional disabilities that could also contribute to UI.

of urine, and 64% had nocturnal enuresis. Diagnosis of the UI type was based on the subject's UI history and simple cystometry. Seventy-five percent of the experimental group and 90% of the control group had urge UI while the remaining 25% and 30%, respectively, had mixed stress and urge UI.

Continence status, or the urinary incontinence frequency ratio, was determined by dividing the number of incontinent voids by the total voiding frequency in a 24-hour period. Thus, if a subject voided eight times during a 24-hour period and four of those were incontinent voids, the urinary incontinence frequency ratio (UIFR) was .5. Similar calculations were done to determine the urinary incontinence volume ratio (UIVR). The PURT treatment produced a reduction in UIFR almost immediately and became most effective by Week 24, i.e., at the end of the 12-week intervention period. As shown in Figure 17.5, the UIFR during the 12-week baseline period averaged .70 and .68 for the experimental and control groups, respectively. During the 12-week treatment period, the experimental group averaged .57 while the control group's incontinence frequency ratio increased to .76. Then during the 12-week posttreatment phase, when project staff withdrew their reinforcing behaviors toward staff, the experimental group's average UIFR was .67 and the control group's average was .75. The UIVR showed a similar pattern during the study.

During the baseline period, both the experimental and control subjects voided an average of 6.8 times per day. Experimental subjects were incontinent an average of 4.8 times per day while the average number of incontinent episodes for the control group was 4.3. During the 12-week treatment period, the experimental group's average frequency of incontinence decreased to 3.9 episodes per day while the average number of incontinent episodes for the control group increased to 5.0 per day.

Thus, PURT reduced incontinence an average of .9 episode per day per subject, which was a statistically significant change from experimental subjects' baseline [$F(1,49) = 7.25$, $p < .001$] and also represented significantly better performance than that of the control group [$F(1,86) = 5.88$, $p < .001$]. These findings are similar to other recent studies except that the PURT data were based on 24-hour toileting rather than 10- to 12-hour toileting programs (Engel et al., 1990; Hu et al., 1989; Schnelle et al., 1989).

Overall, PURT improved continence to some degree in 83% of the subjects; for 33% of the treatment group, continence improved by more than 20%. Subjects who improved most tended to have a larger bladder capacity ($r = .37$) and better mental status scores ($r = .41$). The compliance rate of nursing staff who carried out the treatment was only 70%, which may have dampened the maximum effect of the treatment. The lack of more dramatic results could also be due to changes in voiding patterns from those originally monitored. Data from our pilot study, however, showed that voiding patterns 3 months after the original monitoring were very similar to the original patterns observed. Therefore, it is unlikely that this kind of change affected the results.

FIGURE 17.5. Urinary incontinence frequency ratio for the experimental and control groups over time.

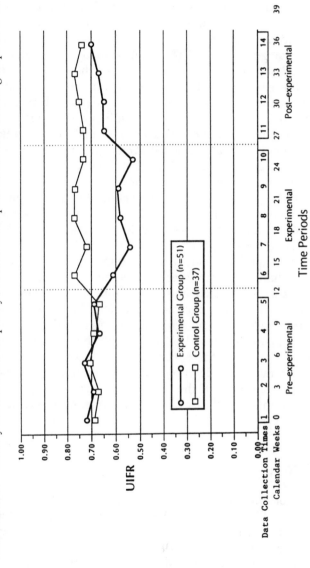

Note: UIFR calculated by dividing the number of incontinent voids by the total number of voids in a 24-hour period.

181

The improvement in continence did not significantly affect the incidence of urinary tract infections (UTI), skin rash, or skin breakdown—these tended to remain infrequent (at or below 10%) throughout the study. This probably reflects the superior level of general care given to these residents. It is interesting to note, however, that when we originally evaluated residents for UTIs, 62% of the control group and 55% of the experimental group had a UTI, as determined by laboratory culture.

Psychosocial status was evaluated in fewer than half of the sample because of the severity of their cognitive impairment. Among those evaluated, no significant changes were found in mood during the study. This may be attributed to the low magnitude of the change in UI status or to the insensitivity of the instrument. Statistically significant improvements, however, were achieved from experimental subjects' baseline measures of behavioral capabilities for elimination [$F(1,49) = 2.34$, $p < .05$], motor achievement [$F (1, 49) = 2.72$, $p < .05$], and dependency status [$F(1,49) = 4.27$, $p < .001$], indicating an increase in subjects' initiation of toileting behaviors and a decrease in dependency.

Direct costs of labor, supplies, and linen were examined for both incontinence and toileting care. Data from 425 timed observations indicated that staff spent an average of 6.37 minutes toileting subjects and 4.03 minutes changing them after they became wet. The overall cost, however, was $.89 for each episode of toileting care and $1.62 for changing patients after they became incontinent. Linen and supply costs decreased with toileting care, while labor costs showed a modest increase. Table 17.4 compares PURT costs with those in four other studies. As Table 17.4 shows, there were some variations in the cost per UI episode, which may have been related to the degree of dependency of nursing home residents and the number and type of supplies used in managing residents. In all cases, however, toileting residents was less costly than UI care.

DISCUSSION

A major goal of nursing is to individualize care to meet patient needs. We found that PURT was an effective noninvasive, individualized approach for decreasing UI among debilitated nursing home patients who were largely unable to provide caregivers with meaningful cues to their voiding needs. Some of our subjects commented that knowing when staff were coming to toilet them greatly enhanced their sense of control. Others said that even small degrees of success were important to their self-esteem. It is clear, however, that staff compliance is crucial to success and that the issues of introducing and maintaining programs such as PURT in nursing homes are complex.

TABLE 17.4 Cost Comparison of Toileting and UI Care across Studies

Investigators	Length of day measured (hr)	Minutes/ UI episode	Cost/UI episode ($)	Minutes/ toileting episode	Cost/ toileting episode ($)	Cost difference ($)
Creason (1987)	12	9.08	1.64	5.56	.56	-1.08
Cella (1988)	?	4.16	.38[a]	—	—	—
Schnelle et al. (1988)	12	5.55	.90	—	.72	-.18
Hu et al. (1989)	14	—	1.68	—	—	-.50[b]
Colling et al. (current study)[c]	24	4.03	1.62	6.37	.89	-.73

[a]Aide time only.
[b]Laundry and supplies only.
[c]Also reported in Colling, Ouslander, Hadley, Eisch, & Campbell (1992).

First, there must be careful selection of residents to receive a particular type of UI program. While almost all incontinent residents can benefit from a treatment program, a number of factors must be taken into account prior to instituting the treatment. The UI guidelines recently published by the Agency for Health Care Policy and Research[2] describe in detail the type of assessment all residents should receive, as well as the indications for use of the many treatment options available. These guidelines can be used by clinicians in nursing homes to decide on treatment for this population.

Second, information about UI should be given to all professional staff and aides. The practice of having experienced aides teach new aides how to carry out clinical activities should be questioned, as it tends to reinforce the status quo. Aides in our study possessed adequate information about applying PURT, but at the same time they expressed very positive attitudes about caring for incontinent patients and believed that it was "just part of their job to change residents." Some aides also commented that unless residents could be kept completely dry, then it was not worth their effort. From our many hours of observation of aide staff, the standard for UI care appeared to be that nursing aides changed or toileted residents "regularly," but the frequency and method of UI management were decided by the aide.

We believe that toileting should be done at night as well as during the day since in this study output was actually a little higher at night than during the daytime or evening shifts. Some residents needed more frequent toileting than the usual two times at night when aides made their rounds, while others needed fewer. However, we found that aides at night were especially resistant to changing their routines to accommodate individual resident voiding times. In addition, most of the professional staff did not supervise aides closely to ensure compliance with the PURT treatment. Thus, a change in philosophy is needed: care should be based on specific patient needs rather than organized for the convenience and efficiency of aide staff.

Finally, the negative incentives in the reimbursement system for continence management must be removed so that care that emphasizes residents' integrity and quality of life is rewarded financially. The PURT program showed an average cost saving of $.73 per incontinent episode. This saving, however, was due to savings in supplies and linen; labor costs actually increased. Facilities might consider targeting toileting programs to those patients who cause particularly high costs for linen and supplies but will not need high labor intensity, in order to maximize cost

[2]More information can be obtained from the Agency for Health Care Policy and Research—(301) 443–4100.

savings (as long as these decisions are compatible with the wishes and rights of residents). Cost and response among residents can be compared. Decreasing UI by even one episode per day for the persons whose incontinence costs most would result in considerable savings to the institution over a year's time. Another possibility is to shift a portion of the cost savings to increase staff, which would pay for the time needed for toileting activities. This shift might in turn lead to greater staff compliance with an individualized routine, and thus increase PURT's effectiveness even further.

ACKNOWLEDGMENTS

The authors thank the following individuals, without whom this study could not have been completed: Margaret McCreedy, R.N., M.N., C.A.N.P., Mary Knight, M.S., R.N., Kathleen Brinknan, R.N., M.S.N., Jacqueline Hudepohl, R.N., M.S., Margaret Lockwood, R.N ., Ed.D., Geraldine Bleifuss, R.N., M.S., G.N.P., Judy Harke, R.N., M.S., G.N.P., Kristin Richgels, R.N., M.S., and Barbara Brozovic, R.N., M.S., F.N.P., who served as clinical nurse specialists; Tom Owen, Ph.D., and Barbara Stewart, Ph.D., for assistance with statistical analyses; Teri Yielding and Laura Hodsen for secretarial support; and the staff at the four nursing homes for their cooperation.

REFERENCES

Azrin, N. H., & Foxx, R. M. (1971). A rapid method of toilet training the institutionalized retarded. *Journal of Applied Behavior Analysis, 4*(2), 89–99.

Cella, M. (1988). The nursing costs of urinary incontinence in a nursing home population. *Nursing Clinics of North America, 23*, 159–168.

Clay, E. C. (1980). Habit retraining: A tested method to regain urinary control. *Geriatric Nursing, 1*, 252–254.

Colling, J., Ouslander, J., Haldey, B. J., Eisch, J., & Campbell, E. (1992). The effects of patterned urge response toileting on urinary incontinence among nursing home residents. *Journal of the American Geriatrics Society, 40*, 135–141.

Collins, R. W., & Plaska, T. (1975). Mowrer's conditioning treatment for enuresis applied to geriatric residents of a nursing home. *Behavior Therapy, 6*, 632–638.

Creason, N. S. (1987, June). Costing urinary incontinence in nursing homes. *Contemporary LTC*, 84–90.

Creason, N., Grybowski, J., Burgener, S., Whippo, C., Weo, S., & Richardson, B. (1989). Prompted voiding therapy for urinary incontinence in aged female nursing home residents. *Journal of Advanced Nursing, 14*, 120–126.

Engel, B. T., Burgio, L. D., McCormick, K. A., Hawkins, A. A., Schene, A. A., & Leahy, E. (1990). Behavioral treatment of incontinence in the long-term setting. *Journal of the American Geriatrics Society, 38*, 361–363.

Grosicki, J. P. (1968). Effect of operant conditioning on modification of incontinence in neuropsychiatric geriatric patients. *Nursing Research, 17,* 304–311.

Hadley, B. J., Wood, J., McCracken, A., & Warshaw, G. (1988). *The Hadley, Wood, McCracken (HWM) Behavioral Capabilities Rating Scale for Older Adults.* Final Report. Washington, DC: American Association of Retired Persons.

Hu, T., Igou, J. F., Kaltreider, D. L., Yu, L., Rohner, T. J., Dennis, P. J., Craighead, W. E., Hadley, E. C., & Ory, M. G. (1989). A clinical trial of a behavioral therapy to reduce urinary incontinence in nursing homes—Outcomes and implications. *Journal of the American Medical Association, 261*(18), 2656–2662.

Johnson, D. E. (1980). The behavioral systems model for nursing. In J. Riehl & C. Roy (Eds.), *Conceptual models for nursing practice* (2nd ed.). New York: Appleton-Century-Crofts.

Kane, R. L., Ouslander, J. G., & Abrass, I. B. (1989) *Essentials of Clinical Geriatrics.* New York: McGraw Hill.

Katz, S., Ford, A. B., Moskowitz, R. W., Jackson, B. A., & Jaffe, M. (1963). The index of ADL: A standardized measure of biological and psychosocial function. *Journal of the American Medical Association, 185,* 914–919.

McNair, D. M., Lorr, M., & Droppleman, L. F. (1971). *Profile of mood states.* San Diego, CA: Educational and Industrial Testing Service.

Ouslander, J. G., Urman H. N., & Uman, G. C. (1986). Development and testing of an incontinence monitoring record. *Journal of the American Geriatrics Society. 34,* 83–90.

Pollock, D. D., & Liberman, R. P. (1974). Behavior therapy of incontinent and demented inpatients. *The Gerontologist, 14,* 488–491.

Pfeiffer, E. (1975). A short portable mental status questionnaire for the assessment of organic brain deficit in elderly patients. *Journal of the American Geriatrics Society, 23,* 106–112.

Schnelle, J. F., Sowell, V. A., Hu, T., & Traughler, B. (1988). Reduction of urinary incontinence in nursing homes: Does it reduce or increase costs? *Journal of the American Geriatrics Society, 36,* 34–39.

Schnelle, J. F., Traughler, B., Sowell, V. A., Newman, D., Petrilli, C., & Ory, M. (1989). Prompted voiding treatment of urinary incontinence in nursing home patients: A behavior management approach for nursing home staff. *Journal of the American Geriatrics Society, 37,* 1051–1057.

Spiro, L. (1978). Bladder training for the incontinent patient. *Geriatric Nursing, 4*(3), 28–35.

Wagner, B. R., & Paul, G. L. (1970). Reduction of incontinence in chronic mental patients: A pilot project. *Journal of Behavior Therapy and Experimental Psychiatry, 1,* 29–38.

[18]

Selecting Patients for Toileting Programs: A Computerized Assessment and Management System

John F. Schnelle, Joseph G. Ouslander, Daniel R. Newman, M. Patrick McNees, Marilyn White, and Barbara M. Bates-Jenson

It is estimated that half of nursing home patients are incontinent of urine (Ouslander, Kane, & Abrass, 1982). Most are frail and thus unable to toilet independently; many also have significant cognitive impairments. Thus surgical, biofeedback, and muscle retraining procedures have limited usefulness with these patients. There are two major approaches to decreasing incontinence among these patients: scheduled or timed-voiding protocols and prompted voiding programs (Schnelle, 1990). We focus here on prompted voiding.

Prompted voiding comprises three major elements. First, as in other toileting programs, there has to be systematic contact with patients, either on a 2-hour or 3-hour schedule. Second, prompted voiding involves a communication protocol, because with the prompted voiding process, aides not only make systematic contact with the patients, but talk to the patients according to a very detailed but simple protocol. The aide checks the patient for wetness or dryness, and then asks the patient: "Mrs. X, are you wet or are you dry?" Next the aide gives the patient feedback about the accuracy of the answer. The crucial point is whether the patient was correct in the answer. Even with very impaired patients, an effort is made to get the patients to recognize their condition. Finally, after that communication, the aide prompts the patient to request toileting assistance, but does not take the patient to the toilet unless he or she says she will try to go. There are two reasons for this: (1) the aim is to get patients to take some initiative and responsibility for their own condition; (2) more importantly, this avoids the wasted effort of trying to toilet patients who say they will not try to go. It is much more efficient, not to mention more humane, to find out from the patient whether he will go. At the conclusion of the contact, patients who toilet successfully are praised for staying dry and for requesting toileting assistance.

Ten articles recently reviewed by a panel on incontinence guidelines present studies of 428 nursing home residents and report a 36% improvement in the patients' continence rate after implementation of prompted voiding (AHCPR, in press). Thus, the consensus seems to be that this system works. It has been replicated, and it can be done. There is also consensus that it is not easy to make it work. In our work in eight nursing homes in Tennessee and Florida, we spent 2–4 weeks working with patients and training staff, motivating and encouraging them. We had an intense training program that was so expensive it was not cost effective, but it did not work in any case. Before we went in, the patients in these eight nursing homes were wet about 31% of the time. That is to say, they were wet at about 1 out of every 3 or 4 hourly checks. When our research team went in and implemented a prompted voiding program, we reduced that percentage to 15%—a figure that has been reported by other people as well. Thus we cut the incontinence rate by half. We then gave a big motivational appeal and said to staff, "We're leaving you the patients, do a good job. We really appreciate being here, and we'll see you." Two weeks later, we came back and made another check, and the patients were wet just about the same amount that they were before, at the baseline point. Therefore, training is not in itself sufficient to get aides to carry out a prompted voiding program.

Only about 25% to 33% of nursing home residents are appropriate for a prompted voiding program. Other residents do not benefit much from such a program, and it is therefore critical to be able to distinguish those who can benefit from those who cannot. It is impossible to maintain a toileting program in a nursing home without making this distinction. The assessment and management system described below not only makes it possible to identify suitable patients but also allows one to set a performance standard that will ensure that nursing aides manage the incontinence program well. We conclude with a brief description of a computerized system for assessment and management.

ASSESSMENT

First the assessment is done over a 6-day period. During this assessment period, patients are checked and prompted every 2 hours, from 7 o'clock in the morning until 7 o'clock at night. Thus, six checks are made each day, one every 2 hours, so in 6 days a total of 36 checks are made. A patient's functioning is evaluated in terms of (1) responsiveness, which is defined as how well the patient responds to questions about whether he or she is wet or dry and to prompts to toilet; (2) the patient's wet frequency, which is self-explanatory; (3) the volume of incontinence episodes; and (4) the patient's toileting ability, based on the percentage of "appropriate" voids, that is, voids made when the patient went to the bathroom on the toilet or a bedpan. To calculate the appropriate toileting percentage, you divide the number of appropriate voids by the total number of voids—appropriate plus inappropriate. A rating of 100% reflects total continence; zero indicates total incontinence. Fifty percent means that half the time a patient goes to the bathroom on the toilet and half the time he is incontinent, and so on. The patient's toileting habits can be rated based on this percentage: 100% is excellent; average ability is 66–75%; poor ability is 0–65%. In general, residents who are most responsive will show the following profile: (1) more than 75% of the wet/dry questions answered accurately; (2) incontinence frequency of 1 episode or less per day; (3) incontinence volumes that average less than 50 cc; and (4) appropriate toileting rates above 75%. These four dimensions will indicate which patients are appropriate for a prompted voiding program and which are not.

Next, standards are set for how wet or how dry patients should be if a toileting program is running well, using a "control chart," which is absolutely fundamental to statistical quality control. Statistical quality control, which is widely used in manufacturing, is implemented in several steps. First, the average and normal variability of work performance outcomes are described by taking repeated samples of work outcomes and comparing them to established standards. It is assumed that all work processes have some variability, but that abnormal variation between the samples and job standards indicates a breakdown in the work system. Thus, the purpose of statistical quality control is to determine whether outcome variability is normal or excessive (Schnelle et al., 1990; Wetherill, 1977).

Basically, a control chart resembles a Cartesian graph with the y-axis representing the "work outcome measure." If it is an incontinence program, the work outcome measure is the percentage of patients wet, ranging from 0 to 100. For example, when prompted voiding is done on a consistent schedule, during each shift, how many wet patients would you expect to find if your program is successful, marginal, or inefficient? The control chart provides this information by giving you an average. It may indicate that between 10% and 20% of the patients should be wet, on average, if everything is going well; if 30% are wet, that is marginal; if 50% are wet, that is poor. The purpose of a control chart is to establish what is good, what is normal, what is marginal, and what is poor. The x-axis of the control chart is the samples of work, in this case, the time points at which patient wetness is assessed. To establish how well a program is working, find out how many patients are wet, and then you can make a quick determination about whether the aides are performing the tasks or not, and whether the patients are responding or not.

In a recent study we used statistical quality control to assess how well a prompted voiding program was carried out by nursing staff in four nursing homes. Figure 18.1 illustrates the control chart used in this study. Eighty-one patients were initially enrolled in the program and 36 of these were assessed to be responsive to prompted voiding. The staff were instructed to maintain the prompted voiding program for these 36 patients. The quality control process involved first setting standards for how dry the patients should be if toileted every 2 hours. This standard was determined during a trial period of 4 days in which prompted

FIGURE 18.1.   Example of a control chart.

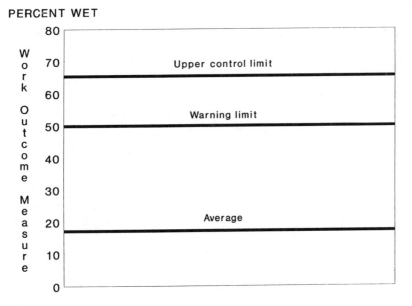

voiding was performed every 2 hours. The percentage of patients who were found wet at each check during this period was calculated and set as the level of wetness one would expect if prompted voiding procedures were done consistently every 2 hours. Overall, the average expected wetness for these patients was 18%.

Next, the ranges of acceptable and unacceptable wetness levels were determined by calculating the standard deviation for wetness level and setting two standard deviations as a "warning limit" and three standard deviations as an "upper control limit." The standard deviation for this sample was 16%, indicating that as long as less than 50% [a mean of 18% + (2 × the standard deviation of 16%)] of the patients were found to be wet on any given check, the toileting procedures were working within appropriate limits. However, wetness checks revealing more than 50% of the patients to be wet would indicate that the program was not working as expected. Observations above the upper control limit of 66% [18% + (3 × 16%)] would indicate that the incontinence level was unacceptable.

Then a control chart was used to continually assess how well these standards were met (Schnelle, Newman, Fogarty, Wallston, & Ory, 1991). The control checks indicated that 50% of the samples were above the expected percent wet but only one or two samples were above the "warning" or "upper" limits. That is to say, the patients were within the limits of "control," suggesting that in fact they were being toileted by staff on a 2-hour schedule and were responding to the program (Schnelle et al., 1991).

Computerization

The assessment system—identifying patients who are appropriate for prompted voiding, setting standards, and constructing a control chart— is best done with a computer. During the assessment period, the aide or assessment nurse carries a printout of the data form, filling in information for each patient. At the end of the day, the aide or assessment nurse goes to the computer and enters the data into the computer. In our recent study, for example, on the first assessment day we made a round at 7 A.M., checked a patient, and found the patient "W"—wet. When asked his status, the patient correctly answered that he was wet. We prompted the patient and were successful in toileting him—for this we marked "yes." The volume of his continent void as measured by a toileting insert was 120 cc, and the volume of his incontinent void as measured by a diaper he was wearing was 246 cc. Every 2 hours we made a round, prompted the patient, and recorded the data; and at the end of a day, we came back and entered it. It is a very simple procedure:

you call the program up on the screen, take the numbers off your sheet and enter them.

At the end of 6 days, there is a final assessment summary sheet, which is too big to put on the screen at one time, but will tell you what the patient did during that 6-day period. Most importantly, it will give you a rating of the patient's toileting abilities, which, as noted earlier, is based on the percentage of appropriate voids. You also get a printout that shows the patient's bladder storage ability, as estimated by frequency of wets per day; another printout shows his average volume per incontinence episode, once again using a categorical system, good, marginal, or poor; and finally, another printout shows his responsiveness over the week.

The printout says the patient has a certain toileting ability, a certain bladder storage ability, and a certain mental responsiveness. Based on these data, you make treatment recommendations. For example, we recommend prompted voiding or we recommend check and change. You can override the data, if you want to. The nurse can override it if he/she doesn't agree with it, and decide to assess further. But the computer will give you the basic information about which patients are appropriate for which regimens. It will tell you to put people on prompted voiding who have either excellent or marginal toileting ability or either excellent or marginal bladder storage ability. It will also tell you to put people there who appropriately toilet, in other words, who void on the toilet or bedpan 60% of the time or more, and who are wet fewer than two times a day. More importantly, the printout gives you a control chart that will allow you to manage nursing aides in the implementation of the program after the assessment period.

MANAGEMENT

Once you know which patients belong on the toileting program and which do not, the major issue is compliance. The control chart allows you to monitor the standard deviations of the work output percentage, and this information will tell you whether or not the aides are administering the appropriate treatments. In our recent study, during assessment, we found the compliance rate was excellent, because we designated specially trained aides to do it. However, the compliance rate that is important for quality control is the rate after the 6-day assessment period. For example, if during the 6-day assessment period, the average wetness rate is 10% and afterwards this percentage begins to escalate one or two standard deviations, say to 32%, then you know that something is wrong. The control chart allows you to keep track of the average wetness of the patients and thereby run the toileting program effectively.

Seven patients out of 15 that we assessed at the Mary Conrad Center in Anchorage, Alaska, were chosen for a prompted voiding program. These seven patients had an average wetness rate of 10%; two standard deviations above that was 32% and three standard deviations above that was 44%. Two standard deviations tells you that if you sample a group of patients who are on a program of prompted voiding and find that 32% are wet, that's unusual. It doesn't tell you why, but it says it's unusual. If you sample a group of patients and find that 50% are wet, that's very unusual. That should not happen very often, by chance, if prompted voiding is being done on a consistent schedule. The first time that we made a round on these seven patients, nobody was wet. The second time, nobody was wet. The third time we made a round, about 14% were wet. The fourth time, nobody, the fifth time, nobody, etc.; you see how the control chart works.

Once you have a control chart, you are set to monitor program quality. On the basis of our research, we suggest that a nurse make two weekly control rounds to sample patient wetness. The nurse should enter into the computer how she found each patient, wet or dry. That takes about 2 minutes per data entry. With the data entered, the computer may tell you that "too many people are wet." Or it may tell you, "everybody's all right, go on." The computer will also give you an individual patient summary. It gives you a record of all the control checks for all the individual patients, and flags patients who are excessively wet. In other words, the group might be in control (i.e., the group control chart will look good), but there might be an individual patient who does not look good. The computer will also give you a schedule for future control checks.

The computer will analyze all the data that you have collected in the last 3 weeks or over a year, or however long you have been using the program, and tell you when the main problems occur. For instance, Wednesday at 9 A.M., you have more wetness than at any other time, so a quality assurance nurse should look at what happens on Wednesday at 9 A.M. You also can identify factors affecting the variability. You can run assessments that will tell you how the program is going by hour of day, by day of week, or by individual staff. You can do an analysis of wet checks by aide, which gets into the area of management. As shown in Figure 18.2, on the bottom of the control chart you see the aides' names, and above each aide's name you see the percent of times a patient the aide was taking care of was found wet. You also see an

FIGURE 18.2. Analysis of wet checks by 11 aides.

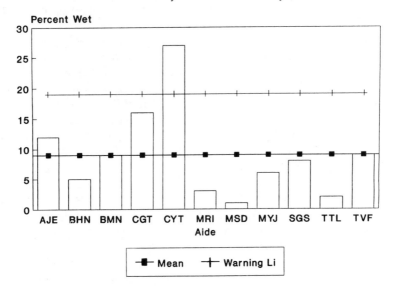

average and the variability; for example, you may find that aide CYT is having a problem. Aide CYT should be looked at. On the other hand, aide MRI looks fine—she/he probably should get a compliment. Basically, you can do an analysis just as in a car factory. I want us to give people as much respect as we do cars. You do not have to look through a hundred charts, or spend 18 hours doing a quality assurance study. You press a button, and say, we have a problem at this time, on this floor, at this day, with this aide. That is the basis of a management system.[1]

ACKNOWLEDGMENT

This research was supported by the National Institute of Aging and the National Center for Nursing Research Grant #5 U01 AG05270-02 to Dr. J. F. Schnelle.

[1]The computer program can be used on DOS-based computers with graphic capability and minimum of 20 megabyte hard drive. Software is available from Dr. John Schnelle, Borun Center for Gerontological Research, UCLA School of Medicine, CHS-32-144, 10833 Le Conte Ave., Los Angeles, CA 90024-1687, or Dr. Patrick McNees, North Rim Systems, 6040 Yukon Road, Anchorage, AK 99516. Write for cost information and details of training system.

REFERENCES

Agency for Health Care Policy and Research. (in press). *Urinary incontinence in the adult, practice guidelines.* Washington, DC: U.S. Government Printing Office.

Ouslander, J. G., Kane, R. L., & Abrass, I. B. (1982). Urinary incontinence in elderly nursing home patients. *Journal of the American Medical Association, 248,* 1194–1198.

Schnelle, J. F. (1990). Treatment of urinary incontinence in nursing home patients by prompted voiding. *Journal of the American Geriatrics Society, 38,* 356–360.

Schnelle, J. F., Newman, D. R., Abby, J., Dray, R., Petrilli, C. O., & Hadley, E. (1990). Urodynamic and behavioral analysis of incontinence in nursing home patients. *Behavior, Health and Aging, 1,* 43–49.

Schnelle, J. F., Newman, D. R., Fogarty, T. E., Wallston, K., & Ory, M. (1991). Assessment and quality control of incontinence care in long-term nursing facilities. *Journal of the American Geriatrics Society, 39,* 165–171.

Wetherill, G. B. (1977). *Sampling inspection and quality controls* (2nd ed.). New York: John Wiley.

[19]

Reduction of Incontinence Among Elderly in a Long-Term Care Setting

Diane A. Smith, Diane Kaschak Newman,
B. Joan McDowell, and Louis D. Burgio

Urinary incontinence (UI) is considered the second leading cause of institutionalization of the elderly, and it is a serious and distressing problem for all whom it affects. Among the 1.5 million residents of nursing facilities in the United States, 50% or more experience incontinence episodes frequently, generally more than once per day (NIH Consensus Conference, 1989). Fecal incontinence, physical and mental immobility, decubitus ulcers, and urinary tract infections commonly are associated with UI (Yu et al., 1990).

A large part of the incontinence seen in nursing homes is related to the effects of institutionalization and inconsistent toileting. Many incontinent nursing home residents are managed with indwelling or external catheters and absorbent products, even though such devices increase the risk of urinary tract infection and skin breakdown. Planned toileting programs and frequent checks for dryness significantly improve incontinence symptoms for many individuals. Prompted voiding or toileting, in which staff remind residents to void and praise their success, can be particularly effective with cognitively impaired persons.

The effectiveness of toileting schedules is strongly affected by the intervals between toileting. Schnelle et al. (1989; Schnelle, 1990) have described prompted toileting techniques that were successful among certain residents; in one study the schedule of toileting began with an hourly schedule and subsequently shifted to every 2 hours; in a second study the schedule was every 2 hours. In that second study, Schnelle (1990) identified those residents most likely to be successful with prompted voiding. Successful residents were those whose baseline incontinence frequency was typically less then four times per 12-hour period and who could recognize the need to void and do so successfully when given toileting assistance. Burgio, Engel, McCormick, Hawkins, and Schieve (1988), however, noted the conflict between adherence to a 2-hour toileting schedule and inadequate nursing time in the real world. They used a 3- to 4-hour schedule individualized to each resident. The study was conducted over a long period of time, and a variety of management strategies were instituted to ensure staff compliance with toileting schedules (Burgio, Jones, & Engel, 1990).

As many nurse managers in long-term care know, a major factor in dealing with incontinence is getting staff to follow protocols. As continence management specialists at a life care community, we were asked to implement a program that would help reduce incontinence and would also be easy for the staff to manage. Most of the studies in the literature used research staff to accomplish the toileting regimens; thus, the major question for our project was, "Can regular staff accomplish toileting?" Additional questions were, "Can every resident be successful?"; "Can this work with the demented, frail elderly?"; and "What components are necessary?" We decided to stage interventions to make it possible to determine which were most useful. It was also important to incorporate staff management techniques into the program so that the long-term care unit would be able to maintain the program once the study was completed. The challenge was to design a program that would take techniques found successful in research studies and implement them in the real-world environment of a long-term care facility.

METHOD

Setting

The study was conducted in a 68-bed skilled nursing section of a life-care community outside Philadelphia, PA. For two years prior to the study, the community had had a continence program for outpatient residents, and inservice programs on the assessment and behavioral treatment of UI had been given to staff on several occasions. The study was confined to an area of the nursing home whose patients were primarily demented and frail elders. This area generally was served by consistent staff, including a permanent charge nurse on both the day and night shifts and many permanent nursing assistants. Both of the charge nurses, the assistant director of nursing, and the director of nursing were involved in the development and implementation of the study. The study's protocol also was approved by the medical director. Since the majority of the study participants were demented and unable to give consent, informed consent was obtained from the party responsible for each resident.

Participants

Because the facility's administration requested that the number of residents involved in the study be limited so as not to burden staff, it was decided to include only 10 control and 10 treatment residents. The control and treatment groups were matched according to their levels of incontinence. The groups were also comparable in age, degree of dementia, and functional status (see Table 19.1).

All residents in the treatment group were evaluated prior to the study for acute or transient causes of incontinence and to establish bladder function. (Control group residents were not evaluated since they were not to receive treatment.) The evaluation included urethral catheterization for post-void residual, testing for urinary tract infection, rectal exam to detect fecal impaction, and drug screening for sedatives and hypnotics. A bedside cystometrogram was performed to evaluate bladder function and capacity and to determine the presence or absence of detrusor contractions. Regimens for the regulation of bowel function were established when needed prior to implementation of the study. Two of the 10 treatment group residents were found to have urinary tract infections and were treated and retested before entering the study. Seven had unstable bladders, as determined by the presence of urine leakage around the catheter at the time of bedside testing. No resident tested

TABLE 19.1   Comparison of Treatment and Control Groups

	Treatment group	Control group
Age (mean)	92.4	90.3
Mini Mental State Exam[a] (mean)	7.0	8.5
Functional status (1 person assist)	60%	50%
Percent incontinent	80%	80%

[a]Folstein, Folstein, & McHugh, 1975.

was found to have a post-void residual of more than 100 cc, and none had fecal impaction at the time of the examination. The use of hypnotics and sedatives was minimal, and no changes were necessary in the patients' drug regimens. All examinations were performed by continence management specialists who were nurse practitioners with master's degrees.

Phases

The study was in four phases. Phase One was a baseline phase in which staff recorded bladder and bowel behavior for both the treatment and control groups. During Phase Two, treatment group residents were placed on a pad and pant system called "Promise"^{TM} and had a commode placed next to the bed. This phase addressed the functional causes of incontinence. Phase Three incorporated the addition of prompted toileting for the treatment group. Phase Four added an anticholinergic medication intended to increase the treatment group patients' ability to comply with prompted voiding. Recording continued for both groups across all four phases.

The study took place over a $3\frac{1}{2}$-month period. The first three phases each lasted approximately 4 weeks, but Phase Four was halted after one week. In Phase One, which established the baseline incontinence rate, staff were asked to document incontinence (wet checks) on an individual bowel and bladder recording form for each of the treatment and control group residents. The form was kept at the resident's bedside and was used to record incontinent episodes as well as changes, toiletings, and checks.

During Phase Two, the Promise^{TM} pad and pant system was implemented along with a commode by the bed. The Promise^{TM} pad and pant system is a disposable, close-to-the-body system for incontinence management that includes two components: a form-fitting washable pant made of lightweight stretchable mesh; and a disposable, body-contoured protective pad with a moisture-proof backing available in four sizes and at four protection levels—light, standard, heavy, and overnight. The pad and pant system was implemented because it was a dignified system and facilitated toileting. The bedside commode was used because most of the treatment residents needed assistance getting to the bathroom, and it was thought that this would make the job easier. Staff were instructed to care for the residents in the usual manner and record incontinence episodes, changes, and any toileting.

Incontinence rates of the treatment and control residents were publicly posted, and feedback was given to the staff on their compliance in using the bladder and bowel recording forms. While information about compliance was given to all staff, charge nurses were given specific information on individual residents and individual shift compliance. This pattern of information feedback was used throughout the study. The continence management specialist also attended staff meetings throughout the study and gave general reports on the status of the study, information about upcoming phases, and shift compliance.

Phase Three involved the use of prompted toileting, a technique by which the resident is prompted to void and praised for successful responses. The nursing assistant was given a schedule to adhere to, and the resident was prompted according to this schedule. The technique was taught at several in-services, and staff were asked to give return demonstration of the procedure. During these return demonstrations, it was noted that despite prior in-services on pivot transfer, many staff members were unable to perform this. Therefore, the continence management specialist also taught every nursing assistant and nurse individually the technique of transferring. One nursing assistant took approximately seven sessions to produce a successful transfer; this came as a revelation to the researchers. Clearly, one barrier to the use of a toileting protocol might be the inability of staff to transfer residents to the commode successfully.

The establishment of the prompted toileting schedule involved choosing a time table that the researchers felt would be successful in achieving dryness and modifying it enough so that staff could comply with the toileting schedule. The initial schedule included having the residents prompted upon waking, before and after meals, and before bed. Staff were asked to accomplish toileting in between their other activities rather than at specific times of the day because this would be easier to remember and would flow with routine resident care. Staff used a different recording form in this phase; the form indicated the steps in prompted toileting and served as documentation of staff compliance and individual resident incontinence rates. This form is shown in Figure 19.1.

At one week into Phase Three, the toileting schedule was modified. It was found that staff could not discriminate between "after arising" and "before breakfast," or between "before dinner" and "after lunch." Compliance rates were poorest before breakfast and before lunch. The schedule was therefore altered to include the following times: upon waking (a night shift responsibility), after breakfast and after lunch (a day shift responsibility), and after dinner and before bed (an evening shift responsibility). This schedule proved to be the easiest to adhere to, and by the end of Phase Three, overall staff compliance was 90.6%.

The researchers abandoned Phase Four after only one week. This phase involved administration of oxybutynin in small doses (2.5 mg

FIGURE 19.1.   Bladder/bowel program prompted voiding form.

BLADDER / BOWEL PROGRAM
PROMPTED VOIDING FORM

Date: _____   Name: _____
                                       Room: _____

Column 1	Column 2	Column 3	Column 4	Column 5
Time Prompted	Wet?	Dry?	Toileted?	Bowel Movement

DIRECTIONS:

Prompt resident to void at these times:
• 6 - 6:30 am
• After Breakfast
• After Lunch
• After Dinner
• Before Bed

PROMPTING STEPS:
1. Approach resident; wait 3 seconds for resident to ask to be taken to the toilet
2. If resident asks to go say, "Thank you for letting me know"
3. Take resident to toilet or commode
4. If resident voids, praise resident
5. Tell resident when you will be back

Note. From "Prompted Voiding Form," by D. A. Smith & D. K. Newman, 1990. Copyright 1990 by Golden Horizons, Inc. Reprinted by permission.

bid), and the charge nurse noted lethargy and delirium in all of the treatment group residents and therefore asked that the drug be discontinued. A possible explanation for the lethargy and delirium was the average age of the treatment group—92.4; side effects such as delirium are much more commonly found in the frail elderly.

During these phases the control group's incontinence rate was monitored but standard care was not altered. The control group was not put on a toileting regimen.

RESULTS

Group Incontinence Rates

Throughout the study, treatment and control group incontinence rates were calculated daily. The assessments were performed between 1:30 and 2:00 P.M. by the charge nurse. They did not coincide or interfere with the post-lunch toileting for the treatment group since the toileting was done between 12:30 and 1:30 P.M. The assessment technique was simple. A list of residents was compiled, and a check was performed to see if each resident was wet or dry. The number who were wet was divided by the total number and then multiplied by 100 to find the percentage of incontinence in the group. This assessment was performed on both the treatment and control groups. The group incontinence rate reflects the overall status of incontinence in the long-term care facility.

Throughout the study the control group stayed at about the same rate—80% incontinent. The treatment group declined in overall incontinence from 80% to slightly over 20% (see Figure 19.2). Daily percentages were averaged to weekly rates, which were then averaged for a phase percentage.

Individual Rates

Individual incontinence rates in the treatment group were determined on a daily basis from 24-hour bladder records kept for each subject (in contrast to the once per day assessment used to estimate group rates above). The percentage of times the individual was incontinent was calculated and averaged weekly. These rates declined steadily. Even during baseline, when staff were not asked to toilet residents, rates began to decline sporadically, resulting in a reduction of the overall individual incontinence rates from an average of 80% to an average of 73% during Phase One. A further decline in individual incontinence rates was noted during Phase Two, when the rate dropped to 69%.

FIGURE 19.2.   Group incontinence rates.

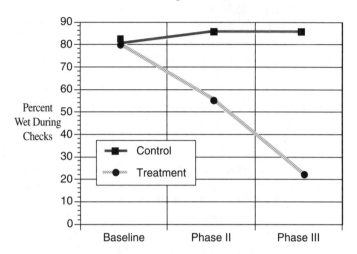

FIGURE 19.3.   Average reduction of individual incontinence rates in treatment group.

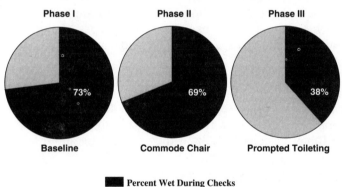

However, the largest decline in incontinence rates occurred during Phase Three—the prompted toileting phase. By the end of this phase the overall individual incontinence rate was 38%, which represented a 42% reduction in incontinence. A summary of the changes can be seen in Figure 19.3.

DISCUSSION

This small study involved the use of prompted voiding on a scheduled basis. Rather than fixing specific toilet times during the day, the schedule incorporated the activities of the staff. Every shift and every nurse or nursing assistant was given responsibility for the continence program. A bedside commode was implemented to make toileting easy, and attempts were made to facilitate staff compliance. Staff were asked at the end of the study which aspects of the program they felt were most important, and the most frequent response was that the addition of the commode chair had been vital to their ability to toilet residents. They also cited the pad and pant system as useful, since the product was easy to use and was dignified. Team work was noted as important, and learning to transfer residents properly was described as a crucial component of the intervention program.

The small number of residents in the study presents a problem in generalizing results to other groups. Also, the long-term care facility asked for the program and therefore made every effort to facilitate it; implementation might be more difficult in other situations. However, the results are very promising.

Based on these results, clinicians should carefully consider the following points in treatment of incontinence in the nursing home:

1. Prompted voiding is usually suggested only for patients who are not severely demented, but in this study success was seen even with very demented patients. Therefore, prompted voiding should be tried since it seems useful for many types of patients.
2. The commode chair and the pad and pant system can facilitate toileting.
3. The physical environment should be arranged to make toileting easier.
4. Staff who are asked to toilet should first demonstrate their ability to transfer patients who need a one- or two-person assist, because staff may hesitate to toilet if they are unsure about transferring.

ACKNOWLEDGMENTS

This research was supported by the Frank Morgan Jones Fund, Scott Health Care, a unit of Scott Paper Company. The authors would like to thank Foulkeways Gwynedd Life Care Community and their excellent staff.

REFERENCES

Burgio, L., Engel, B. T., McCormick, K., Hawkins, A., & Schieve, A. (1988). Behavioral treatment for urinary incontinence of elderly inpatients: Initial attempts to modify prompting and toileting procedures. *Behavioral Therapy, 19*, 345–357.

Burgio, L. C., Jones L. J., & Engel, B. (1990). Studying incontinence in an urban nursing home. *Journal of Gerontological Nursing, 4*, 40–45.

Folstein, M. F., Folstein, S. E., & McHugh, P. R. (1975). "Mini-Mental State": A practical guide for grading the cognitive state of patients for clinicians. *Journal of Psychiatric Research, 12*, 189–198.

National Institutes of Health Consensus Development Conference. (1989). Urinary incontinence in adults. *Journal of the American Medical Association, 261*, 2685–2690.

Schnelle, J. F., Traughler, B., Sowell, V. A., Newman, D., Petrilli, C. O., & Ory, M. (1989). Prompted voiding treatment of urinary incontinence in nursing home patients. *Journal of the American Geriatrics Society, 37*, 1051–1057.

Schnelle, J. F. (1990). Treatment of urinary incontinence in nursing home patients by prompted voiding. *Journal of the American Geriatrics Society, 38*, 356–360.

Yu, L. C., Rohner, T. J., Kaltreider, D. L., Hu, T., Igou, J., & Dennis, P. J. (1990). Profile of urinary incontinent elderly in long-term care institutions. *Journal of the American Geriatrics Society, 38*, 433–439.

[20]

Skin Alterations in Elderly Women Using Disposable Adult Incontinence Briefs

Leigh A. Bertholf and Sue Popkess-Vawter

The skin makes up 15–16% of total body weight, provides protection from the environment, and is the first line of defense against external injury and infection (Delancy & North, 1983; Dossey, 1983; Hogstel, 1983). The skin is also responsible for regulation of body temperature, sensory reception, and storage of water and fats (Delancy & North,

1983). Preventive care and early detection of skin problems are critical in retention of proper skin functioning.

The elderly person's integumentary system has already been compromised by nature. There is a significant decrease in skin turgor with aging, and often the skin has a transparent, tissue-like appearance. Sebaceous and sweat gland secretions decrease, and the dermis becomes less elastic and loses collagen; elastic fibers shrink. Body fat decreases, especially in the extremities, and bony prominences have a sharp, angular appearance (Fitzsimmons, 1983).

Urinary incontinence often accompanies aging, immobility, loss of mental alertness, and debilitation. Incontinence increases the potential for skin impairment because it serves as a medium for bacterial growth (Hogstel, 1983). Not only impaired skin integrity, but also odors and interference with social interactions are associated with urinary incontinence. In an effort to reduce odor, encourage social interaction, and promote skin integrity, disposable briefs were developed. However, because of the plastic outer liner, continued use of disposable incontinence briefs may interfere with the skin's ability to serve as a protective barrier and lead to formation of decubitus ulcers.

Phipps (1984), Byrne and Feld (1984), and Mangieri (1982) summarized the commonly accepted classifications for decubitus ulcers. The stages have defining characteristics to identify the progression of the decubitus ulcer, as shown below:

Stage I: This is the stage of transient circulatory disturbance when pressure is applied, blocking the blood flow to the tissue. As pressure is released, reactive hyperemia of the skin occurs, displayed as a bright red flush. This pressure sore involves the superficial epidermal and dermal layers. The surrounding tissue is inflamed and swollen.

Stage II: These sores are shallow, full thickness skin injuries that involve adipose tissue. There is complete loss of the dermal and epidermal layers. The epidermis can be broken by either a blister or a superficial ulcer.

Stage III: These ulcers have progressed into muscle tissue. Necrotic tissue must be removed before healing will take place.

Stage IV: The epithelial, adipose, and muscle tissue have necrosed; underlying bone or joint structures are involved.

Carpenito (1983) suggests the following skin integrity index:

Stage 1: Transient circulatory disturbance that disappears after pressure is removed.

Stage 2: Reddened or blanched area with no breakdown in skin that does not disappear after pressure is removed.

Stage 3: Erythema and edema with blister or skin break.

Stage 4: Full thickness lesion extends to subcutaneous fat, may have serosanguinous drainage.

Stage 5: Full thickness lesion extends to deep fascia, muscle, and bone.

Currently, impaired skin integrity is recognized as a nursing diagnosis. The nursing diagnosis statement, "impaired skin integrity: pressure ulcer related to patient's inability to move," gives a clearly defined etiology; however, this etiology does not describe the phenomenon that occurs with the use of disposable adult incontinence briefs. Moisture becomes trapped between the skin and the plastic outer layer of the brief, resulting in a continually moist environment. If the brief is left on for a long period, the outer skin develops a shriveled white appearance similar to that of hands left too long in dishwater. This skin is very fragile and susceptible to trauma.

Unfortunately, only a few studies have examined the effects of the disposable incontinence brief on skin integrity (Beber, 1980; Boulton & Kazemi, 1984; Haecker, 1985; Hu, Kaltreider, & Igou, 1989). On four long-term chronic care units at a Department of Veterans' Affairs Medical Center, Boulton and Kazemi (1984) compared the effectiveness of disposable incontinence briefs to reusable diapers, to determine if use of the disposable brief would increase or decrease redness, rashes, ulcerations, and pressure sores on the abdomen, hips, genitals, buttocks, and upper thighs. Prior to the study, reusable diapers were used exclusively in the facility. Thirty-two incontinent male subjects, aged 47–87 years, were measured the day before the study began for redness, rashes, ulcerations, and pressure sores. Eight had skin impairments prior to the study. All subjects then wore only disposable briefs during the study period and were evaluated again at the end of 4 weeks. All had completely healed or improved significantly by the end of the study.

Beber (1980) compared the effects on skin integrity of disposable adult incontinence briefs and reusable diapers for controlling incontinence. The 19-week study included 276 totally incontinent subjects in seven different nursing homes divided into two matched groups. The control group subjects were maintained on their usual regime, which consisted of the use of disposable bed pads, frequent clothing and bedding changes, and reusable cloth diapers. The test group wore the incontinence brief as the only incontinence care product. Pre- and post-tests were used to evaluate skin integrity.

Each week each subject's skin was examined by registered nurses and assigned a numerical grade for skin condition: 0 was excellent, 1 good, 2 fair, and 3 poor. Each individual was given an overall skin impairment score. After data gathering was complete, staff were asked about the physiologic and psychological impacts and the performance of the brief compared to products normally used.

The researchers found no significant differences in skin integrity between the two groups. Both groups showed a trend toward better skin conditions as the study progressed. The major difference between the control and test groups was the staff's perception of improved quality of life related to increased mobility and reduced embarrassment among patients who wore the disposable briefs.

Haecker (1985) also looked at the effects of disposable briefs. Pressure sores and other skin lesions were measured prior to the study, and six subjects were found to have existing skin problems. Of these six, only one could wear the disposable incontinent brief for the entire 4-week research period. The other five complained of "burning" and the legs "cutting into them." At the end of the study period, 22% of the subjects were found to have some type of alteration in skin integrity, as compared to 6% of the subjects prior to using the disposable product. Haecker (1985) listed the following characteristics of the skin problems: blisters, rash, wheals, open lesions, and redness. These characteristics differ only slightly from the list given by Carpenito (1983).

Hu, Kaltreider, and Igou (1989) examined three issues related to the use of disposable incontinence briefs: cost differences between a disposable brand and reusable cloth diapers; overall quality of care afforded by each product, according to such measures as bedding protection and containment of odor and urine; and the skin condition of residents using disposable briefs and cloth diapers. The research was conducted in a rural Pennsylvania nursing home that offered both skilled and intermediate care; the 22 subjects were incontinent at least once per day. Reusable gauze diapers were compared to "Promise," a disposable brief distributed by Scott. Care remained the same for the two groups, including routine washing but no special perineal care unless skin breakdown occurred. The skin was assessed before the study, once a week during the study, and following the study, using a skin assessment instrument designed by the researchers. Five skin conditions were checked for: erythema, rash, excoriation, blister, and skin breakdown; they were coded according to intensity levels: 1 = slight, 2 = moderate, 3 = moderately severe, 4 = severe. The mean scores for the Promise group improved from 1.22 to 1.09 while the cloth diaper group deteriorated from 1.13 to 1.43. The difference between the two groups was significant at the .01 level.

The purposes of the study reported here were to further explore the effects of disposable incontinence briefs on alteration in skin integrity and to attempt to determine whether capillary refill time can be used as an indicator of risk for development of skin alteration.

METHOD

Skin integrity, dimension (size) of skin alteration, location of impairment, and capillary refill time were compared for a group wearing disposable diapers (Group A), a group wearing gauze diapers (Group B), and a continent group (Group C).

Sample/Setting

Thirty elderly women over the age of 65 were assessed for level of skin integrity prior to the study. All the women were confined to wheelchairs for no longer than 2-hour intervals, and none had any areas of skin impairment. All the women were Caucasian. Three groups of ten were constructed using purposive selection, according to their room location within the care center, to keep the groups separate and allow for better control. The subjects in Groups A and B were totally incontinent, and Group C was continent.

Intervention

Following the selection of subjects, nursing personnel were notified and given directions for caring for the three groups. Group A wore the disposable incontinence briefs at all times except when soiled or if skin breakdown began. Pericare was done after each episode of incontinence using a disposable, lanolin-moistened washcloth. Group B wore the gauze diaper except when soiled or if skin breakdown began. Pericare was done after each episode of incontinence using a disposable, lanolin-moistened washcloth, and all diapers were changed when soiled. Group C wore no incontinence brief and pericare was not performed other than at normal bath times because these subjects were continent. The disposable lanolin washcloth currently being used within the facility had been used for over a year's time without any adverse reaction to its use; it contained no alcohol.

Data Collection

The three groups were evaluated by the investigator every 8 hours for 72 hours (for a total of 9 observations) using the Bertholf Skin Assessment Instrument to monitor changes in skin integrity. This instrument allows recording of capillary refill time and assessment of skin integrity using a gradient scale (i.e., 1 = normal, 2 = reactive hyperemia, 3 = erythema, 4 = excoriation, 5 = blister, 6 = decubitus), with an anatomic model for identification of areas of skin impairment. The coccyx was assessed for capillary refill time in an effort to determine if this could be a predictor of alteration in skin integrity. The skin was blanched at the coccyx using the thumb, and the time for the return of color was measured. The subjects were checked at 7 A.M., 3 P.M., and 11 P.M. These times were identified as the best assessment times after Bertholf (1986) identified that assessment after meals may lead to identifying redness over pressure areas because subjects have been sitting up in a wheelchair for a prolonged period of time.

Following the skin assessments, frequency of occurrence of skin alterations, location, and increase or decrease in the size of the affected area, capillary refill time, and any other pertinent data were recorded. The subjects were monitored every 2 hours by the primary nurse when routine rounds were made. Early signs of skin impairment, beginning with excoriation, were immediately reported to the investigator by the primary nurse. Excoriation was used as an indicator because of the frequent occurrence of erythema and reactive hyperemia in the elderly, often a result of being immobile and sitting in a sustained position for up to 2 hours. If a subject developed excoriation, the experimental treatment was withdrawn, but data continued to be collected on the subject.

RESULTS

Significant differences in skin integrity between Group A, wearing disposable incontinence briefs, Group B, wearing gauze diapers, and Group C, wearing no incontinence protection, were expected within 72 hours. Differences at Observations 7 (56 hours), 8 (64 hours), and 9 (72 hours) were significant at the .05 level using analysis of variance (ANOVA) with repeated measures. On the average, patients wearing disposable briefs (Group A) showed signs of erythema, those wearing gauze diapers were rated in the "reactive hyperemia" range, and the controls (Group C) were normal (see Table 20.1). Two clients in Group A wearing disposable briefs were withdrawn from the study as a result of decubitus formation. In Group B, wearing gauze diapers, one subject developed a blister on the buttock.

Differences in the dimension of skin alteration were also expected between Group A (disposable briefs), Group B (gauze), and Group C (control). Differences in dimension were significant at Observations 7, 8, and 9 at the .01 level using ANOVA. At each of these observations,

Group A had the largest dimension of skin alteration, Group B a smaller
amount, and Group C almost no skin alteration (see Table 20.1).

Differences in capillary refill time were also expected between the
three groups. Capillary refill was assessed at each of the observations
during the 72-hour assessment period. However, no significant differences were found among the three groups of subjects. Readings of 0
indicated that the skin color was too pale to measure any change in skin
capillary refill. Other readings ranged from 1 to 3 seconds. Slight
hyperemic skin color made the most easily measured readings.

Pearson correlation coefficients were calculated to determine if there
was any relationship between stage of skin alteration, dimension of
alteration, and capillary refill. There was a clustering effect between
capillary refill time, stage, and dimension as predictors of skin impairment approximately 16–26 hours prior to impairment. The skin was
blanched and immeasurable or measured 0. This pale immeasurable
area was the same area that would later develop alteration. The clustering occurred at Observations 4 and 5 prior to skin impairment developing at Observations 7, 8, and 9. The correlations seen between stage of
skin alteration, dimension, and capillary refill at Observations 4, 5, and 6
suggest that capillary refill time could be useful in developing a risk
index to predict skin alteration. Capillary refill time is measurable, and

TABLE 20.1   Mean Skin Integrity and Dimension Scores at Observations
7, 8, and 9 for Groups A, B, and C

	Observation		
	7	8	9
Skin integrity[a]			
Group A (disposable diapers) (n = 10)	3.0	3.5	3.6
Group B (gauze diapers) (n = 10)	1.8	1.8	1.8
Group C (control) (n = 10)	1.2	1.0	1.1
F statistic	3.59[b]	5.78[c]	5.99[c]
Dimension (cm)			
Group A (n = 10)	1.1	1.2	1.2
Group B (n = 10)	0.4	0.3	0.3
Group C (n = 10)	0.2	0.0	0.1
F statistic	6.78[d]	13.68[d]	10.78[d]

[a]Scale: 1 = normal to 6 = decubitus
[b]$p < .05$
[c]$p < .01$
[d]$p < .001$

staff and consumers could be shown how to measure it and how to assess skin integrity and intervene to protect the client from decubitus formation.

When observed every 8 hours, Group A displayed an unusual phenomenon that appeared as shriveled, moist, and pale skin. Two of the subjects with this condition were identified as having a decubitus ulcer within 8–16 hours after the initial observation of this phenomenon. A third subject was observed to have this shriveled skin, but no decubitus ulcer had developed by the end of the study. This phenomenon occurred only in the coccyx area and only within Group A, wearing disposable incontinence briefs. Interestingly, only one of the subjects who developed a decubitus ulcer was taking a diuretic. This was significant because it is widely accepted that diuretics place the individual at greater risk for decubitus development (McCormick, Scheve, & Leahy, 1988).

DISCUSSION

The use of adult disposable incontinence briefs has been increasing ever since their introduction into the market. Hospitals and nursing homes have greatly increased their use of these products. They are convenient for nursing staff since fewer hours are spent rinsing soiled linens and changing bedding. Also, the briefs are no longer used only in institutions such as nursing homes and hospitals; the general consumer can now buy them at the nearest grocery store or drug store. For many, they have become a convenient solution to stress incontinence and they have freed many elderly from fear of leaving their homes in case an episode of incontinence might occur.

The data from this study, however, indicate that continued use of adult disposable incontinence briefs affects skin integrity. In this study, the disposable incontinence briefs were worn continuously for a 72-hour period. This study used a small population and observed these individuals over a short period of time. Skin protocols had been well established and were followed closely. If skin alteration of this magnitude (i.e., decubiti formation) can occur in this short period of time using well-established protocols, the potential for impairment under circumstances where no written skin care protocols exist is frightening.

Moisture, heat, and pressure compromise the integrity of the protective outer layer of skin, which is the first and one of the most effective defense mechanisms for the elderly. These briefs provide a constantly warm, moist environment; they hold more urine than gauze does, and the plastic outer liner allows for no evaporation of moisture from the skin.

The briefs should not be used in lieu of bowel and bladder training but, rather, as an adjunct to this procedure. Also, the briefs should not be worn continuously. A period to allow for evaporation of moisture from the skin is needed. Nurses should also be meticulous about removing urine from the skin, so each incontinence episode should be followed by a thorough skin cleansing. Constant vigilance should be maintained to assess for changes occurring in the skin. Many nursing homes are unable to hire enough professional staff, and therefore much of the assessment is the responsibility of the nurses' aides. Skin assessment in-services need to be available to teach, not only about decubitus prevention and care, but also about signs of changes in skin integrity such as the pale, moist, shriveled skin that is so fragile.

Disposable incontinence briefs have freed many from the embarrassment of incontinence and allowed them to maintain dignity and continue to socialize with others. Prior to this, many were tied in wheelchairs or kept out of certain areas in nursing homes because of fears that they would be incontinent on upholstery or carpeting. These products can be an asset to the individual but they must be used properly.

REFERENCES

Beber, C. (1980). Freedom for the incontinent. *American Journal of Nursing, 80,* 482–484.

Bertholf, L. (1986). *Potential for skin impairment related to the use of disposable adult incontinence briefs.* Unpublished manuscript.

Boulton, S., & Kazemi, M. (1984). Evaluating disposable briefs. *American Journal of Nursing, 84,* 1413–1439.

Byrne, N., & Feld, M. (1984). Preventing and treating decubitus ulcers. *Nursing 84, 14,* 55-57.

Carpenito, L. (1983). *Nursing diagnosis: Application to clinical practice.* Philadelphia: J. B. Lippincott.

Delancy, V., & North, C. (1983). Skin assessment. *Topics in Clinical Nursing, 5,* 5–10.

Dossey, L. (1983). The skin, what is it? *Topics in Clinical Nursing, 5,* 1–4.

Fitzsimmons, V. (1983). The aging integument: A sensitive and complex system. *Topics in Clinical Nursing, 5,* 32–38.

Haecker, S. (1985). Disposable versus reusable incontinence products. *Geriatric Nursing, 6,* 345–347.

Hogstel, M. (1983). Skin care for the aged. *Journal of Gerontological Nursing, 9,* 431–437.

Hu, T., Kaltreider, D., & Igou, J. (1989). Incontinence products: Which is the best? *Geriatric Nursing, 10,* 184–186.

Mangieri, D. (1982). Saving your elderly patient's skin. *Nursing, 12,* 44–45.

McCormick, K., Scheve, A., & Leahy, E. (1988). Nursing management of urinary
    incontinence in geriatric inpatients. *Nursing Clinics of North America, 23,*
    231–263.
Phipps, M. (1984). Staging care for pressure sores. *American Journal of Nursing,*
    84, 999–1004.

[21]

Graded Exercise: Effect on Pressures Developed by the Pelvic Muscles

Molly C. Dougherty, Kevin R. Bishop,
Ruth A. Mooney, Phyllis A. Gimotty, and
Bradford Williams

Urinary incontinence affects between 15% and 30% of community-dwelling women and over 50% of women in hospitals and nursing homes (Diokno, Brock, Brown, & Herzog, 1986; Ouslander, 1990). Low-cost and low-risk techniques for self-management of urinary incontinence are important in the care of the elderly. Exercise of the muscles that support the bladder (Delancey, 1988) and contribute to urethral pressure (Gosling, Dixon, Critchley, & Thompson, 1981) has long been recommended by health professionals to improve postpartal restitution (Noble, 1982) and pelvic relaxation (Kegel, 1948), enhance sexual response (Kline-Graber & Graber, 1978), and manage stress urinary incontinence (SUI) (Wells, 1990). However, Wells found that in 22 studies in which pelvic muscle exercise was used in the treatment of SUI, exercise prescriptions varied widely. Wells therefore pointed to the importance of clearly describing the exercise prescription and using objective outcome measures. Our earlier research addressed some of these issues (Dougherty, Abrams, & McKey, 1986; Dougherty, Bishop, Mooney, & Gimotty, 1989). The purpose of this study was to determine the intensity and duration of pelvic muscle exercise necessary to significantly increase intravaginal pressure in healthy, aging women.

METHOD

Sample

The sample was recruited through posters in health and exercise centers, presentations to women's groups, and newspaper advertising in Gainesville, FL, and the surrounding area. Contacts with potential subjects focused on the potential health benefits of pelvic muscle exercise and the need for healthy women volunteers. Parous women, 35 years of age and over, who were in normal health and living in the community were studied. Before entry into the study, subjects gave informed consent and demonstrated the ability to relax the gluteal and abdominal muscles while contracting the pelvic muscles. Women who did not achieve a 5 mm Hg maximum intravaginal pressure during voluntary contractions of the pelvic muscles were excluded from the study. The 5 mm Hg limit was set on the assumption that women who could not achieve at least 5 mm Hg pressure did not have sufficient voluntary control of the pelvic muscle to achieve a training effect. An earlier study indicated that failure to control abdominal pressure contributed to higher variance in the pelvic muscle variable; therefore, women who could not maintain abdominal pressure increases at 5 mm Hg or less during pelvic muscle contractions were also excluded. Subjects received $50 for completing 12 weeks of pelvic muscle exercise at home and making five visits to the research site.

Intervention

The intervention was a graded program (increased every 3 weeks) of regular (3 times per week, every other day) pelvic muscle exercise at home lasting 12 weeks. Principles of exercise physiology (Astrand & Rodahl, 1977) were incorporated in the exercise program and included (1) testing and training the same activity; (2) regular training; (3) using an assessment interval (3 weeks) sufficient for training to have an effect; (4) developing endurance through repeated, sustained (12-second) contractions; and (5) developing strength through a burst of intense activity when initiating a contraction. The exercise program began with sessions requiring 15 repetitions of a 12-second contraction of the pelvic muscles. Ten repetitions were added every 3 weeks, resulting in 45 repetitions during the final (fourth) interval. An audio cassette tape recording was provided to guide the exercise sessions. The subjects received a telephone call from the project staff each week to monitor progress, and they submitted a written record of their exercise each week.

Measurements

Measures were taken at baseline and after Exercise Level 1 (15 repetitions), Exercise Level 2 (25 repetitions), Exercise Level 3 (35 repetitions), and Exercise Level 4 (45 repetitions). Subjects returned to the research site after each 3 weeks of exercise at home (5 visits total) and a repeat assessment was performed, as described below. For the baseline assessment, the subject assumed a modified (head elevated 20o) lithotomy position on the examining table. A bimanual examination was performed and the subject was coached through 4–5 pelvic muscle contractions. If needed, further coaching was done until the subject demonstrated the ability to contract the pelvic muscles while relaxing the abdominal and gluteal muscles.

For each measurement session an audio tape led the subject through a relaxation sequence of 3.3 minutes. Large muscle groups and the muscles of the hands and face were sequentially tightened and relaxed; special attention was directed to relaxation of the abdominal muscles. Instructions for pelvic muscle contractions were designed to (1) give hard, steady contractions, (2) deter retightening the muscle during the contraction, (3) begin the contraction at the sound of the tone provided, (4) end the contraction at the sound of a second tone, and (5) ensure full relaxation during the 15-second rest period. The audiotape provided cues to begin and end each of 10 contractions, which were recorded on the equipment. If problems arose, or the subject experienced difficulties during the assessment, the audio tape was stopped and the problems were corrected before proceeding.

Custom-fitted intravaginal balloon devices (IVBD) were used to measure the pressures developed by the pelvic muscles (Abrams et al., 1986; Dougherty et al., 1986). At the baseline assessment, an alginate (from Healthco International, Boston, MA) impression of the vagina was obtained; this impression was used to match an IVBD from a series of 11 sizes to the subject (Samples, Dougherty, Abrams, & Batich, 1988). The

IVBD was positioned in the distal one-third of the vaginal space. To monitor abdominal pressure, a $0.25 \times 1 \times 2$ cm posterior balloon device (PBD) was fabricated and positioned in the posterior fornix of the vagina. Water soluble lubricant was used to facilitate placement, and the comfort of the subject was assured before proceeding. One or two contractions were recorded to familiarize the subject with the procedure and to inspect the integrity of the system. When the assessment was completed, the measuring devices were removed.

The water-filled PBD and IVBD were attached to strain gauge pressure transducers (Bell & Howell, Chicago, IL) and a dual-channel strip-chart recorder (Cole-Parmer Instrument Co., Chicago, IL). The baseline for the system was established at atmospheric pressure and was calibrated with a mercury manometer (W.A. Baum, Copiague, NY) prior to collection of data.

Analog and digital data were obtained on the IVBD and PBD during 10 contractions representing maximum, sustained contractions of the pelvic muscles for 12 seconds and the corresponding abdominal pressure. The data were obtained at baseline and at the four exercise levels.

Tracings reflecting the pressures developed by the pelvic muscles during relaxation and contraction and the abdominal pressures were also obtained. The pressure curves for one subject at baseline and after 12 weeks of exercise are shown in Figure 21.1. The data were recorded simultaneously on a Compaq computer (Compaq Computer Corporation, Dallas, TX) using the acquisition portion of the ASYSTANT+ software (Macmillan, New York, NY).

Outcome variables were characteristics of the pressure curves: (1) maximum pressure, (2) minimum pressure, and (3) sustained pressure. Maximum pressure (mm Hg) was obtained by subtracting the resting pressure from the maximum pressure attained during each of 10 contractions and averaging the differences. Minimum pressure and sustained pressure required bracketing the 10 seconds representing maximal effort during the 12-second contraction, for each of 10 contractions. Minimum pressure was obtained by selecting the minimum value within the 10-second bracket for each contraction and averaging the 10 values. Sustained pressure was calculated by (1) obtaining the average pressure for 200 points over the 10-second bracket for each contraction, and (2) averaging the values obtained for the 10 contractions.

RESULTS

Of the 120 women who entered the study, 85 completed it. The subjects were between 35 and 78 years of age (mean 52.6; SD 10.6) and had given

FIGURE 21.1   Pelvic muscle pressure curves for one subject at baseline and
                  after 12 weeks of pelvic muscle exercise.

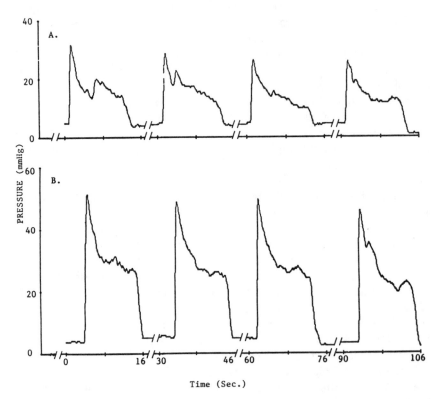

Time (Sec.)

Note: A = baseline; B = after 12 weeks of pelvic muscle exercise.

birth at least once (1 birth $n = 21$; 2 births $n = 27$; 3 births $n = 18$; more
than 3 births $n = 19$). Only 18 subjects reported having done any pelvic
muscle exercise before participating in the study; 58 reported never or
rarely experiencing urinary incontinence. Occasional leakage ($n = 13$) or
urge symptoms ($n = 9$) were reported. Several women reported having
had a hysterectomy ($n = 11$) or other pelvic surgery ($n = 18$), although
none reported having had surgery for incontinence. Nearly half ($n = 41$)
were premenopausal; the others had achieved menopause naturally or
as a result of surgery. On average, the subjects completed 33.5 (SD 7.1)
pelvic muscle exercise sessions out of the prescribed 36 sessions.

Improvement in maximum pressure, minimum pressure, and sustained pressure occurred at all exercise levels (see Figure 21.2 and Table
21.1). Multivariate analysis of variance showed that the differences
between exercise levels were statistically significant for all three outcome

FIGURE 21.2 Intravaginal pressures during voluntary contractions of the pelvic muscles at baseline and 4 levels of exercise ($N = 85$).

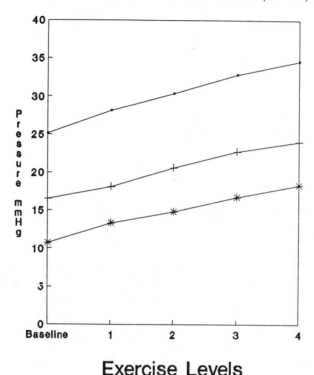

Exercise Levels

Note: Level 1 = 15 Repetitions, Level 2 = 25 repetitions, Level 3 = 35 repetitions, Level 4 = 45 repetitions.
Note: Maximum pressure . . .; sustained pressure + + +; minimum pressure * * *.

variables [maximum pressure F (4,81) = 18.4, p = .0001; sustained pressure F (4,64) = 12.2, p = .0001; and minimum pressure F (4,79) = 16.5, p = .0001]. That is, pressures increased significantly as exercise increased. When changes were examined across exercise levels, significant increases were found to occur in minimum, maximum, and sustained intravaginal pressure at Exercise Levels 1, 2, and 3, but only minimum pressure increased significantly at Exercise Level 4 (Table 21.2).

To examine the effects of parity and age, the women were categorized as para one (n = 21) or para greater than one (n = 64). They were also categorized by age into those 35–54 and those 55 years or older, which ensured postmenopausal status. The mean age of the younger group (n

TABLE 21.1   Pressures (mm Hg) for Outcome Variables at Four Exercise Levels[a]

Exercise level	Repetitions	Pressure					
		Maximum		Sustained		Minimum	
		Mean	SD	Mean	SD	Mean	SD
	n	85		68		83	
Baseline		25.1	11.7	16.5	9.2	10.7	7.2
Level 1	15	28.5	14.3	18.1	11.8	13.3	10.5
Level 2	25	30.4	16.0	20.6	13.9	14.8	11.7
Level 3	35	32.8	16.4	22.7	13.5	16.7	11.4
Level 4	45	34.5	17.5	24.0	15.0	18.3	13.0

[a]n is less than 86 when analysis of pressure curves was not possible for all subjects.

= 49) was 45.5 years (SD = 5.3), and the mean age of the older group (n = 36) was 63.3 years (SD = 6.4). When the pressure curve data were analyzed with age (<55 and $\geq$ 55) and parity (1 and >1), using multivariate analysis of variance, significant interactions between exercise level and age category were found for maximum pressure [$F_{(4,77)}$ = 3.21, p = .02], sustained pressure [$F_{(4,61)}$ = 4.25, p = .004], and minimum pressure [$F_{(4,75)}$ = 3.76, p = .008]. Women in the two age categories were relatively equal at baseline on all the outcome measures, but the younger group showed greater improvement by Exercise Level 4 (Table 21.3).

DISCUSSION

The greatest improvements in maximum pressure and minimum pressure occurred from baseline to Exercise Level 1; familiarity with the exercise procedure and increased ability to relax and concentrate at the research site may have accounted for this. In previous research, a 5 mm Hg change in maximum pressure was defined as clinically significant (Dougherty et al., 1989); a clinically significant change was not found at Level 1 in this study, however.

A consistent although small increase in the pressure variables occurred at both Level 2 and Level 3 exercise. The 5 mm Hg or greater increases were found by Level 2 for maximum pressure and for all three

TABLE 21.2 Changes (mm Hg) in Outcome Variables Across Exercise Levels[a]

Exercise level		Pressure					
		Maximum		Sustained		Minimum	
		Mean	F	Mean	F	Mean	F
	n	85		68		83	
Level 1–Baseline		3.4	11.7^b	1.6	6.7^b	2.6	12.7^b
Level 2–Level 1		1.9	5.5^b	2.5	5.3^b	1.5	5.1^b
Level 3 –Level 2		2.3	13.3^b	2.1	12.6^b	1.9	9.3^b
Level 4 –Level 3		1.8	3.0	1.3	2.4	1.6	5.3^b
Total change		9.4		7.5		7.6	
Percent change		37.5		45.5		71.0	

[a]n is less than 86 when analysis of pressure curves was not possible for all subjects.
[b]$p < .03$.

variables by Level 3. Significant improvement did not occur in maximum pressure or sustained pressure at Level 4. It may be that 35 repetitions per session represent the optimal exercise intensity, and 45 repetitions are demotivating, or it is possible that subjects lessened their exercise effort as the end of their commitment neared.

Wells (1990) found that pelvic muscle exercise prescriptions varied widely in published studies. Our results indicate that improvement occurs at much lower levels of exercise intensity than are usually reported in the incontinence literature. However, important questions about the relationship among continence mechanisms, pelvic muscle function, and exercise remain. Parity did not significantly affect performance on the exercise protocol, but age was significantly related to improvement. Although the older age group improved, increases in pressure curve variables were more gradual, suggesting that women age 55 and over may need more time or a more intense exercise intervention to obtain the desired results.

Better understanding of the pressure curves may contribute to improved behavioral management of incontinence. Maximum pressure may represent fast-twitch fibers and may be important in quickly increasing urethral pressure during events such as coughs or sneezes that

TABLE 21.3 Mean Pressures (mm Hg) for Outcome Variables by Age Category Before and at End of Exercise Protocol[a]

Age category	Exercise level	Pressure		
		Maximum	Sustained	Minimum
n		85	68	68
35–54	Baseline	24.5	16.8	12.1
	Level 4	35.8	27.5	21.8
55 or older	Baseline	25.5	16.2	9.7
	Level 4	30.6	19.6	13.6

[a]n is less than 86 when analysis of pressure curves was not possible for all subjects.

increase abdominal and bladder pressure and lead to involuntary urine loss. The muscle fibers of the external urethral sphincter are predominantly slow-twitch fibers capable of maintaining tone over prolonged periods without fatigue (Gosling et al., 1981). The activity of periurethral muscles may be better represented by sustained pressure and minimum pressure. Contractions that emphasize gradual, sustained effort may be indicated, because, as Balliet (1989, p. 190) notes: "Slower, smaller, weaker and fatigue-resistant motor units are not necessarily recruited before larger, faster, stronger and more easily fatigued motor units."

Clinicians may use the results from this study to teach pelvic muscle exercise and monitor the progress of women during an exercise intervention. Characteristics of the exercise intervention that appeared to contribute to improvement were these:

1. Begin with moderation, for example, 15 repetitions per session.
2. Increase the number of repetitions by 10 every 3 weeks.
3. Exercise every other day.
4. Build up to 35 repetitions per session.
5. Build the intensity of exercise over 12 weeks.
6. Isolate the pelvic muscles during exercise by assuming a posture that permits relaxation of the abdominal, gluteal, and quadraceps muscles.
7. Concentrate on each contraction.
8. Relax completely between contractions.
9. Rest for 1–3 minutes between each set of 10 contractions, or as needed.

10. Give a strong, maximum effort with each contraction.
11. Hold each contraction firm and steady. Do not retighten during a contraction. If concentration and hold are lost, relax completely and begin another contraction.

The research protocol included other elements that also may have contributed to success. For example, a preliminary assessment of the pelvic muscles was carried out, and the women returned for periodic pelvic muscle assessments. They also kept records of their exercises. It is not clear to what extent such records and assessments contributed to improvement, but it may be important to incorporate a clear pelvic muscle exercise plan, periodic clinical assessment, and follow-up and record keeping by the women.

The results of the study suggest that early gains reflect learning and that graded, regular exercise is needed to build the muscles. Older women respond to exercise more gradually than women 35–54 years of age, who experience improvement after 6 weeks and 25 repetitions per session. In two earlier studies employing the methods described here, reproductive-age women (mean = 34 years) (Dougherty et al., 1989) and reproductive-age women (mean = 36 years) with genuine SUI (Ferguson et al., 1990) carried out a graded pelvic muscle exercise protocol for 6 weeks, with significant improvements in maximum pressure (Dougherty et al., 1989) and in pressure curve variables and urine loss (Ferguson et al., 1990). Yet not all women improve with pelvic muscle exercise (Bishop, Dougherty, Mooney, Gimotty, & Williams, 1991). Though the reasons for failure to improve are not entirely clear, age is a factor. Therefore, clinicians should be careful to avoid offering false assurances about improvement: research-based statements may help to place the potential outcomes of exercise into perspective for women.

ACKNOWLEDGMENTS

This research was supported by a grant, "Managing Lower Urinary Tract Dysfunctions in Aging Women" (NR 1115), from the National Center for Nursing Research, National Institutes of Health. Co-investigators Robert Abrams and Christopher Batich provided expertise in physiology and in materials science and engineering, respectively.

REFERENCES

Abrams, R. M., Batich, C. D., Dougherty, M. C., McKey, P. L., Lin, Y. C., & Parker, J. (1986). Custom-made vaginal balloons for strengthening circum-vaginal musculature. *Biomaterial, Medical Devices, and Artificial Organs, 14,* 239–248.

Astrand, P. O., & Rodahl, K. (1977). *Textbook of work physiology* (2nd ed.). New York: McGraw-Hill.

Balliet, R. (1989). Facial paralysis and other neuromuscular dysfunctions of the peripheral nervous system. In R. P. Di Fabio, S. V. Paris, E. J. Protas, & A.F. VanSant (Eds.), *Manual of physical therapy*. New York: Churchill Livingstone.

Bishop, K. R., Dougherty, M. C., Mooney, R. A., Gimotty, P. A. & Williams, B. (1991). *Age, parity, and adherence: Factors affecting pelvic muscle performance*. Manuscript submitted for publication.

Delancey, J. O. L. (1988). The anatomy and mechanics of structures around the vesicle neck: How vesicle neck position might affect its closure. *Neurourology and Urodynamics, 7*(3), 161–165.

Diokno, A. C., Brock, B. M., Brown, M. B., & Herzog, A. R. (1986). Prevalence of urinary incontinence and other urologic symptoms in the non-institutionalized elderly. *Journal of Urology, 136*, 1022–1025.

Dougherty, M. C., Abrams, R. M., & McKey, P. L. (1986). An instrument to assess the dynamic characteristics of the circumvaginal musculature (CVM). *Nursing Research, 35*, 202–206.

Dougherty, M. C., Bishop, K., Mooney, R., & Gimotty, P. (1989). The effect of circumvaginal muscle (CVM) exercise. *Nursing Research, 38*, 331–335.

Ferguson, K. L., McKey, P. L., Bishop, K. R., Kloen, P., Verheul, J. B., & Dougherty, M. C. (1990). Stress urinary incontinence: Effect of pelvic muscle exercise. *Obstetrics and Gynecology, 75*, 671–675.

Gosling, J. A., Dixon, J. S., Critchley, O. D., & Thompson, S. A. (1981). A comparative study of the human external sphincter and periurethral levator muscles. *British Journal of Urology, 53*, 35–41.

Kegel, A. H. (1948). Progressive resistance exercise in the functional restoration of the perineal muscles. *American Journal of Obstetrics and Gynecology, 56*, 238–248.

Kline-Graber, F., & Graber, B. (1978). Diagnosis and treatment procedures of pubococcygeal deficiencies in women. In J. LoPiccolo & L. LoPiccolo (Eds.), *Handbook of sex therapy* (pp. 227–239). New York: Holt.

Noble, E. (1982). *Essential exercises for the childbearing year: A guide to health and comfort before and after your baby is born* (2nd rev. ed.). Boston: Houghton Mifflin.

Ouslander, J. G. (1990). Urinary incontinence in nursing homes. *Journal of the American Geriatrics Society, 38*, 289–291.

Samples, J. T., Dougherty, M. C., Abrams, R. M., & Batich, C. D. (1988). Dynamic characteristics of the circumvaginal muscles. *Journal of Obstetric, Gynecologic and Neonatal Nursing, 18*(3), 194–201.

Wells, T. J. (1990). Pelvic (floor) muscle exercise. *Journal of the American Geriatrics Society, 38*, 333–337.

[22]

Pelvic Muscle Exercise for Elderly Incontinent Women

Carol A. Brink, Thelma J. Wells, Carolyn M. Sampselle, Robert Mayer, and Ananias C. Diokno

This chapter reports a study of the effectiveness of pelvic muscle exercise (PME) as a treatment for urinary incontinence in elderly women (Wells, 1990). The data presented are part of a larger study conducted between 1982 and 1987 on 338 community-living women residing in Michigan (Wells, Brink, & Diokno, 1987; Diokno, Wells, & Brink, 1987). The study sought to identify the characteristics of urinary incontinence, to compare the effectiveness of specific behavioral exercises and pharmacologic treatments, and to explore the relationship of selected factors to pelvic muscle strength.

Pelvic muscle exercise (PME), a learned technique of perivaginal muscle contraction and relaxation, is directed at the muscles of the levator ani and, in particular, the pubococcygeus (Kegel, 1948). It is believed that through exercise these muscles increase in size and strength, exerting a greater force on the urethra, thus increasing closure pressure. Figure 22.1 displays a model that describes the effect of pelvic muscle exercise on urine control and identifies key intervening variables. In this model, relevant exercise components are techniques such as contraction time and exercise frequency, as well as teaching methods, with or without a resistive device. Exercise adherence is essential and directly affects pelvic muscle strength. Urogenital structure refers to anatomic dynamics such as urethral hypermobility. Health includes variables such as age, parity, previous bladder surgery, and physical status.

The study reported here was designed to determine:

1. What happens to pelvic muscle strength following a PME protocol?
2. Does pelvic muscle strength affect incontinence; i.e., is wetting reduced?
3. What factors explain differences in posttreatment muscle strength?

METHOD

The sample included community-dwelling women, 55 years of age and older, self-described as having uncontrolled urine loss, who were able to self-toilet and willing to participate and keep diary records. One hundred fifty-one women met the diagnostic criteria of having pure or predominantly stress incontinence and were assigned to the PME program. Eighty-six completed the study and constituted the final sample. The 43% attrition rate was due primarily to failure to complete the treatment program.

Intervention

The exercise protocol defined an exercise unit as a 10-second contraction followed by a 10-second relaxation. Ninety to 160 exercises were to be done daily for 6 months. Women were taught in a three-step program

FIGURE 22.1.   Pelvic muscle exercise and urine control model.

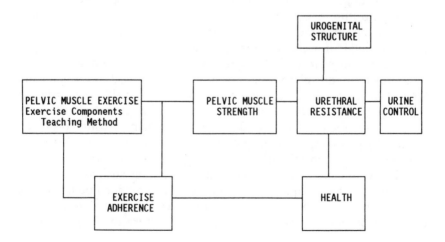

that represented different learning phases. Privacy, quiet, concentration, and "tuning into pelvic muscles" were emphasized in the first step. Stopping the urine stream while voiding was taught as an awareness technique during this step. The exercise itself was to be done while sitting on a firm chair with the feet flat on the floor and the knees apart. Clients were to squeeze as if to stop urine flow with a sensation of closing and lifting, or pulling inward, and to hold at least briefly. Step 2, "controlling pelvic muscles," moved beyond the quick contractions to the 10-second holding goal. Building muscle strength for a steady, sustained contraction was emphasized. Step 3 explored individual lifestyles and focused on incorporating the exercise into one's life routine, emphasizing exercise reminders, time for practice, and distracting or facilitating factors.

Data Collection

Evaluation measures included a digital test for pelvic muscle strength developed by Brink, Sampselle, Wells, Diokno, and Gillis (1989). In this test, subjects are asked to squeeze as hard as they can around two of the examiner's fingers. Using an integrated concept of pressure sensation and time duration, examiners score the contraction from 0 to 5 along a scale that has greater discrimination at the low or weak pressure end, i.e., 0, .3, .5, 1.0, 1.5, 2.0, 2.5, etc. Analysis of a condensed scale yielded a test–retest reliability of $r = .65$, $p < .01$ ($N = 228$), interrater reliability of $r = .91$, $p < .01$ ($N = 60$), and significant construct validity, based on correlations with selected history and vaginal myography data. Scores for this sample were obtained pre- and posttreatment, as well as at monthly intervals. Only pre- and posttreatment data are discussed here.

Treatment outcome evaluation was limited to subjective self-report, self-recorded diary of wetting, and a simple standing stress test. The self-report involved asking subjects to compare current to previous urine control, noting it as the same, better, or worse. The diary record was computed as the daily mean number of wettings for the week (7 days) preceding the evaluation. Both self-assessment and diary records are common measures in studies such as this one. The simple stress test required the subject to stand with a self-described full bladder, holding a tissue to the urethral meatus, and to cough vigorously one or two times. If the subject experienced involuntary loss of urine upon coughing, this was recorded. Validity of this measure of stress incontinence was supported by comparing the results to subsequent, more precisely instrumented urodynamic stress test findings; the two measures were significantly related ($\chi^2(1) = 15.04$, $p < .01$, $N = 257$).

RESULTS

The subjects' ages ranged from 55 to 89 with a mean of 67.2 years (SD = 8.3). Over two-thirds (69%) were self-referred to the study. The majority (88%) were either married or widowed. They were well educated, with 61% having some college or a graduate degree. Seventy-nine percent perceived their health as good to excellent.

Daily involuntary urine loss was experienced by two-thirds of the women. Eighty-one percent reported urine loss volumes sufficient to pool on the floor, run down their legs or wet their clothing. The majority (64%) had experienced wetting for from 1 to 10 years.

After a six-month PME protocol, outcomes ranged from a gain of 5 to a loss of 4 points on the digital test for pelvic muscle strength. For clarity we adjusted the clinical scoring to single-unit intervals from 1 to 12, that is, from lower to higher pressures. The mean change score was .8, or just below one unit, and the standard deviation of 1.7 suggested considerable variability (see Table 22.1). However, the computed standard error of measurement was .6, indicating a real but rather modest overall gain in pelvic muscle strength. A paired t-test indicated that the scores differed significantly from pre- to postprotocol testing [$t(85) = 4.39, p < .001$].

Further examination revealed that there were two different outcome groups: one with increased strength ($n = 47$) and one without increased strength ($n = 39$). Those who increased in strength did so in a range of 1–5 points with a mean of 2.0 (SD 1.1). Given the standard error of measurement of .6, this represents a measurable increase in strength. In the group who did not increase in strength, outcomes ranged from 0, that is, no change, to a 4-point decrease, with about half (51%) showing no change. The negative group had several outliers but otherwise clustered around .7, close to the standard error of measurement, suggesting that these individuals were probably a "no change" group. Overall, 55%

TABLE 22.1   Pelvic Muscle Strength Pre- and Post-PME Protocol[a]

Digital test	Mean	SD
Preprotocol	3.9	1.9
Postprotocol	4.7	2.2
Change score	0.8	1.7

[a]Paired $t(85) = 4.39, p < .001$

of the PME protocol group improved in pelvic muscle strength, and 45% did not.

There was no statistically significant difference between those who increased in pelvic muscle strength and those who did not in their subjective self-reports of urine control. About the same percentage in both groups reported urine control to be better (70% and 78%) or the same (28% and 22%). Only one person thought her urine control was worse; she was in the group who showed increased pelvic muscle strength.

The findings may reflect the value of attentive support; that is, whether the protocol resulted in increased muscle strength or not, it provided basic bladder health information and encouraged general behavioral change to improve urine control. Alternatively, perhaps subjective self-report is simply a poor measure; response may be affected by a desire to please.

Examination of self-recorded diaries of wetting revealed no statistically significant difference between those who increased in pelvic muscle strength and those who did not (see Table 22.2). Women were not selected for the study on the basis of a predetermined wetting level and initially reported wetting that ranged from daily to monthly or that varied under selected circumstances. Women who reported in their diaries a dry pretreatment status had a minimal history of involuntary urine loss. There were more diary reports of pretreatment dry status in the group who increased in pelvic muscle strength ($n = 10$) than among those who did not increase in strength ($n = 3$). The overall outcomes,

TABLE 22.2   Pelvic Muscle Strength Urine Control Outcome: Diary Report of Wet Status ($N = 49$)[a,b]

	Increased pelvic muscle strength ($n = 31$)		Not increased pelvic muscle strength ($n = 18$)	
Status	n	%	n	%
Dry to wet	4	13	1	6
Wet to more wet	5	16	3	17
Stayed dry	6	19	2	11
Wet to less wet	10	32	5	28
Wet to dry	6	19	7	39

[a]$\chi^2(4) = 2.79$, $p = .59$
[b]Possible outcomes have been ordered to reflect the most negative to most positive treatment response.

however, were similar for the two groups. The percentage of those who reported reduced wetting was 51% for those with increased strength and 67% for those who did not increase in strength. Interestingly, the percentage of women in the group who did not increase in strength who reported a change from wet to dry was greater than in the group who did increase in strength (39% versus 19%).

It is important to note that there were some missing data. Twenty-eight percent of the group with increased pelvic muscle strength and 51% of the group who did not increase in strength did not complete a posttreatment diary. This difference was significant ($p < .05$), pointing to a possible adherence problem in those who did not show increased strength. As a result, the self-recorded diary was not a very adequate measure of urine control outcome.

On the simple stress test, there was a significant difference between the group who increased in pelvic muscle strength and the group who did not [$\chi^2(3) = 11.6$, $p < .01$, $N = 53$] (see Table 22.3). However, it is difficult to explain the difference between the groups. This test was added as a measure during the course of the study and only 62% ($n = 53$) of the sample had complete data on the test; the percentages of the two groups for whom these data were missing were similar, however (36%, 41%). A total of 20 patients had negative outcomes both pre and post; that is, they lost no urine upon coughing. The majority of these (70%) were in the group who increased in pelvic muscle strength. Five women had negative pretreatment scores but had positive scores by the end of treatment; the majority of these (80%) were also in the increased strength group. Thirteen subjects stayed positive from pre- to posttreatment, most in the increased strength group. The expectation that those who began treatment positive would end with a negative score was met

TABLE 22.3 Pelvic Muscle Strength Urine Control Outcome: Simple Stress Test ($N = 53$)[a]

Outcome	Increased strength ($n = 30$)		Not increased strength ($n = 23$)	
	n	%	n	%
Negative to negative	14	47	6	26
Positive to positive	9	30	4	17
Negative to positive	4	13	1	4
Positive to negative	3	10	12	52

[a]$\chi^2(3) = 11.6$, $p < .01$

in only 15 women, 12 of whom were in the group who did not increase pelvic muscle strength.

If we assume a standard performance on the simple stress test—an assumption that is perhaps not warranted—the test is still probably too crude and indirect a measure to relate to pelvic muscle strength. That is, a static measure of pelvic muscle strength that is obtained vaginally while the patient is supine, even though a good measure, probably does not relate well to a dynamic urethral pressure challenge (a cough) in an upright position. However, the data suggest that a pretreatment negative stress test score may reflect minimal dysfunction; a positive test may reflect maximal dysfunction, but this needs further exploration.

To determine why some subjects increased pelvic muscle strength and others did not, exercise adherence, operationalized as the average number of exercises done over the 6-month, six-treatment period, was examined. The difference between groups was not statistically significant (ANOVA, $p = .08$). The group with increased pelvic muscle strength reported a mean of 71.5 exercises per day, in contrast to 56.8 in the group who did not increase strength. The average number of exercises done, however, may not be an adequate operationalization of exercise adherence. Consistency of exercise may be an important factor.

Examining selected relationships, it was reassuring to find that age was not significantly related to pelvic muscle strength gain. The mean ages were similar in the two groups, 67.9 (SD 8.8) and 66.5 (SD 7.7). Thus, age was apparently neither a barrier to nor a facilitator of increased pelvic muscle strength.

The number of vaginal deliveries was minimally correlated with pelvic muscle strength gain ($r = .19$, $p < .05$). Number of vaginal births ranged from 0 to 9. Of those having had vaginal births, the mean was 3.1 (SD 1.8). The low but positive correlation supports the view that vaginal deliveries are not a deterrent to increasing pelvic muscle strength.

DISCUSSION

Urinary incontinence and pelvic muscle strength are complex concepts. This study was an effort to explore these concepts, examine relationships between pelvic muscle exercise and urine control, and develop a model to begin explaining these relationships.

Our PME protocol succeeded in 55% of the women. However, based on subjective self-assessment and diary records, urine control did not significantly differ between those who increased pelvic muscle strength and those who did not. Both groups thought their urine control was better and recorded improvement in their diaries, although the group who did not increase in strength had more subjects who reported progressing from wet to dry status. While the simple standing stress test showed a significant difference between the two pelvic muscle strength groups, the group who did not increase in strength did better than the other group.

Interestingly, while the exercise protocol required 90 to 160 exercises daily, few women reached this goal. However, the higher exercise frequency in the increased pelvic muscle strength group (mean = 71.5) suggests that the standard was appropriate. Methods to increase exercise adherence and ensure proper exercise technique should be explored.

Clearly the urine control outcome measures were problematic. Urogenital structure variables such as hypermobility, operationalized as angle and distance measures derived from cystometrogram data; neurologic status as shown on physical examination; urethral resistance, derived from simultaneous bladder–urethral pressure measures; and pelvic muscle strength obtained from vaginal myography data all hold potential to further explain pelvic muscle strength differences.

ACKNOWLEDGMENTS

This research was supported by the National Institute on Aging (R01 AG03542) and BSRG 2 S07 RR05952-05 from the Biomedical Research Support Program, Division of Research Resources, NIH.

REFERENCES

Brink, C. A., Sampselle, C. M., Wells, T. J., Diokno, A. C., & Gillis, G. L. (1989). A digital test for pelvic muscle strength in older women with urinary incontinence. *Nursing Research, 38,* 196–199.

Diokno, A. C., Wells, T. J., & Brink, C. A. (1987). Urinary incontinence in elderly women: Urodynamic evaluation. *Journal of the American Geriatrics Society, 35,* 940–946.

Kegel, A. (1948). The nonsurgical treatment of genital relaxation. *Annals of Western Medicine and Surgery, 2,* 213–216

Wells, T. J. (1990). Pelvic (floor) muscle exercise. *Journal of the American Geriatrics Society, 38,* 333–337.

Wells, T. J., Brink, C. A., & Diokno, A. C. (1987). Urinary incontinence in elderly women: Clinical findings. *Journal of the American Geriatrics Society, 35,* 933–939.

[23]

Research on Incontinence: Implications for Practice

Thelma J. Wells

Years ago, when I was a graduate student, one of the things I did to keep myself sane was to visit a little old lady in the local nursing home. She was a great support to me—helping me through graduate school; and I like to think I helped her a bit. One day she confided to me that she wet her pants, and said that it was the most devastating experience she had ever had. As an enthusiastic graduate student I said to myself, "I can fix this. I'll just go to the library, look this up in a few books, come back and make this all work out right." And there began my search. I'd like to tell you that I cured that old lady's incontinence, but I didn't; however, she gave me the energy to pursue a cure. And the chapters in this book indicate how far we have come.

Wyman's chapter provides a comprehensive overview of current knowledge in urinary incontinence. Most research has focused on diagnostic evaluation, a limited but logical first step in understanding the complexity of this clinical problem. Wyman acknowledges that we are still in the early days of research on urinary incontinence with significant impediments to progress. It may surprise some clinicians that terminology used for diagnosis and treatment, and especially for behavioral programs, is neither totally agreed on nor fully developed. This difficulty reflects a conceptual issue, that is, what are the bases for both normal urine control and various challenges to this function? Interestingly, the state of our knowledge is dynamic, requiring the clinician to read the current work and to be alert to terms used and sensitive to underlying assumptions and explicit conceptual frameworks. Put simply, there are few established facts and many important questions; the clinician needs to keep an inquiring mind.

Wyman points out neglected areas in urinary incontinence research that may have special value for nursing: cross-cultural dimensions, male experiences, nonelderly experiences, failure to seek help, and standardization of urinary incontinence measures. She concludes with 14 specific recommendations for further research.

Two chapters explore risk: Pearson and Larson abstracted 12 urinary incontinence risk factors from the literature and developed specific risk-reduction interventions for a group of community-living women. They found significant risk reduction for all subjects by 6 months. Clinicians should value the preventive thrust of this interesting work and might try some of the suggested risk-reduction strategies. Taking a different tack, Bertholf and Popkess-Vawter assessed a measure to detect potential skin alteration in response to the use of disposable briefs for urinary incontinence. Interestingly, they found that skin capillary refill time may be a predictor of impending skin impairment.

Three chapters present behavioral treatment techniques for dealing with urinary incontinence in nursing homes. Each of the three presents a discrete technique, related to, but different from the others. Also, the studies vary in design, sample, and measures. These differences may be important; until research shows otherwise, the clinician will be wise to keep these factors in mind when interpreting the results.

Colling et al. describe a study in which the idea of targeting a toileting program to the incontinent individual's wetting pattern has moved into modern times through the use of a heat-sensitive electronic monitor over a 24-hour period with typical nursing home patients. This use of technology holds exciting potential for clinical practice; PURT, or patterned urge response toileting, is a system of prescribing toileting within 30 minutes of the individual's voiding pattern established by use of the monitor. The technique was successful in significantly reducing incontinence. The authors lament a staff treatment compliance rate of only 70% during the treatment program, however; in their view, greater staff compliance might have increased success. While the point is reasonable, 70% staff compliance seems quite impressive given the enormous demands of long-term care nursing and the difficulty created by change in practice. Thus, PURT and its underlying technology hold promise.

Schnelle et al. describe prompted voiding, a technique that requires the aide to approach the patient every 2–3 hours from 7:00 A.M. to 7:00 P.M. for a systematic verbal exchange and pant check and, usually, a toilet visit. Although prompted voiding reduces incontinence by as much as 36%, it has been found difficult to keep the program going when the researchers leave. Therefore, a statistical quality control program was developed to monitor compliance. As a further improvement, the whole program has been adapted to a computer system that sets standards, constructs control charts, and keeps patient records. The authors report a recent successful test of the computer-assisted prompted voiding program. Clinicians should welcome this advancement. Building on an established research base and utilizing helpful technology, the program has carefully evolved and is now ready for general clinical adoption.

Smith et al. demonstrated success with a toileting program based on prompted voiding concepts but differing from the original technique. Rather than a fixed 2–3 hour staff–patient voiding prompt contact, timing was set around established work routines such as patient waking and before meals. In practice this resulted in one less toileting prompt than with the standard prompted voiding technique. The authors argue that the alteration was done to improve staff compliance, which was determined to be 91%. Further differences included adding a pad/pant system and bedside commode to make toileting easier.

The clinician should be mindful of several common points in these three studies. All provide details about careful initial patient assessment. Any treatment program must always be preceded by patient assessment. Urinary tract infections, medication side effects, acute illnesses, and other disorders can cause or make worse urine control problems. While toileting programs will not harm patients, they are a waste of effort without effective screening for appropriateness. Another common theme in these chapters is staff compliance; toileting programs are dependent on aide involvement. To change practice from diapering rounds to toileting programs is a major task—not to be underestimated. Be sure you understand all about the technique, make careful plans, seek helpful resources, and remember change theory.

Two chapters describe pelvic muscle exercise as a technique to improve pelvic muscle strength and enhance urine control. Dougherty et al. explored the intensity, that is, the number of exercises per day, needed for pelvic muscle exercise to significantly increase intravaginal pressure in healthy women with a mean age of 52.6 (SD 10.6). Using a 12-second contract in the contract–relax exercise unit and graded 3-week exercise program, exercise units were increased from 15 to 45 on an every-other-day basis. Optimal exercise intensity for these women appeared to be 35 units every other day. Clinicians will benefit from the helpful suggestions provided for a pelvic muscle exercise program.

Brink et al. offer a model to describe the effect of pelvic muscle exercise on urine control. Their exercise program differed from the Dougherty et al. program in that the contract time per unit was 10 seconds and 90 to 160 units of exercise were done daily for 6 months. Also, the sample differed, being older (mean age 67) and incontinent. Strength was rated subjectively by the clinician rather than using an intravaginal device. Although the treatment protocol was the same for all the women, only 55% increased pelvic muscle strength. Issues of patient compliance and measurement were raised by the authors. This chapter cautions clinicians that while the literature generally supports pelvic muscle exercise as a useful technique to enhance urine control, it remains a complex behavioral technique with, as yet, little specificity to underlying pathology.

The two chapters on pelvic muscle exercise show that there is no established standard for contraction time or frequency of exercises, or for distribution within the frequency pattern, for example, all at one time or sets at fixed times. These and other issues remain to be resolved. The clinician would do best to recognize the potential importance of variance in technique and settle on an established technique such as either of the two presented here or others in the literature.

Where do we go from here? Many of us need to understand better the bases of urinary incontinence. These chapters all assume a very high level of understanding, but most clinicians receive no education about incontinence in undergraduate or graduate work, and many are probably not very familiar with the literature. Therefore, it is important to catch up. Twenty years ago, when I tried to find something in the library, I could find very little; now there is a great deal, and it is important to read it, and to keep up with the development of the research.

These chapters provide us a new way of looking at urinary incontinence—a way of questioning, a way of wondering, a way of noticing differences. There are new measures, clearer protocols, and better questions. Be brave; begin by thinking about your own practice. Be enthusiastic; working to improve practice is challenging but rewarding too. And be patient. Everyone, clinician and researcher alike, is committed to doing a better job. But it takes time to find answers and even more time to change practice. These chapters represent a good start.

Part IV

MANAGING COGNITIVE IMPAIRMENT

[24]

Managing Cognitive Impairment: The Current Bases for Practice

Virginia J. Neelon and Mary T. Champagne

Some time ago, the sports commentator Red Barber was asked about Jack Nicklaus's chances in the Master's tournament. Barber said, "As you get older, you can handle one day. But the mounting, relentless pressure of more than one day finally gets to you." The mounting, relentless pressure—that summarizes what we would like to convey about how hard it is for the cognitively impaired to respond to challenges in the environment.

First we will review the issues underlying the increasing prevalence of acute and chronic cognitive dysfunction in the elderly. From a clinical perspective, there are three problem areas: inadequate understanding, underdetection and misdiagnosis, and inadequate treatment and care. We will then highlight the encouraging progress made in our understanding of the problem over the last 10 years and examine ideas about aging and function—crossing disciplines—that provide a link between what we have learned and how we might use the knowledge to develop interventions. And finally, we would like to call attention to the barriers to change in our practice and urge a commitment to make a difference—to improve care and outcomes for patients with acute and chronic cognitive impairment. What is required is not only knowing about the problem, but doing something about what we know.

Cognitive impairment is most frequently characterized by dysfunction in one or more of the following "higher cortical" functions:

1. perception, which is the ability to attend and meaningfully interpret sensory information;

239

2. thinking, which is a conscious process that refers to awareness and language and knowledge of objects and includes abilities to understand, reason, make decisions, and apply judgment;
3. memory, which is the retention and recall of previous experience and knowledge, including tasks and concepts, and the ability to store new information.

Cognitive impairment is a defining feature of a number of impairments characterized by the term "disturbed information processing." There are six problems or states that, along with other unique and overlapping features, may have impairment in cognitive function as a major manifestation: acute confusion or delirium, dementias, depression and psychosis, mental retardation, brain injury, and terminal state. The discussions in this volume focus for the most part on the first two problems: delirium or acute confusion, and dementia. This chapter will primarily address the problem of delirium or acute confusion, which differs from chronic or progressive impairment by its rapid onset (hours, days, weeks), fluctuating manifestations, abrupt deterioration of present mental status, and potential for reversibility.

There are two major barriers to early detection and treatment of acute confusion. First there is controversy about how to measure it in acutely ill patients, especially older patients. Even the simplest mental status tests require the patient to respond, to perform; and these types of tests are not very well suited to the acute care setting. A second barrier is the controversy about what this syndrome is—and even about what its name is. *Delirium* is the term recommended in the psychiatric evaluation of acute organic brain disorders in medical and surgical patients. The term most commonly used in nonpsychiatric specialties is *acute confusion* or *acute confusional states*.

It is important to differentiate acute confusion from the diagnosis of dementia. Dementia-like syndromes refer to chronic, generally irreversible, and progressive cognitive impairments reflecting loss of previously acquired higher cognitive functions in an alert subject. Acute confusion or delirium is a disturbance in information processing resulting from a reversible, diffuse impairment of higher cortical function, including the loss of attention and alertness.

The diagnostic criteria for delirium formulated in the *Diagnostic and Statistical Manual of Mental Disorders* of the American Psychiatric Association (DSM-III-R) (1987) are these:

1. reduced ability to attend to external stimuli;
2. disorganized thinking, irrelevant or incoherent speech;

3. at least two of the following:
   reduced level of consciousness,
   perceptual disturbances,
   disturbed sleep-wake cycle,
   increased/decreased psychomotor activity,
   disorientation, memory impairment—poor learning and difficulty
   in reporting past events;
4. onset of short duration, symptom fluctuation;
5. evidence of an etiological organic factor or absence of a nonorganic
   mental disorder.

These criteria have some limitations, however. They emphasize extreme, overt behaviors—the so-called delirious state: hallucinations and agitated psychomotor behavior. They undervalue milder or more subtle manifestations—the quiet confused; and they include several items that are frequently associated with acute medical illness or postoperative status in the elderly—sleep/wake disturbance, organic related causes that are commonly present in this population, and reduced level of consciousness.

Confusion is a physiologic assault on the body and mind—it has serious adverse consequences. Patients, particularly elderly patients who already have chronic cognitive impairments, are at higher risk for superimposed acute confusional states during acute illness or after surgical interventions. Dependence on extreme delirium-like manifestations or overlooking acute deterioration of mental status in the chronically impaired and viewing it as part of the dementing process delays diagnosis and intervention and puts the patient at great risk of complications, of higher mortality, of prolonged hospital stays, and of lessened functional recovery at the time of discharge or post-discharge (Fields, MacKenzie, Charlson, & Sax, 1986; Gillick, Serrell, & Gillick, 1982; Levkoff, Safran, Cleary, Gallop, & Phillips, 1988; Lipowski, 1983; Rabins & Folstein, 1982).

Among hospital patients, the incidence and prevalence of acute confusion are reported to be high and increasing. The incidence in postoperative patients has been estimated to range from less than 10% to as high as 70% in some populations (Sadler, 1981; Smith & Dimsdale, 1989; Williams, Campbell, Raynor, Mlynarczyk, & Ward, 1985). Several studies of medical patients have reported incidence/prevalence rates of 25-40% (Foreman, 1989; Gillick et al., 1982; Hodkinson, 1973, 1981; Neelon & Champagne, 1988). We have actually seen an increase in prevalence from the original study that we completed in 1988, where the prevalence rate was 39%, to more than half the population (52%) at the time of admission in a more recent study. And also, nearly half of the patients in our more recent studies have some measurable level of cognitive impairment at discharge. This increase reflects the trend in hospital admissions toward a population that is older and sicker, with a higher prevalence of chronic cognitive impairment, bringing an increased risk of acute confusion.

Differences in the types of patients, the classification systems used to diagnose the problem, and the places where the assessment is done are among the problems in determining just how prevalent acute confusion is in the clinical setting. It is hard to evaluate patients with cognitive impairment. Because the prevalence is highest on admission to an acute care setting, it is important to evaluate patients in the first 24 hours after admission. Yet standard assessment tools are not easy to administer to the cognitively impaired in the acute care setting, and confusion is hard to document; it is often overlooked or missed because of the fluctuating nature of the problem. Thus, many things make for variability in evaluating incidence and prevalence.

Multiple factors lead to the development of acute confusion; and most probably, there is no single pathophysiologic mechanism underlying its varied manifestations. The primary hypotheses focus on factors affecting cerebral oxidative metabolism, impaired synthesis of acetylcholine, and abnormalities in synaptic transmission (Engel & Romano, 1959; Levkoff et al., 1988; Lipowski, 1983). It is also important, however, to discover how environmental factors can provoke so much physiologic derangement in so many patients. As studies begin to accumulate on abnormalities in the chemical milieu of the central nervous system— endorphins, cortisol, interleukens—we are gaining a better sense of how external stress can elicit the biochemical changes that can cause this kind of problem.

Acute confusion presents as a spectrum of nonadaptive psychophysiologic responses characterized by disordered cognition (perception, thinking, and memory); dysfunction of the reticular activating system (attention and wakefulness); and dysfunction of the autonomic nervous system (psychomotor and regulatory functions).

Different presentations are seen in different patients; some patients present almost immediately with cognitive signs and cues, while other patients present with autonomic nervous system disturbances as early cues. In fact, the manifestations may take on different patterns within the same patient.

Given the multiple psychobiologic stressors and the lower reserves of the ill elderly, the real question may be why more patients do not develop acute confusion.

We have made some progress in what we know, even if we have not made much progress in how we use this knowledge. Physiologic and psychosocial research on changes in function with age provide a foundation for understanding the greater risk of cognitive dysfunction and the complexity of its manifestations in elderly patients.

Three ideas about the association of chronic conditions with aging help us understand the increased risk of acute confusional states in the elderly: diminishing reserve capacity, the threshold of functional integrity, and the multifactorial nature of the pathogenesis and manifestations of acute confusion.

The reserve capacity of many organs and systems diminishes with age. Whatever we do with life, as we get older, we lose reserve function. There is not an athlete alive who does not know this. If you measure the elderly at rest, you may not elicit the signs of diminished reserve. What is lost or increasingly at risk is the ability to respond to challenge—to multiple, increasing levels of stressors or load (Johnson, 1985). It is not clear why this is the case. It may take longer to synthesize or store or activate vital biochemical substrates, or the elderly may have less effective mechanisms to remove metabolic wastes. Eventually, these kinds of things take their toll on the function of systems.

From these data, we gain a principle about intervention: conserving reserves—as limited as they may be—and timing the amount and duration of challenge with rest and restoring periods may underlie effective treatment of the cognitively impaired.

A second concept useful for examining the development of acute confusion is the threshold nature of vulnerability (Drachman, 1983). When functional systems, and particularly neuronal function, reach a certain threshold, that is, the point at which reserves are depleted, continued challenge presses these systems beyond functional resources, often causing irreversible damage or failure in the system. This explains the cascade effect that we frequently see with acutely ill elderly patients. That is, you affect or try to intervene in one system but within a short time several other systems—which are also at "threshold"—go into disarray. When you go beyond the threshold of vulnerability, the system truly disintegrates.

Thus there is a second principle we need to incorporate in our intervention framework: preventing challenges to systems when they are most vulnerable for irreversible damage—when they are near threshold. You can extrapolate this principle to understand the vulnerability of the acutely chronically ill, cognitively impaired person.

We are using these principles in trying to understand the development of acute confusion in the clinical setting. We consider acute confusion/delirium to be an extreme manifestation of a spectrum of non-adaptive responses to the cumulative effect of multiple challenges. We have described a spectrum of increasing risk and increasing load (see Figure 24.1). Some patients come in with minimal risk factors, or minimal load, and with these patients there is some margin of safety before you see any kind of disturbed or dysfunctional behavior. This may explain why, with all that is happening to them, they have not become confused. It is because they come in with some kind of protective margin, or reserve capacity. Many other elderly patients are already further along the curve, near the threshold. It does not take much added adversity to cause dysfunction, to bring them to a clinical level of manifestation. The acutely ill elderly with chronic cognitive impairment are at greatest risk. So we are always trying to evaluate where on this curve people are. And the more frequently people travel up this curve, the less likely they are to come back to baseline.

The third principle that can serve as a basis for intervention comes from psychosocial-environmental frameworks that recognize the relationships between environmental stressors and dysfunctional behavior. The concepts of Lawton and Nahemow (1973) play a great part in how people look at the problem of acute confusion and chronic cognitive

FIGURE 24.1.   Spectrum of disturbed information processing.

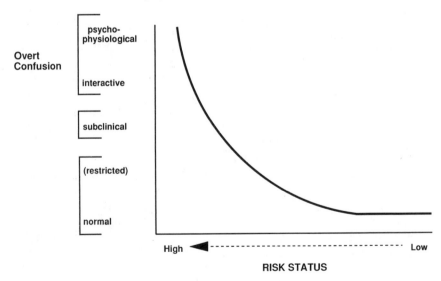

Note: From V. Neelon & M. Champagne (1988), "Acute Confusion in Hospitalized Elders: Patterns and Interventions," grant proposal funded by the National Center for Nursing Research, NIH. Grant #2 R01 NR01339–04.

impairment. Lawton developed a model in which there is a range of environmental press within which the individual functions in comfort and with the potential for maximum performance. The quality of the individual's function and adaptation depends on the characteristics of the person—labeled competence, and a more general phenomenon—called "environmental press."

Competence involves the domains of biological health, sensorimotor function, cognitive skills, and ego strength. Lawton and Nahemow (1973) classified environments on the basis of "demand character": some environments place great behavioral demands on people, and the hospital environment must rank at the top of "pressing" environments. The way a person with a given level of competence performs in an environment with a given press level may be placed on a continuum, from very negative, when press is too little or meaningless, to positive, where rest and function are maximized, back to negative, when press is too great. We are talking not only about a point of negative effect because of too much load, but also about a point where the load or press or the sense of the environment is inadequate to help the person remain either in comfort or perform or function maximally (see Figure 24.2).

Two important principles emerge from this model (Staats, 1984). As Staats notes, at every level of competence, the environmental press can be too little or too great. Further, for patients who have a low level of competence, who are acutely ill and hospitalized, a small change in environmental press may lead to a large change in the degree of adaptation. For example, letting a patient wear some of his own clothes, letting a woman keep her pocketbook, or letting the person have pictures and treasured possessions in the room may have a sizable benefit. However, these same measures might have little or no effect on an individual who is functioning at a higher level of competence, because such small changes would then have an insignificant impact on level of adaptation. This might explain why some of our generally applied interventions, like clocks and calendars, are not very effective with many patients in the hospital setting, because the patients have varied levels of competence and need, and these interventions are not specific to those varied levels.

Although the regulation of patient environments is recognized as a therapeutic domain of nursing, the lack of conceptual understanding that links internal functional integrity and external adaptive performance has limited the development of effective intervention strategies.

The model in Figure 24.3 is based on the concepts of limited reserve, threshold vulnerability, and internal and external press. Using these concepts, we have developed a hierarchy of factors that might relate to the development of acute confusion, and also help to describe patterns

FIGURE 24.2. Environmental press.

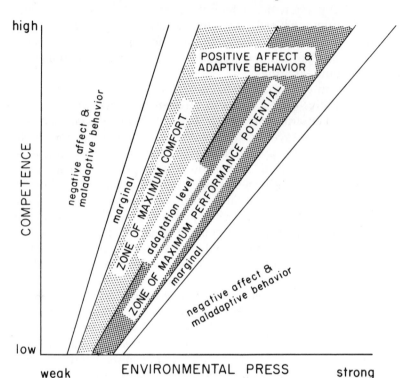

Note: Adapted from M. Lawton & L. Nahemow (1973), "Ecology and the Aging Process" in C. Eisdorfer & M. Lawton (Eds.), The Psychology of Adult Development and Aging. Copyrighted by the American Psychological Association, 1973. Used with permission.

of confusion development (Neelon, Champagne, & McConnell, 1987). We have observed at least three patterns of confusion development. One pattern is seen in patients with low cognitive reserve, who are extremely susceptible to environmentally provoked states. A second pattern is seen in patients with low physiologic reserve, where physiologic factors and efforts to stabilize physiologic factors are key. And finally, a third pattern involves low biochemical reserve, where toxic agents are key in the development of acute confusion.

This framework also indicates how to intervene with people with acute confusion. Basically, at Level 1, those individuals with primary problems in vital function, oxygen-energy components, obviously need as their major interventions ways to stabilize these functions. Similarly,

FIGURE 24.3. Interactive level of information processing: A framework for factor identification in confusion development.

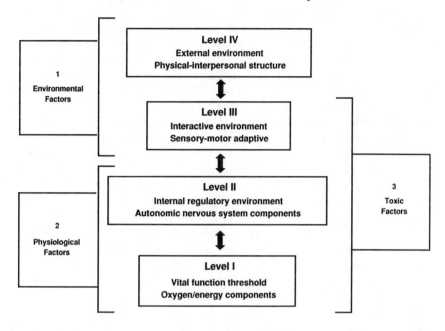

Note: From V. Neelon & M. Champagne (1988), "Acute Confusion in Hospitalized Elders: Patterns and Interventions," grant proposal funded by the National Center for Nursing Research, NIH. Grant #2 R01 NR01339–04.

internal regulatory patterns may be the key for many other kinds of patients, and ways of stabilizing reserve capacity and minimizing challenge to reserves may be the crucial intervention. Level 3 interacts very closely with the environment and involves sensorimotor types of adaptations. Lastly, factors in the environment themselves may impinge on how well somebody can function.

Thus, these concepts are guiding our approaches to interventions, which are broadly divided into two groups: first, modification of factors to prevent or reverse the confusional state, and second, strategies to reduce morbidity during the confusional episode.

Hall and Buckwalter (1987) have also used these concepts, particularly Lawton's competence model, to develop a framework for understanding stresses related to the symptoms and behavior observed in chronically cognitively impaired individuals, including confusion, agitation, combative behavior, and nighttime waking. Adults with dementia exhibit three main types of behavior: baseline, anxious, and dysfunctional. The proportions of each type of behavior change with the progression of the disease. Baseline is a socially accessible state—the person is calm, able to communicate needs and respond to communications from others; he is cognitively accessible—aware of or oriented to the environment (Wolanin & Phillips, 1981). In the anxious state, the person feels stress, he loses eye contact and exhibits avoidance behavior—the person avoids offending stimuli (people, questions, technical press). However, the caretaker can still maintain contact. The dysfunctional state reflects cognitive and social inaccessibility. The patient is unable to communicate effectively with others and is unable to use the environment in a functionally appropriate manner. He may exhibit catastrophic behavior (Wolanin & Phillips, 1981). Here again, one sees the idea of increasing stress or press on the individual, taking him from a normal or adequately performing state into a so-called disabled, anxious state and eventually beyond threshold into disturbed and dysfunctional behavior. Many chronically cognitively impaired patients spend most of their time in this anxious, unstable, and dysfunctional state. They may arise or start their day in a more functional way, but as the press of the environment increases, their activity becomes less and less functional.

The suggestions for intervention are very similar to those we have suggested and Lawton suggests: if you program or structure the environment, that is, program challenges, you can keep the individual in the zone of functional behavior. Several other people are also looking at different methods of structuring activity for cognitively impaired patients, to prevent or minimize dysfunctional behavior. All of these discoveries, links, and frameworks provide some clear guides for effective interventions which protect and promote cognitive integrity (see Table 24.1).

First, increase internal competence; that is, preserve or restore internal reserves and minimize challenge near threshold. Second, optimize the environmental press—and we use the word *optimize* so that

TABLE 24.1 Cognitive Protecting Model

Increase Internal Competence
    Preserve/Restore Internal Reserve
    Minimize Challenge Near Threshold Function

Optimize Environmental Press
    Enhance "Meaningful" Signals and Minimize "Noise"
    Support Positive Cognitive Protecting Behaviors
    Diminish Demands During Acute Illness

---

we recognize the need to define the essential environment that people need to function in. Enhance meaningful stimuli, minimize noise, support positive cognitive behaviors that reduce stress, promote comfort, and enhance performance. And diminish demands during illness.

Wolanin and Phillips (1981) say: "It is our position that, unless confusion is viewed as secondary to some other cause, and treated as such, the frequency, intensity, and amount of confusion that is seen will remain unchanged, and acute confusion will inevitably lead to irreversible confusional states" (p. 101). Nothing we have observed would lead us to think differently from this. If anything, present concerns with costs, unnecessary stress to "old" patients and their families, and the continued tendency to associate the word *demented* with *hopeless* lead to misdiagnosis and undertreatment of confused older patients (Neelon, 1990).

REFERENCES

American Psychiatric Association. (1987). *Diagnostic and statistical manual of mental disorders*, 3rd Ed., Revised, Washington, DC: Author.

Drachman, D. (1983). How normal aging relates to dementia. In D. Samuel (Ed.), *Aging and the brain* (pp. 19–31). New York: Raven.

Engel, G., & Romano, J. (1959). Delirium: A syndrome of cerebral insufficiency. *Journal of Chronic Diseases, 9,* 260–277.

Fields, S., MacKenzie, C., Charlson, M., & Sax, M. (1986). Cognitive impairment: Can it predict the course of hospital patients? *Journal of the American Geriatrics Society, 34,* 579–585.

Foreman, M. (1989). Confusion in the hospitalized elderly: Incidence, onset, and associated factors. *Research in Nursing and Health, 12,* 21–29.

Gillick, M., Serrell, N., & Gillick, L. (1982). Adverse consequences of hospitalization in the elderly. *Social Science and Medicine, 16,* 1033–1038.

Hall, G., & Buckwalter, K. (1987). Progressively lowered stress threshold: A conceptual model for care of adults with Alzheimer's disease. *Archives of Psychiatric Nursing, 1,* 399–406.

Hodkinson, H. (1973). Mental impairment in the elderly. *Journal of the Royal College of Physicians of London, 7,* 305–317.

Hodkinson, H. (1981). Value of admission profile tests for prognosis in elderly patients. *Journal of the American Geriatrics Society, 29,* 206–210.

Johnson, H. (1985). Is aging physiological or pathological? In H. Johnson (Ed.), *Relations between normal aging and disease.* New York: Raven.

Lawton, M., & Nahemow, L. (1973). Ecology and the aging process. In C. Eisdorfer & M. Lawton (Eds.), *The psychology of adult development and aging.* Washington DC: American Psychological Association.

Levkoff, S., Safran, C., Cleary, P., Gallop, J., & Phillips, R. (1988). Identification of factors associated with the diagnosis of delirium in elderly hospitalized patients. *Journal of the American Geriatrics Society, 36,* 1099–1104.

Lipowski, Z. (1983). Transient cognitive disorders (delirium, acute confusional states) in the elderly. *American Journal of Psychiatry, 140,* 1426–1436.

Neelon, V. (1990). Response to "Mental status change in the elderly: Recognizing and treating delirium" by C. Morency. *Journal of Professional Nursing, 6,* 364–365.

Neelon, V., & Champagne, M. (1988). Nutrition and cognitive function in the hospitalized elderly. *Biomedical Advances in Aging '88.* VIIIth International Washington Spring Symposium. George Washington University (Abstract).

Neelon, V., Champagne, M., & McConnell, E. (1987). Acute confusion in the hospitalized elderly: Patterns and early diagnosis. *Nursing Advances in Health: Model, Methods, and Application.* International Nursing Research Conference Abstracts. Kansas City: American Nurses' Association (Abstract).

Rabins, P., & Folstein, M. (1982). Delirium and dementia: Diagnostic criteria and fatality rates. *British Journal of Psychiatry, 140,* 149–153.

Sadler P. (1981). Incidence, degree, and duration of postcardiotomy delirium. *Heart & Lung, 10,* 1084–1092.

Smith, L., & Dimsdale, J. (1989). Postcardiotomy delirium: Conclusions after 25 years? *American Journal of Psychiatry, 146,* 452–458.

Staats, D. (1984). Physical environments. In C. K. Cassel & J. R. Walsh, (Eds.), *Geriatric medicine: Medical, psychiatric and pharmacological topics. 2,* 436–447.

Williams, M., Campbell, E., Raynor, W., Mlynarczyk, S., & Ward, S. (1985). Reducing acute confusional states in elderly patients with hip fractures. *Research in Nursing & Health, 8,* 329–337.

Wolanin, M., & Phillips, L. (1981). *Confusion, prevention and care.* St. Louis: Mosby.

[25]

Clinical Assessment of Confusion

Patricia E. Hadley Vermeersch

Confusion is a multidimensional problem (Foreman, 1986, 1987; Vermeersch, 1986, 1990; Wolanin & Phillips, 1981), and these multiple dimensions have made both definition and measurement difficult. Differences in conceptualization have driven instrument development in a variety of directions—focusing, for example, on cognitive change, functional tasks, or behavior patterns. Two themes, however, are consistent: (1) confusion is perceived by nurses as multidimensional, and (2) it is diagnosed based on observation of multiple patient behaviors. An instrument to measure confusion in hospitalized adults should therefore (1) reflect the nurse's perception of the phenomenon as multidimensional; (2) supply the nurse with objective and consistent patient behaviors descriptive of the presence and level of confusion; (3) have demonstrated validity and reliability; and (4) be clinically useful, that is, address phenomena of direct clinical nursing relevance, be brief and easy to use, and directly facilitate use of one or more aspects of the nursing process (Nagley, 1984; Vermeersch, 1990; Wolanin & Phillips, 1981).

Two new instruments have begun to address the inadequacies of older instruments. The NEECHAM Confusion Scale developed by Champagne, Neelon, and McConnell (1987) is an observational scale developed deductively from information processing theory and is designed to measure acute confusion in the hospitalized elderly. The Clinical Assessment of Confusion, also an observational scale, was developed inductively from the behaviors nurses use to describe confusion. It is also designed to measure confusion in hospitalized adults. This second scale, which was developed by the author, currently exists in two forms.

Table 25.1   Clinical Assessment of Confusion-A with Visual Analogue Scale of Confusion

1. Patient   _____
2. Nurse   _____
3. Date   _____ Time _____

Directions: Under each category circle the number for each behavior the patient has exhibited. Next, sum the numbers for each category and for the total scale.

Cognition

1. Extreme forgetfulness	4
2. Forgetfulness	3
3. Decreased ability to concentrate	3
4. Altered conceptualization	3

(Maximum = 13) Sum __

General behavior

5. Noisy	3
6. Not recognizing limitations of illness	3
7. Restless	3
8. Difficulty relating to others	3
9. Antagonistic	3
10. Withdrawn	2
11. Irritable	2
12. Demanding	2
13. Apathetic	2

(Maximum = 23) Sum __

Motor activity

14. Speech slurred	3
15. Altered voluntary motor response	3
16. Absence of any meaningful response	3
17. Altered involuntary motor response	2
18. Little body movement	2

(Maximum = 13) Sum __

Orientation

19. No idea of place	4
20. Calling people from past	4
21. Calling someone known to him/her by another name	4

(Maximum = 12) Sum __

Table 25.1 *Continued*

___

Psychotic/neurotic behaviors

22. Delusional	....	4
23. Paranoid ideation	....	4
24. Talking to people not actually present	....	4
25. Behavior regressed, repulsive, and/or repetitive	....	4

(Maximum = 16) Sum __

(Maximum = 77) Total score __

Additional behaviors:

Visual Analogue Scale of Confusion[a]
Directions: On the line place a "/" indicating your overall assessment of the patient's level of confusion.

___

No Confusion   Severe Confusion
___

[a]Adapted with permission from Nagley, S. J. (1984). Prevention of Confusion in Hospitalized Elderly Persons. *Dissertation Abstracts International, 45*(06B), 1732. (University Microfilms International No. 8420848)

The Clinical Assessment of Confusion-A (CAC-A) is a 25-item observational scale developed in a two-phase study. That study has been described in detail elsewhere (Vermeersch, 1990). Briefly, in Phase One of the study, 228 medical-surgical nurses rated 141 patient behaviors as more or less important in determining the presence of confusion in hospitalized adults. On the basis of these ratings, the 25-item observational scale was developed. Factor analysis was then used to identify five underlying dimensions of confusion: cognition, general behavior, motor activity, orientation, and psychotic/neurotic behavior. To reflect more accurately the importance each item carried in the diagnosis of confusion, the items on the scale were weighted using the average importance rating given to the item by the 228 nurses.

The resulting instrument is scored by summing the weights of behaviors nurses check as present within each dimension of confusion, and by summing for a total score. It is assumed that the higher the score, the greater the confusion. No training beyond the printed directions is considered necessary for use of the instrument. The CAC-A is presented in Table 25.1.

In Phase Two of the study, the validity and reliability of the CAC-A were determined from 305 observations made on 129 medical or surgical patients by 24 nurses. Concurrent validity was determined by comparing CAC-A scores with the global ratings of confusion given patients on the Visual Analogue Scale of Confusion (VAS-C). Each dimension of the CAC-A correlated with the VAS-C rating at .50 or above. Multiple regression indicated that the dimensions of the CAC-A explained 53% of the variance in the VAS-C ratings ($r = .73$), with all five dimensions contributing significantly ($p = .05$) to the relationship. Interrater reliability of the CAC-A was measured using Pearson's r for 23 pairs of observations; the r was .88, a value adequate for the study sample.

The fact that the CAC-A measures a concept of direct clinical nursing relevance was evidenced by the validity and reliability results of both phases of the study. Also, the study nurses reported to the investigator that the CAC-A was easy for them to use since it required little if any training (directions were printed on the CAC-A form) and took less than 5 minutes to complete once the nurse had used it with one or two patients. There were, however, questions about the meaning of some items (for example, "altered conceptualization"). The clinical utility of the CAC-A was thus only partially established by the study. Also, because the study did not examine whether or how the CAC-A facilitated the nursing process, no conclusions could be drawn regarding this aspect of clinical utility.

Written and verbal comments from the nurses participating in the study raised some issues about the content validity of certain subscales and pointed to problems in deciding how to evaluate the severity and duration of certain behaviors. As a result, the CAC-A was expanded and modified, and a new scoring procedure was developed. This resulted in the CAC-B, a 58-item instrument with one general screening item and seven subscales: cognition; general behavior; motor activity/speech motor ability/sensory acuity; orientation; behaviors that threaten the safety of the patient; psychotic/neurotic behaviors; and ability to interact/perform ADL/speech content. All items on the CAC-B are evaluated by checking one of three boxes: not present, present intermittently, or present continuously. Items are given a corresponding score of 1, 2, or 3 except for two items ("intact but lacks knowledge or understanding of situation or illness" and "pleasant, cooperative"), which are reverse scored. As with the CAC-A, the assumption is that the higher the score, the more confused is the patient. No training beyond the written directions is considered necessary for use of the instrument, which takes approximately 10 minutes to complete. The CAC-B is presented in Table 25.2.

The CAC-B was reviewed by a panel of three experts for content validity, inclusiveness, and areas needing improvement or modification. Content validity was determined using the method described by Lynn (1986) in which the content validity index (CVI) is "derived from the

TABLE 25.2   Clinical Assessment of Confusion-B

PART I: Initial assessment: Level of consciousness

1. Circle one of the following:
    a. Alert and not confused at any time.
    b. Alert but confused sometimes, at any level.
    c. Alert but confused continuously, at any level.
    d. Alert but unable to interact due to medical diagnosis or treatment (e.g., aphasia of some kind, paralysis such that the patient cannot communicate verbally or in writing with words, intubated, etc.).
    e. Lethargic, difficult to arouse. May or may not be confused at some level.
    f. Comatose, responds only to deep painful stimuli or does not respond to any stimuli.

Directions: Circle the appropriate number for each item. Next, sum the numbers for each category and for the total scale. *Please note:* if your patient is comatose you should not complete Part II of the assessment.

PART II: Patient behaviors

Item	Not present	Present intermittently	Present continuously
A. Cognition			
2. Intact but lacks knowledge or understanding of situation or illness.	3	2	1
3. Minor forgetfulness: some short-term memory loss but does not interfere with patient's understanding of situation or illness.	1	2	3
4. Extreme forgetfulness: short- and long-term memory loss; poor retention—no carryover of information or learning; interferes with patient's understanding of situation or illness.	1	2	3
5. Decreased ability to concentrate, short attention span.	1	2	3
6. Altered conceptualization.	1	2	3
7. Uses poor judgment.	1	2	3
			Total _____
			(Max. 18)

TABLE 25.2 *Continued*

B. **General behavior and affect**

8. Pleasant, cooperative.	3	2	1
9. Does not recognize limitations of his/her illness.	1	2	3
10. Has difficulty relating to others.	1	2	3
11. Restless, agitated, anxious, or nervous.	1	2	3
12. Frightened.	1	2	3
13. Angry, antagonistic, demanding, noisy, or irritable.	1	2	3
14. Withdrawn or unusually quiet, depressed, teary eyed, crying.	1	2	3
15. Apathetic, unmotivated.	1	2	3

Total _____
(Max. 24)

C. **Motor activity/speech motor ability/sensory acuity**

Altered voluntary motor response:

16. Change in muscular tension.	1	2	3
17. Alteration in posture.	1	2	3
18. Unsteady gait.	1	2	3
19. Increased amount of motor activity during sleep.	1	2	3
20. Little body movement.	1	2	3
21. No movement in some extremities.	1	2	3

Altered speech motor ability:

22. Answers slowly or with difficulty.	1	2	3
23. Speech slurred or garbled.	1	2	3

Decreased sensory acuity:

24. Vision.	1	2	3
25. Hearing.	1	2	3
26. Sensation.	1	2	3

Total _____
(Max. 33)

D. **Orientation**

27. Disoriented to any sphere, but reorients easily.	1	2	3

TABLE 25.2 *Continued*

Disoriented to person; does not re-orient easily:			
28. Calls someone known to him/her by another name.	1	2	3
29. Patient thinks you are someone else.	1	2	3
Disoriented to place; does not re-orient easily:			
30. Some idea of place (hospital, nurse) but not larger context (name of hospital, city, season for admission).	1	2	3
31. No idea of place including immediate environment, e.g., uses wrong bed or drawer, loses room.	1	2	3
Disoriented to time; does not re-orient easily:			
32. Some idea of time: can indicate season, year, current event but not day, month.	1	2	3
33. No idea of time: cannot indicate season, or current event.	1	2	3
34. Calling people from past.	1	2	3
35. Talks about the past as if it were the present.	1	2	3

Total _____
(Max. 27)

E. **Behaviors that threaten the safety of the patient**			
36. Uncooperative, rebellious, difficult to manage, threatening to leave.	1	2	3
37. Attempting to get out of bed inappropriately.	1	2	3
38. Pulling at tubes, dressings.	1	2	3
39. Allowing meal tray to remain untouched.	1	2	3
40. Removing clothing or bedclothes.	1	2	3
41. Incontinent of bowel.	1	2	3
42. Incontinent of bladder and/or Foley in place.	1	2	3

TABLE 25.2 *Continued*

43. Disregards personal cleanliness.	1	2	3
			Total _____
			(Max. 24)

F. Psychotic/neurotic behaviors

44. Delusional, hallucinations, illusions.	1	2	3
45. Paranoid ideation.	1	2	3
46. Behavior regressed.	1	2	3
47. Behavior repetitive, including verbal behavior.	1	2	3
48. Confabulation.	1	2	3
49. Combative, hostile.	1	2	3
50. Watching others and confusing their actions for his/her own.	1	2	3
			Total _____
			(Max. 21)

G. Ability to interact/perform ADL/speech content

51. Little eye contact.	1	2	3
52. Not interacting.	1	2	3
53. Distracts easily.	1	2	3
54. Egocentric.	1	2	3
55. Yelling.	1	2	3
56. Speaking incoherently.	1	2	3
57. Able to perform some daily activities alone or with help.	1	2	3
58. Unable to perform any daily activities, even with help.	1	2	3
			Total _____
			(Max. 24)

GRAND TOTAL _____
(Max. 171)

Please rate your patient's overall level of confusion for this shift by placing a "/" on the line below.

No Confusion   Severe Confusion

[a]Adapted with permission from Nagley, S. J. (1984). Prevention of Confusion in Hospitalized Elderly Persons. *Dissertation Abstracts International, 45*(06B), 1732. (University Microfilms International No. 8420848)

content relevance of the items on an instrument using a four-point ordinal rating scale" (Lynn, 1986, p. 384). The results yielded an overall CVI of 0.88 (most items judged valid), with individual subscales ranging from 0.67 to 1.00 (all subscales judged valid), and individual items ranging from 0.33 to 1.00 (all items judged valid by at least one expert). No single item was judged by all experts as invalid, and no additional items were suggested. Thus, no items or subscales were dropped from the CAC-B, but three items were reworded to enhance clarity. Based on the ratings and comments of the panel, the scale was considered sufficiently inclusive.

The CAC-B was then tested for reliability on adult medical-surgical units at three New Jersey hospitals. Three hundred seventy-five observations were made by 22 nurses on 149 patients. Reliability was measured using Cronbach's alpha and interrater correlations. Cronbach's alpha was .95 for the overall scale of 58 items, and interrater reliability using 20 paired observations was $r = .69$. Factor analysis was performed to look for patterns in the patients' behaviors. Although no clear behavior patterns emerged from the data, the results did confirm the multidimensional nature of confusion.

The results of these two studies raise several conceptual and practical issues in regard to the measurement of confusion in hospitalized adults. These can be summarized as follows:

1. No single behavior or dimension is sufficient for the diagnosis of confusion; it is the pattern across dimensions that leads the nurse to decide whether confusion exists and at what level. The structure of the CAC-B suggests that at least seven domains should be assessed: cognition, general behavior, motor activity (including speech), orientation, behaviors that threaten the safety of the patient, psychotic/neurotic behaviors, and the ability to perform activities of daily living.

2. A single score cannot capture behavioral patterns since various combinations of behaviors may be reflected by the same score. Without knowing the particular behavioral pattern of the patient (i.e., how the patient scored on the subscales), the nurse cannot determine if a change has occurred or how best to intervene. Thus, repeat measures are needed, and changes in subscale scores may be a better indicator of confusion than the total score.

3. Nurses perceive confusion as both a dichotomous phenomenon (i.e., confused or not) and a continuous phenomenon (i.e., ranging from slight confusion to severe confusion). Critical behavior patterns may exist that allow the nurse to classify the client as confused or not confused. A continuum of severity may also exist that can guide the

nurse to decide when and how to intervene. Two instruments are therefore needed—a brief scale to screen for the existence of confusion and another, longer scale to monitor confusion once it has been identified.

4. A diagnosis of confusion depends on accurate interpretation of the patient's behavior, which in turn depends on some form of interaction with the patient and some amount of time spent with the patient. This suggests that confusion may be most accurately assessed at the conclusion of a shift rather than on admission or at the beginning of the shift.

5. Confusion has the quality of duration; that is to say, the length of the confused episode has some importance for the nurse. Any scale that measures confusion should therefore provide some means of determining the duration of the confusion.

6. Nurses make a diagnosis of confusion based on more than just behavior; that is, risk factors such as poor vision and hearing are likely to influence the nurse's decision making. Whether these risk factors should be part of a screening tool and/or part of a monitoring tool has yet to be determined.

The Clinical Assessment of Confusion Scale now exists in two forms, the CAC-A and the longer CAC-B. Although both scales have been used in research, the results are not yet conclusive in regard to the validity, reliability, and sensitivity of the scales. The author therefore feels it is premature to use either scale for clinical decision making (Vermeersch, 1990, 1991). It is appropriate, however, to use them in clinical trials, with the following recommendations:

1. Use the CAC-A as a screening instrument and the CAC-B as a more in-depth assessment once confusion has been identified. Table 25.3 provides a suggested method of interpreting scores on the CAC-A and CAC-B.

2. Use either the CAC-A or CAC-B concurrently with another, more established measure such as the Mini-Mental State Exam (MMSE) or a psychogeriatric nurse's evaluation. Interpret the scores in light of the second measure.

3. Evaluate patients on admission and on a regular basis, i.e., once a shift, to establish baseline behavior patterns and to note changes in patterns.

Our understanding of confusion is still largely incomplete; we lack consensus on the nature of the phenomenon, how to measure it, and how to treat it. The lack of consensus, our imperfect tools, and the few

TABLE 25.3 Measured Level of Confusion from the VAS-C, with Corresponding Score Ranges from the CAC-A[a] and CAC-B[b]

Measured level from VAS-C in mm	Range of scores from CAC-A	Range of scores from CAC-B
Confusion possible (1–9mm)	2–8	66–80
Mild confusion (10–39mm)	9–14	81–100
Moderate confusion (40–69mm)	15–28	101–120
Severe confusion (70–100mm)	>28	>120
Maximum possible	77	167

[a]N = 305 observations (129 patients)
[b]N = 375 observations (149 patients)

interventions available should not, however, deter us from pursuing greater understanding. Confusion remains a troubling clinical problem for nurses in all settings. The Clinical Assessment of Confusion Scales A and B are offered as catalysts for further work on this problem, in both research and practice.

ACKNOWLEDGMENTS

The research reported here was partially supported by the Alpha Mu Chapter of Sigma Theta Tau, the Frances Payne Bolton School of Nursing Alumni Association, the Rutgers University Research Council and the College of Nursing, Rutgers, The State University of New Jersey.

REFERENCES

Champagne, M., Neelon, V., & McConnell, E. (1987). Acute confusion in the hospitalized elderly: Patterns and early diagnosis (abstract). In A. M. McLane (Ed.), *Classification of nursing diagnoses: Proceedings of the seventh conference* (pp. 293–294). St. Louis: Mosby.

Foreman, M. D. (1986). Acute confusional states in the hospitalized elderly: A research dilemma. *Nursing Research, 35,* 34–38.

Foreman, M. D. (1987). Reliability and validity of mental status questionnaires in elderly hospitalized patients. *Nursing Research, 36,* 216–220.

Lynn, M. R. (1986). Determination and quantification of content validity. *Nursing Research, 35,* 382–385.

Nagley, S. J. (1984). Prevention of confusion in hospitalized elderly persons. *Dissertation Abstracts International, 45*(06B), 1732. (University Microfilms International No. 8420848)

Vermeersch, P. E. H. (1986). Development of a scale to measure confusion in hospitalized adults. (Doctoral dissertation, Case Western Reserve University, 1986). *Dissertation Abstracts International, 47*(09B), 3709.

Vermeersch, P. E. H. (1990). The Clinical Assessment of Confusion-A. *Applied Nursing Research, 3,* 128–133.

Vermeersch, P. E. H. (1991). Response to "The cognitive and behavioral nature of acute confusional states." *Scholarly Inquiry for Nursing Practice, 5,* 17–20.

Wolanin, M. O., & Phillips, L. R. (1981). *Confusion: Prevention and care.* St. Louis: Mosby.

[26]

Acute Confusional States in the Hospitalized Elderly

Marquis D. Foreman

Acute confusion, also known as delirium, is a significant health problem afflicting 20–80% of hospitalized elderly patients (Cavanaugh, 1983; Foreman, 1989; Gillick, Serrell, & Gillick, 1982; Lipowski, 1983; Williams et al., 1979; Williams, Campbell, Raynor, Mlynarczyk, & Ward, 1985). Despite this prevalence, 37–72% of elderly patients who become acutely confused are never recognized by physicians or nurses as suffering from an acute confusional state (Knights & Folstein, 1977; Lucas & Folstein, 1980; Palmateer & McCartney, 1985). Hence, clinicians fail to diagnose and treat the condition. Although many factors contribute to the failure to accurately diagnose and treat acute confusion in elderly patients, the limited knowledge about acute confusional states is a major factor (Foreman, 1986; Levkoff, Besdine, & Wetle, 1986).

The two studies reported here (Foreman, 1989, 1991) were undertaken to provide information for improving the diagnosis and treatment of acutely confused elderly patients, by answering the following questions:

1. What is the incidence of acute confusion in the hospitalized elderly?
2. When, during the course of hospitalization, is an acute confusional state likely to develop?
3. Are the clinical features of acute confusion actually observed in patients experiencing an acute confusional state?
4. Which clinical features of acute confusion facilitate the accurate identification or diagnosis of this condition?
5. What causes acute confusion in this patient population?

STUDY ONE

METHOD

Sample

For admission to the first study, patients were required to be 60 years of age or older, able to speak and understand English, hospitalized within the previous 24 hours, and willing to participate in the study. Patients were excluded if they were admitted for any surgical procedure; had changes in cognitive function attributable to alcoholism, a diagnosis of dementia, or a score less than 24 on initial mental status testing; were unconscious, or were unable to see, hear, and/or verbally communicate.

Measures

Variables considered important in the development of acute confusion in the hospitalized elderly were identified through an extensive review of the literature on acute confusion, delirium, and cognitive impairment (Foreman, 1986). Vague, imprecise, and/or redundant variables were eliminated, and those remaining were categorized according to Levine's (1967, 1971) conservation principles (see Table 26.1).

Four instruments were used to examine factors associated with acute confusion in this sample—Folstein's Mini-Mental State Examination; the

TABLE 26.1 Variables Associated with Acute Confusion Categorized by Levine's Four Conservation Principles[a]

Conservation Principle	Variable
Energy	Serum albumin
	Serum glucose
	Total lymphocyte count
	Body temperature
	Mean arterial pressure
	Heart rate
	pH
	Serum creatinine
Structural integrity	Serum sodium, potassium, and calcium
	Hemoglobin
	Blood urea nitrogen
	pO_2
Personal integrity	Sensory status
	Medications
	Orienting objects
Social integrity	Presence of significant others
	Nurse perception of acute confusion

[a]Levine, 1967.
Note. From "Acute Confusion in the Hospitalized Elderly: A Research Dilemma," by M. D. Foreman, 1986, *Nursing Research, 35,* 34–48. Copyright 1986 by the American Journal of Nursing Company. Reprinted by permission.

Clinical Assessment of Confusion-A; a visual analogue scale for confusion, and a visual analogue scale for depression. The Mini-Mental State Examination (Folstein, Folstein, & McHugh, 1975), commonly referred to as the MMSE, consists of 11 questions, requires 5–10 minutes to complete, and is valid and reliable for elderly patients (Anthony, Le-Resche, Niaz, Von Korff, & Folstein, 1982; Foreman, 1987, 1989). Answers are scored as either right or wrong; the total score ranges from 0 to 30 and is a weighted sum of the correct responses (Folstein et al., 1975). A score less than 24 is considered evidence of confusion (Anthony et al., 1982).

The Clinical Assessment of Confusion-A (CAC-A) (Vermeersch, 1990) is a checklist of 25 behaviors associated with varying degrees of acute confusion; the greater the number of behaviors observed, the more severe the confusion. The patient is evaluated on the basis of the presence or absence of each behavior. The score is the total number of observed behaviors, and any four or more behaviors are considered evidence of confusion. Reliability and validity testing has been conducted with various samples (Foreman, 1989; Vermeersch, 1986, 1990).

The Visual Analogue Scale for Confusion (VAS-C) (Foreman, 1989; Nagley, 1986; Vermeersch, 1990) is a 10-cm horizontal line, with anchors of "no confusion" (0 cm) and "severe confusion" (10 cm); staff nurses and the investigator independently placed a "slash" through the line at a point indicating their perception of the patient's degree of confusion. To calculate the degree of confusion, the distance from the respondent's mark to the "no confusion" end of the scale was measured in centimeters. The VAS-C has been demonstrated as a valid and reliable measure of confusion (Foreman, 1989; Nagley, 1984, 1986; Vermeersch, 1986, 1990).

Because behavioral manifestations of depression appear similar to the symptoms of acute confusion (Kane, Ouslander, & Abrass, 1984; Zarit & Zarit, 1983), the Visual Analogue Scale for Depression (VAS-D) (Aitken, 1969) was used to discriminate between acutely confused and depressed patients. The VAS-D is a 10-cm horizontal line representing an affective continuum, anchored with "I am not depressed" on the left end (0 cm), and "I am as depressed as I can possibly imagine myself being" on the right (10 cm). Subjects placed a "slash" through the line at the point indicating their feelings at the moment. The degree of depression was determined by measuring the distance in centimeters from the respondent's mark to the left anchor. The psychometric properties of the VAS-D have been reported by Foreman (1987).

Procedure

Seventy-one patients, selected within 24 hours of admission to the hospital and meeting the criteria specified above, were interviewed daily by the investigator for a maximum of 8 days, or until discharged or acutely confused. During the interview, which lasted approximately 20–30 minutes, the MMSE, CAC-A, VAS-C, and VAS-D were administered. Questions were also asked to elicit information about variables considered important in the development of acute confusion (see Table 26.1). Data on medications administered and the results of selected laboratory tests were obtained from each patient's hospital record.

To assure that all instances of acute confusion were detected, the nurses caring for subjects were requested to routinely assess mental status once each shift using the CAC-A and VAS-C. Also, if any change was observed in the subject's level of alertness, psychomotor behavior, and/or orientation, the nurses were asked to complete a VAS-C, CAC-A, and MMSE.

Subjects were classified as acutely confused on the basis of the combined criteria of the CAC-A and MMSE administered by the investigator. That is, to be considered acutely confused, subjects had to score less than 24 on the MMSE (Anthony et al., 1982) and exhibit four or more of the behaviors on the CAC-A (Vermeersch, 1990).

The values of the variables in Table 26.1 on the day each subject developed an acute confusional state were used for the analysis (range = Day 2 to Day 6, mode = Day 2). To assure comparability, the values of variables from Day 2 were used for subjects who did not become acutely confused.

RESULTS

The majority of the 71 subjects were female and black; their mean age was 74 years (see Table 26.2). Of the 71 subjects, 38% ($n = 27$) developed an acute confusional state within 6 days of admission to the hospital.

TABLE 26.2 Characteristics of the Sample (Study 1)

	Not acutely confused $n = 44$		Acutely confused $n = 27$		All subjects $n = 71$	
Characteristic	n	%	n	%	n	%
Gender						
Female	26	59.1	19	70.4	45	63.4
Male	18	40.9	8	29.6	26	36.6
Race						
Caucasian	20	45.5	11	40.7	31	43.7
Black	24	54.5	13	48.1	37	52.1
Hispanic	0	0.0	3	11.1	3	4.2
	M	SD	M	SD	M	SD
Age	72.93	7.35	74.78	8.13	73.63	7.65
Education	11.43	2.96	9.33	2.45	10.63	2.94
Depression[a]	.03	.15	.89	.93	.36	.72

[a]Depression is measured on a scale from 0 (not depressed) to 10 (as depressed as can imagine being).
Note: From "Confusion in the Hospitalized Elderly: Incidence, Onset, and Associated Factors," by M. D. Foreman, 1989, *Research in Nursing & Health, 12,* 21–29. Copyright 1989 by John Wiley & Sons, Limited. Reprinted by permission.

Nineteen of the 27 patients developed acute confusion by the second day, an additional 4 by the fourth day, and another 4 by the sixth day. No new instances of acute confusion were identified after the sixth day of hospitalization.

Age, gender, race, and reasons for hospitalization did not differ significantly between patients who did and did not become acutely confused. However, patients who became acutely confused had significantly less education [$t(69) = 3.09$, $p = .003$] and reported significantly greater depression [$t(69) = -6.02$, $p = .001$]. Because lower levels of education and higher levels of depression can be expressed as lower scores on the MMSE (Anthony et al., 1982), these variables were analyzed further to determine if this was the case. The analysis indicated that scores on the MMSE were not related to the level of education or depression.

In most of the research to date, only single agents associated with the onset of acute confusion have been examined. Yet in a patient population hospitalized for acute exacerbations of multiple chronic illnesses for which they are receiving myriad complex medical therapies, multiple rather than single agents are likely to be operative. Therefore, a statistical approach for examining the simultaneous effects of multiple agents as illustrated in Table 26.1 was used in this study. There were a number of missing values for pH, pO2, hemoglobin, serum calcium, and total lymphocyte count; therefore these variables were excluded from the analysis. The statistical approach used was multivariate analysis of variance, or MANOVA. The MANOVA was statistically significant [multivariate $F(14,48) = 37.88$, $p \leq .001$] indicating that, in fact, multiple agents were associated with the onset of acute confusion. To identify the specific agents involved, a stepwise discriminant function analysis was performed. Discriminant function analysis provides an equation of the combination of variables that maximizes the differences between groups (Tabachnick & Fidell, 1983)—in this instance, the combination of variables that maximized the differences between those patients who did and did not become acutely confused. The standardized discriminant equation was significant [$x^2(13) = 137.61$, $p = .0001$], and included the following agents (listed in descending order of importance):

$D =$ 2.13 (creatinine) + 2.03 (nurse ratings of confusion) + 1.50 (orienting objects) – 1.41 (potassium) + 1.08 (glucose) + .91 (sodium) + .90 (blood urea nitrogen) – .63 (interactions with significant others) + .45 (medications) – .30 (mean arterial pressure).

The weight or relative importance of each variable is indicated by the standardized discriminant function coefficient (the number preceding each variable in the equation). Values of each variable for a given patient can be inserted into the equation, multiplied by the weight or standard-ized coefficient, for that variable, and then summed. The score for the patient indicates group membership, or whether the status of the patient is such that an acute confusional state might develop.

Since statistical significance is necessary but not sufficient for meaningful discrimination between groups, the accuracy of the equation in classifying patients as either confused or not confused was evaluated. On the basis of the equation, 94% of the subjects (see Table 26.3) were correctly classified as either acutely confused or not confused—with 93% of the acutely confused subjects and 95% of the subjects who were not confused correctly classified. There were few false-positive and false-negative classifications (5% and 7%, respectively).

In this sample, the equation shows that the development of an acute confusional state, as indicated by the discriminant equation, was associ-ated with azotemia, being perceived by nurses as confused, more orient-ing objects in the immediate environment, hypokalemia, hyperglyce-mia, hypernatremia, fewer interactions with significant others, receiving more medications, and hypotension. This profile of the acutely confused elderly patient provides guidelines for the nursing care of such patients, guidelines that are discussed below in conjunction with the report of the second study.

TABLE 26.3 Classification of Subjects as Acutely Confused or Not Confused on the Basis of the Discriminant Equation (Study 1)[a]

	Predicted group membership			
	Not confused		Acutely confused	
Actual group membership[b]	n	%	n	%
Not confused (n = 40)	38	95.0	2[c]	5.0
Acutely confused (n = 27)	2[d]	7.4	25	92.6
Total (n = 67)	40		27	

[a]Four cases were excluded from this analysis as a result of at least 1 missing discriminant variable.
[b]Actual group membership as determined by the MMSE < 24 and CAC-A ≥ 4.
[c]False-positive misclassifications.
[d]False-negative misclassifications.
Note: From "Confusion in the Hospitalized Elderly: Incidence, Onset, and Associated Factors," by M. D. Foreman, 1989, Research in Nursing & Health, 12, 21–29. Copyright 1989 by John Wiley & Sons, Limited. Reprinted by permis-sion.

STUDY TWO

While there is general agreement on the defining characteristics of acute confusion (American Psychiatric Association, 1987; Foreman, 1986, 1989; Nagley & Dever, 1988; Williams et al., 1979, 1985), there has been little research to support the contention that these features are in fact fundamental dimensions of acute confusional states (see Table 26.4). Thus, Study Two was conducted to determine whether the clinical features of acute confusion are actually observed in patients experiencing acute confusion and whether these clinical features are diagnostic, that is, whether they facilitate accurate identification of an acute confusional state.

METHOD

The sample selection criteria for this study were similar to those described in the preceding study. Two hundred thirty-eight patients were enrolled in the study; the majority were female and Caucasian, with a mean age of 72 years (see Table 26.5).

TABLE 26.4 Clinical Features of Acute Confusion

Feature	Acute confusion
Onset	Acute/subacute—depends on the cause
Course	Short, diurnal fluctuations in symptoms, worse at twilight, in dark, and upon awakening
Duration	Hours to less than 1 month
Alertness	Fluctuates; hypervigilant to stuporous
Attention	Reduced ability to maintain and shift
Orientation	Generally impaired, but fluctuates in severity
Memory	Recent and immediate impaired
Thinking	Disorganized, distorted, fragmented, slow or accelerated
Perception	Distorted, illusions, hallucinations, and delusions
Psychomotor behavior	Variable, hypo- and hyperkinetic or mixed
Sleep–wake cycle	Reversed
Associated features	Variable affective changes, symptoms of autonomic hyperarousal

Note: From "Acute Confusional States in the Hospitalized Elderly: A Research Dilemma," by M. D. Foreman, 1986, *Nursing Research, 35,* 34–38. Copyright 1986 by the American Journal of Nursing Company. Reprinted by permission.

TABLE 26.5   Characteristics of the Sample (Study 2)

Characteristic	Not acutely confused $n = 125$		Acutely confused $n = 113$		All subjects $n = 238$	
	n	%	n	%	n	%
Gender						
Female	64	51.2	78	69.0	142	59.7
Male	61	48.8	35	31.0	96	40.3
Race						
Caucasian	79	63.2	37	32.7	116	48.7
Black	43	34.4	56	49.6	99	41.6
Hispanic	3	2.4	20	17.7	23	9.7
	M	SD	M	SD	M	SD
Age	70.78	7.35	72.93	8.13	71.63	7.65
Education	12.42	2.96	8.55	2.45	10.68	2.94

Note: From "The Cognitive and Behavioral Nature of Acute Confusional States," by M. D. Foreman, 1991, *Scholarly Inquiry for Nursing Practice, 5,* 3–16. Copyright 1991 by Springer Publishing Company, Inc. Reprinted with permission.

Procedure

The data collection instruments used in the previous study also were used here, with two differences in the data collection procedure. First, responses on the MMSE were recorded as "correct," "incorrect," "I don't know," "unable to respond," or "refuses to answer." This scoring scheme was used to allow greater understanding of the type of impairment, that is, affective versus cognitive, since it is known that various patterns of responses are associated with different cognitive and affective states. For example, a majority of "I don't know" and "refuses to answer" responses are associated with depression rather than acute confusion (Foreman, 1991).

Second, the Clinical Assessment of Confusion Form B (CAC-B) was utilized rather than Form A. The CAC-B (Vermeersch, 1988) is a checklist of 58 rather than 25 behaviors. In addition, the behaviors are rated as: "not present," "present intermittently," or "present continuously," rather than merely present or absent. As with Form A, observation of a minimum of four behaviors is considered evidence of confusion (Vermeersch, 1988).

RESULTS

Of the 238 subjects, 47.5% ($n = 113$) developed acute confusion within 6 days of admission to the hospital; the modal onset of acute confusion was the second day; no new cases of acute confusion were identified after the sixth day of hospitalization. Exploratory factor analysis of the items on the MMSE and CAC-B was used to determine whether the clinical features of acute confusion identified in the literature were actually observed in patients experiencing an acute confusional state (Tabachnick & Fidell, 1983). The factor analysis was specifically used to see if aspects of cognition and psychomotor behaviors would cluster into subgroups similar to those listed in the literature, for example, orientation, memory, and thinking, among others (see Table 26.4).

A five-factor solution derived from maximum likelihood factor analysis with varimax rotation accounted for 29.8% of the total variance and met the criteria for an acceptable factor analytic solution (Gorsuch, 1983). The five factors that approximated the clinical features identified in the literature were: (1) cognition; (2) orientation; (3) perception; (4) motor behavior; and (5) higher integrative functions (see Table 26.6 for factor items).

To determine whether these clinical features were diagnostic of acute confusion, that is, whether they accurately differentiated between patients who did and did not become acutely confused, stepwise discriminant function analysis was used. The equation, a combination of variables that maximized the differences between patients who did and did not become acutely confused, was significant [$\chi^2(9) = 51.4$, $p = .001$]:

D = 1.45 (spell WORLD backwards) + .85 (speech slurred or garbled) − .82 (serial 7s) + .58 (draw pentagon) + .51 (general behavior pleasant and cooperative) − .40 (able to perform some ADLs) + .37 (minor forgetfulness) + .29 (calling people from past) + .24 (name three objects).

In other words, the clinical features representing the factors of cognition, perception, and higher integrative functions accurately discriminated acutely confused from nonconfused patients. However, level of alertness and orientation, aspects upon which nurses rely almost exclusively for diagnosing acute confusion (Pompei, Cassel, & Foreman, 1991), were not in the equation.

The adequacy of the equation was indicated by the fact that it correctly classified 90.3% of the subjects as either acutely confused or not con-

TABLE 26.6 Factors with Item Loadings (Study 2)

	Factors				
Items	1	2	3	4	5
Factor 1: Cognition					
Does not recognize limitations of illness	.75[a]	.01	-.02	.03	-.02
Intact cognition	.75	.08	.05	-.05	-.04
Floor/unit	.64	.18	.11	.09	.15
Extreme forgetfulness	.57	.05	.13	.09	.06
Date	.53	.34	.23	.10	.16
Speech garbled	.51	.08	-.19	.29	.25
Serial subtraction by 7s	.49	.21	.33	-.02	.18
Minor forgetfulness	.44	-.01	.35	.07	-.20
Calls people from past	.36	.11	.14	.07	.13
Some idea of time	.36	.11	.09	.16	-.09
Altered conceptualization	.31	.07	.30	.07	.03
Name 3 objects	.25	-.02	-.03	.03	-.04
Factor 2: Orientation					
Season	.09	.73	.12	.09	-.01
Hospital	.15	.70	.08	-.03	-.08
Year	.09	.68	.13	.10	.09
Month	.14	.64	.13	.04	.05
Day	.18	.57	.04	-.01	.12
State	.27	.53	.12	.16	-.05
County	.49	.51	.05	.06	-.06
City	-.10	.38	.15	.04	-.01
Disoriented, does not reorient	-.07	.30	-.06	.21	.21
Disoriented, but does reorient	.12	.41	.15	-.07	-.05
Factor 3: Perception					
Draws pentagon	.18	.07	.64	.07	.03
Write complete sentence	.03	.29	.59	-.10	-.02
Follows 3-stage command	.03	.06	.58	.23	.20
Spells WORLD backwards	.27	.20	.56	-.05	.14
Close your eyes	-.07	.35	.55	-.13	-.04
Impaired concentration	.24	-.01	.42	.45	.01
Impaired vision	.05	.24	.32	.26	-.01
Factor 4: Motor Behavior					
No movement	.20	.08	-.03	.71	-.03
Answers slowly	.10	.17	-.13	.61	-.05
Little eye contact	.07	-.03	.32	.49	-.12
Restless	.02	-.08	.29	.45	.13
Increased motor activity	-.06	.24	-.10	.45	.29
Little movement	.01	.18	-.14	.44	.33

TABLE 26.6 *Continued*

Items	Factors				
	1	2	3	4	5
Altered posture	−.06	.06	.03	**.41**	.12
Calls by another name	.22	.32	.35	**.39**	−.08
Factor 5: Higher Integrative Functions					
Poor judgment	.02	−.01	.10	.05	**.82**
Impaired hearing	.02	−.01	.17	.13	**.73**
Pleasant/cooperative	−.07	−.11	−.05	.07	**−.62**
Able to perform some ADLs	−.18	.06	.14	.06	**.27**
No ifs, ands, or buts	.13	−.02	−.04	.02	**.25**

ᵃItems Loading on (belonging to) a factor are in bold type.
Note: From "The Cognitive and Behavioral Nature of Acute Confusional States," by M.D. Foreman, 1991, *Scholarly Inquiry for Nursing Practice, 5,* 3–16. Copyright 1991 by Springer Publishing Company, Inc. Reprinted by permission.

fused; however, there were more correct classifications of the nonconfused group (99%) than the acutely confused group (80%) (see Table 26.7).

DISCUSSION

The incidence of acute confusion was 38% in the first study and 47% in the second; these rates are comparable to those reported in the literature (Cavanaugh, 1983; Sadler, 1979; Williams et al., 1979, 1985). This high incidence rate supports the view that acute confusion is a significant and highly prevalent health problem for acutely ill elders—a problem that warrants greater attention from clinicians and researchers alike (Foreman, 1986, 1989). It is difficult to understand why such a prevalent problem with such serious consequences often fails to attract the attention of nurses and physicians. The answer to this question may be found in the discovery in this second study that alertness and orientation, on which clinicians rely heavily for identifying confusion, are not by themselves diagnostic of acute confusion in acutely ill hospitalized patients.

In this sample, the onset of acute confusion occurred most frequently around the second day of hospitalization, no later than the sixth. More precise information about the timing of onset of an acute confusional

TABLE 26.7 Classification of Subjects as Acutely Confused or Not Confused on the Basis of the Discriminant Equation (Study 2)

	Predicted group membership			
	Not confused		Acutely confused	
Actual group membership	n	%	n	%
Not confused ($n = 125$)	124	99.2	1[a]	.8
Acutely confused ($n = 113$)	22[b]	19.5	91	80.5
Total ($n = 238$)	146		92	

[a]False-positive misclassifications.
[b]False-negative misclassifications.
Note: From "The Cognitive and Behavioral Nature of Acute Confusional States," by M. D. Foreman, 1991, Scholarly Inquiry for Nursing Practice, 5, 3–16. Copyright 1991 by Springer Publishing Company, Inc. Reprinted with permission.

state can assist in focusing efforts at detection of the problem and improving surveillance methods. Assessment should be routine, to enable prompt detection of any change in cognition, and systematic, so that every assessment is performed similarly. Time of onset can also assist in identifying the cause. Acute confusion developing rather precipitously after admission to the hospital may indicate the cause to be some combination of stresses related to hospitalization and the associated physical illness. In contrast, acute confusion developing later in the course of hospitalization may indicate the cause to be iatrogenic or nosocomial. Thus, knowing precisely the onset helps to narrow the search for the cause.

The clinical features observed in acutely confused patients in these two studies were similar to those identified in the literature. However, the five factors in acute confusion identified in the second study—cognition, orientation, perception, motor behavior, and higher integrative functions—accounted for only one third of the confused behavior observed in these patients, indicating that there is much more to acute confusion than is represented by these factors. The missing pieces may come as we learn more about the experience of acute confusion from the patient's perspective—a perspective about which we still have little information.

Although these five factors do not represent the entire picture of confused behavior, they are extremely accurate in identifying a state of acute confusion. However, as noted above, the behaviors most heavily relied upon by nurses—alertness and orientation—are not diagnostic. It is not surprising that alertness and orientation lack diagnostic utility, as all patients experience the fatigue that accompanies acute illness and the disorienting characteristics of the environment and activities of hospitals. In other words, lack of alertness and disorientation are certainly aspects of acute confusion, but they are not sufficient in and of themselves; acute confusion is more—certainly much more than not being alert or oriented. Therefore, in addition to being routine and systematic, the assessment of cognitive functioning should be comprehensive, to ensure that aspects of cognition other than alertness and orientation are assessed. To be comprehensive and systematic, a mental status questionnaire such as Folstein's Mini-Mental State Examination can be used in combination with a behavioral rating scale such as the CAC by Vermeersch.

These findings on the causes of acute confusion clearly indicate that human beings are complex organisms who cannot be divided into unrelated components. That is, these findings support a holistic approach to patient care by indicating that the causes of acute confusion are multifactorial and span all aspects of human life. Given the specific causal agents identified in the first study, recommended guidelines for the prevention and treatment of acute confusion include these: (1) administer medications judiciously and intelligently; (2) maintain or reestablish normal physiologic functioning; (3) create an environment that promotes orientation; and (4) assist patients in accurately interpreting and finding meaning in their environment. These guidelines for the prevention and treatment of acute confusion have great potential for improving the outcomes of hospitalization for acute illness among the elderly.

ACKNOWLEDGMENTS

These studies were supported by National Research Service Awards, a predoctoral fellowship, #5 F31 NU05837, funded by the Division of Nursing, and a postdoctoral fellowship, #1 F31 NR06180, funded by the National Center for Nursing Research. Support for the studies also was provided through a Critical Care Research Grant, funded by the American Association of Critical Care Nurses. I would like to acknowledge the assistance of the nursing staffs of the general medical units of the University of Illinois Hospital and Rush–Presbyterian–St. Luke's Medical Center, Chicago, IL.

REFERENCES

Aitken, R. C. B. (1969). Measurement of feelings using visual analogue scales. *Proceedings of the Royal Society of Medicine, 67,* 989–993.

American Psychiatric Association. (1987). *Diagnostic and statistical manual of mental disorders* (3rd ed., rev.). Washington, DC: Author.

Anthony, J. C., LeResche, L. A., Niaz, U., Von Korff, M. R., & Folstein, M. F. (1982). Limits of the "Mini-Mental State" as a screening test for dementia and delirium among hospitalized patients. *Psychological Medicine, 12,* 397–408.

Cavanaugh, S. (1983). The prevalence of emotional and cognitive dysfunction in a general medical population: Using the MMSE, GHQ, and BDI. *General Hospital Psychiatry, 5,* 15–24.

Folstein, M. F., Folstein, S. E., & McHugh, P. R. (1975). "Mini-Mental State": A practical guide for grading the cognitive state of patients for clinicians. *Journal of Psychiatric Research, 12,* 189–198.

Foreman, M. D. (1986). Acute confusion in the hospitalized elderly: A research dilemma. *Nursing Research, 35,* 34–38.

Foreman, M. D. (1987). Reliability and validity of mental status questionnaires in elderly hospitalized patients. *Nursing Research, 36,* 216–220.

Foreman, M. D. (1989). Confusion in the hospitalized elderly: Incidence, onset, and associated factors. *Research in Nursing & Health, 12,* 21–29.

Foreman, M. D. (1991). The cognitive and behavioral nature of acute confusional states. *Scholarly Inquiry for Nursing Practice, 5,* 3–16.

Gillick, M. R., Serrell, N. A., & Gillick, L. S. (1982). Adverse consequences of hospitalization in the elderly. *Social Science and Medicine, 16,* 1033–1038.

Gorsuch, R. L. (1983). *Factor analysis.* Hillsdale, NJ: Lawrence Erlbaum Associates.

Kane, R. L., Ouslander, J. G., & Abrass, I. B. (1984). *Essentials of clinical geriatrics.* New York: McGraw-Hill.

Knights, E. B., & Folstein, M. F. (1977). Unsuspected emotional and cognitive disturbance in medical patients. *Annals of Internal Medicine, 87,* 723–724.

Levine, M. E. (1967). The four conservation principles of nursing. *Nursing Forum, VI,* 45–59.

Levine, M. E. (1971). Holistic nursing. *Nursing Clinics of North America, 6,* 253–264.

Levkoff, S. E., Besdine, R. W., & Wetle, T. (1986). Acute confusional states (delirium) in the hospitalized elderly. *Annual Review of Gerontology and Geriatrics, 6,* 1–26.

Lipowski, Z. J. (1983). Transient cognitive disorders (delirium, acute confusional states) in the elderly. *American Journal of Psychiatry, 140,* 1426–1436.

Lucas, M. J., & Folstein, M. F. (1980). Nursing assessment of mental disorders on a general medical unit. *Journal of Psychiatric Nursing and Mental Health Services, 18*(5), 31–33.

Nagley, S. J. (1984). *Prevention of confusion in hospitalized elderly persons.* Unpublished doctoral dissertation. Case Western Reserve University, Cleveland, OH.

Nagely, S. J. (1986). Predicting and preventing confusion in your patients. *Journal of Gerontological Nursing, 12*(3), 127–131.

Nagley, S. J., & Dever, A. (1988). What we know about treating confusion. *Applied Nursing Research, 1,* 80–83.

Palmateer, L. M., & McCartney, J. R. (1985). Do nurses know when patients have cognitive deficits? *Journal of Gerontological Nursing, 11*(2), 6–16.

Pompei, P., Cassel, C. K., & Foreman, M. D. (1991) [Early detection, evaluation, and treatment of delirium in the hospitalized elderly.] Unpublished data. University of Chicago, Chicago, IL.

Sadler, D. P. (1979). Nursing assessment of postcardiotomy delirium. *Heart & Lung, 10,* 1084–1092.

Tabachnick, B. G., & Fidell, L. S. (1983). *Using multivariate statistics.* New York: Harper & Row.

Vermeersch, P. E. H. (1986). *Development of a scale to measure confusion in hospitalized adults.* Unpublished doctoral dissertation. Case Western Reserve University, Cleveland, OH.

Vermeersch, P. E. H. (1988). *The Clinical Assessment of Confusion Form B.* Unpublished manuscript.

Vermeersch, P. E. H. (1990). The Clinical Assessment of Confusion-A. *Applied Nursing Research, 3,* 128–133.

Williams, M. A., Campbell, E. B., Raynor, W. J., Mlynarczyk, S. M., & Ward, S. E. (1985). Reducing acute confusional states in elderly patients with hip fractures. *Research in Nursing & Health, 8,* 329–337.

Williams, M. A., Holloway, J. R., Winn, M. C., Wolanin, M. O., Lawler, M. L., Westwick, C. R., & Chin, M. H. (1979). Nursing activities and acute confusional states in elderly hip-fractured patients. *Nursing Research, 28,* 25–35.

Zarit, S. H., & Zarit, , J. M. (1983). Cognitive impairment. In P. M. Lewinsohn & L. Teri (Eds.), *Clinical geropsychiatry: New directions in assessment and treatment* (pp. 38–80). New York: Pergamon.

[27]

Use of the NEECHAM Confusion Scale to Assess Acute Confusional States of Hospitalized Older Patients

Virginia J. Neelon, Mary T. Champagne, Eleanor McConnell, John Carlson, and Sandra G. Funk

Among the hospitalized elderly, the development of acute confusion/ delirium or worsening of chronic cognitive impairment delays recovery, increases morbidity, and increases mortality (Gillick, Serell, & Gillick, 1982; Levkoff, Safran, Cleary, Gallop, & Phillips, 1988; Lipowski, 1983; Rabins & Folstein, 1982; Weddington, 1982; Williams et al., 1985). Acute confusion is a syndrome of diffuse impairment of the central nervous system. Multiple factors lead to the development of acute confusion and, most probably, there is no single pathophysiologic mechanism underlying the varied manifestations. The primary hypotheses focus on factors affecting cerebral metabolism and impaired neurochemical transmission (Engel & Romano, 1959; Levkoff, Besdine & Wetle, 1986; Wolanin & Phillips, 1981). Because the key features in all acute confusional states are global cognitive dysfunction, disturbed attention and/ or arousal, and psychomotor disturbances, a common pathologic mechanism involving lesions in cortical cholinergic systems and cerebral oxygen consumption is probable.

Three clinical issues play into the problem of morbidity of acute confusion in the hospitalized elderly. First, our understanding of the pathophysiological mechanism(s) of delirium-like syndromes is still fragmentary. Second, the problem often goes undetected until the patient presents with the most severe, extreme signs of acute confusion or delirium, partly because many clinicians continue to accept cognitive deterioration as an expected and unchangeable consequence of old age. And finally, evaluation of cognitive function and cognitive changes in the acutely ill hospitalized patient suffers from inadequate measurement tools for use at the bedside.

There are certain minimum requirements for a scale to be effective as a bedside assessment tool. First of all, the scale must be sensitive to early cues to disturbed information processing. Also, it must allow evaluation during usual bedside nursing activities. That is, it must incorporate the data base the nurse already obtains when she spends time with a patient. Finally, it must be performed in a rapid, meaningful manner like other vital function nursing assessments, and be performed with minimal demand and stress on the patient's functional status.

We developed the NEECHAM Confusion Scale for rapid and unobtrusive assessment of the patient's cognitive function and behavioral performance, in order to detect early cues to the development of acute confusion and to monitor recovery.

The NEECHAM has advantages over standard mental status examinations for monitoring acute cognitive changes during hospitalization because it can be rapidly scored by the nurse at the bedside using a structured data base that is derived during routine nursing assessments. Because the NEECHAM places a minimal response burden on the patient, testing can be repeated at frequent intervals to monitor changes in the patient's status.

The NEECHAM evaluates nine information processing, performance, and vital function items (see Table 27.1). The items are divided into three levels of assessment. Level 1 evaluates responsiveness to meaningful information: attentiveness, ability to follow complex commands, and orientation and memory. Scores range from 0 to 14 points. Level 2 evaluates the integrity of sensory-motor behavior and speech; scores range from 0 to 10 points. Level 3 evaluates physiological control and stability, including vital function, oxygenation, and continence; scores may range from 0 to 6 points. This last area has not typically been involved in scales that look at confusion or cognitive impairment, but it was our intention to begin to look at what kinds of associated factors might indicate early changes and thus dictate or give direction to interventions for the physiological problems that might be occurring.

The NEECHAM can be completed within minutes after the nurse walks into a room. The nurse immediately observes how the patient turns to her, how he responds to her, whether he anticipates what she wants to do with him. She goes in to take a temperature, and the patient turns his head and opens his mouth. (There are multiple opportunities

TABLE 27.1 The NEECHAM Confusion
Scale—Three Subscales With a Total of
Nine Items

Level 1:	responsiveness
	Attention
	Motor processing
	Verbal processing
Level 2:	behavior
	Appearance
	Motor performance
	Verbal performance
Level 3:	physiologic control
	Vital function
	Oxygen saturation
	Continence

---

to evaluate attentiveness at the nurse's hands when interacting with
a patient.) The scale makes it possible to look at beginning changes in
this attentiveness, including slowed or short attentiveness and
hyperattentiveness to meaningless items. To illustrate, we measure oxygen saturation with a pulse oximeter. It has a very nice colored screen,
and we have had some patients who simply focus on what's on that
screen and actually repeat the numbers over and over again. This is an
example of hyperattentiveness to meaningless things.

One item on the scale relates to recognition, interpretation, and action—the ability to follow a complex command. Again, when they are
working with patients, nurses have many indications of how well
patients can follow a complex command. This is not simply following an
order, it involves listening to what is being asked or happening, interpreting it, and then processing and acting on it. We frequently use
the ability of the patient to understand and learn how to use call bells to
contact the nurse. That can be quite a challenge today, the way the new
nurse call bells are put on beds; but nevertheless, it is a very effective
and useful way to monitor the patient's changing condition.

Another area on the scale is motor behavior. Some patients present
first, not with obvious cognitive function changes, but with behaviors
that may be more related to sensory-motor changes. We look for tremor
or the way a patient can rest in bed, certain kinds of movements or
position. We also measure a number of physiologic parameters, including oxygen saturation, which we examine noninvasively, with an oximeter. When we started using them, oximeters were not very common,
but now almost every unit in the hospital has an oximeter, so it is

easy to use this kind of instrument to evaluate oxygen status. There are, however, certain caveats in interpreting oxygen saturation. First, the nurse is usually evaluating to determine risk, and the way a person is at risk may differ when he is resting in bed compared to when he is challenged, that is, after he has gone to the bathroom and come back again. Further, oxygen saturation simply measures the ability to carry oxygen, not how well certain parts of the body are being perfused, so a patient can have normal oxygen saturation while cerebral perfusion is inadequate. Also an anemic person can maintain a very high saturation at rest, and may even do so under significant physiologic challenge. But nevertheless, tissue oxygenation is threatened.

We also monitor bladder control and note four states—maintains bladder control, incontinent of urine in the last 24 hours, incontinent now, or has indwelling or intermittent catheter. This item is difficult because the measurement of it is very closely related to nursing care and time spent with the patient. Thus, it ends up being sometimes more an appearance item than a measure of autonomic function or integrated control. That is, if it is a busy floor, the incontinence may not be related to the patient's problem but to a staffing problem.

The NEECHAM total score is calculated by summing the scores for the three levels; total scores can range from 0 (minimal responsiveness) to 30 (normal function). Total scores of 0 to 19 indicate moderate to severe confusion, scores of 20 to 24 indicate mild or early development of confusion, and scores above 24 are classified as "not confused." The scale has shown high internal consistency (Cronbach's alpha = .85) and high interrater (.96) and test–retest reliability (.96) in stable subjects.

METHOD

The study reported here was designed to determine the clinical validity of the NEECHAM Confusion Scale by comparing scores on the NEECHAM with scores on six other clinical measures of cognitive impairment and acute confusion: Folstein's Mini-Mental State Exam (MMSE), the DSM-III criteria for delirium, the clinical record of mental status problems and psychiatric problems, patient self-report of confusion, and the primary nurse's report. The study was part of a larger ongoing study of patterns of development and etiology of disturbed information processing and acute confusion in the hospitalized elderly.

A convenience sample of 158 patients newly admitted to the medical wards was selected. Patients admitted to the study had to be age 65 or over, speak English, and give informed consent (informed consent by a close family member was accepted for patients who had severe cognitive impairment on admission). Patients who were unable to assume an upright position were excluded from the study.

Data Collection Instruments

Patients were followed on a daily basis throughout hospitalization and interviewed at four weeks postdischarge. Direct assessment of subjects, review of records, and interviews with nursing staff were used to obtain data on demographic characteristics, vital function, orthostatic ability, oxygen saturation, nutritional status, activity, sensory-motor function, cognitive status, episodes of acute confusion, environmental factors, and severity of illness.

Cognitive status and acute confusion were measured by the NEECHAM Confusion Scale (Champagne, Neelon, McConnell, & Funk, 1987; Neelon, Funk, Carlson, & Champagne, 1989), the MMSE (Folstein, Folstein, & McHugh, 1975), the DSM-III (American Psychiatric Association, 1980), patient self-report, and the primary caregiver nurse's evaluation. Medical and nursing records of mental status and psychiatric problems were also recorded. Patients were scored as positive on the DSM-III if six of the eight criteria were positive and as positive on the MMSE if the score was less than 24.

Functional status was evaluated using the Katz Index of Activities of Daily Living (ADL) (Katz, Ford, Moskowitz, Jackson, & Jaffee, 1963), the OARS Instrumental ADL scale (Duke University Center for the Study of Aging and Human Development, 1978), and the nurse's response to Level of Care Needs Instrument (Neelon & Champagne, 1988, adapted from Johnson, 1984).

Severity of illness was measured by the APACHE-II Severity of Disease Classification Index (Knaus, Wagner, & Draper, 1985), oxygen saturation by a noninvasive pulse oximeter, and vital function by standard clinical measurements. Laboratory measures were gathered from the medical record.

The admission history of mental status problems and psychiatric problems was gained from the admission record and thus these were recorded prior to the NEECHAM. Also, we instituted the nurse report of confusion. A check form was placed on the patient's door as soon as we admitted the patient to the study. The nurses then checked the form each shift, or more than once each shift, indicating whether they thought this patient was confused or not confused (see Table 27.2). Many times, however, because of the busyness of the situation, the form was not checked, and we had to contact the nurse to ask, "Did you think this patient was confused?" Thus, nurse report has some problems as an assessment tool.

TABLE 27.2 Nurse Report of Patient Confusion

Instructions: When taking vital signs at 6:00 A.M., 2:00 P.M., and 10:00 P.M. please record whether the patient is confused or behaving differently than before. If patient has a confusional episode at other times, please record this episode.

Time	None	Mild to moderate	Severe	Comments
Code	(2)	(1)	(0)	
6:00 A.M.				
Other				
2:00 P.M.				
Other				
4:00 P.M.				
Other				

We also used self-report. Patients, however, do not usually volunteer that they are confused, although we had some who did. Patients who understand that their confusion is related to physiology tend to volunteer: "I'm not right, I'm getting in trouble, I think I'm not breathing well." But most patients do not volunteer. We asked the patient how he or she felt, in a way that seemed meaningful to that patient; therefore, our language changed with different patients. We asked, "Do you feel confused, or mixed up, or have you recently felt confused, etc.?" Responses were coded as 0 (no response), 1 (high level of confusion), 2 (some confusion), and 3 (no confusion). A score from 0 to 2 was considered self-report of confusion; only 3 was considered no confusion. Interestingly, when we looked at patients who gave no response, we found that they tended to have low scores on the NEECHAM; thus in our experience, "no response" tends to be an indication that the patient is in trouble.

RESULTS

On admission, 39.2% of the patients had NEECHAM scores indicating some level of confusion: 24.7% ($n = 39$) showed mild or early confusion (scores of 20–24) and 14.5% ($n = 23$) showed moderate to severe confusion (scores less than 20). The remaining 60.8% of patients had scores above 24 and were classified as "not confused." We also looked at scores on the other two major clinical indicators that people use in the clinical setting. Using a score below 24 as the cutoff on the Mini-Mental State Exam, 60.1% of our patients were classified as having some cognitive dysfunction on admission. However, a large proportion of our sample had minimal formal education, which can affect scoring on mental status tests. Also, the Mini-Mental is not always easy to administer to an acutely ill population.

Approximately 13% of our patients (13.3%) had 6 or more positive items on the DSM-III, and were thus classified as confused. Similar percentages were identified by the nurses as confused (13.9%) and were classified as having a psychiatric diagnosis (13.3%). Although these percentages were similar, the patients were not necessarily the same. Also, similar percentages of patients were identified as confused using the mental status problem indicator and self-report (22.8% and 22.2%, respectively). Clearly, the MMSE classified by far the greatest percentage as having some level of cognitive impairment on admission (60.1%) (see Table 27.3).

We examined rank order correlations of the NEECHAM scores (using the three categories of severe confusion, early confusion, and not confused) with the other clinical indicators of confusion. Substantial associations were seen with mental status problem (Rho = .63, $p < .0001$), DSM-III positive on 6 or more 8 items (Rho = .62, $p < .0001$), and the MMSE (<24 = cognitive impairment; Rho = .50, $p < .0001$). Slightly

TABLE 27.3 Number and Percentage of Patients Classified as Having Cognitive Problems on Seven Clinical Indicators at Admission

Indicator	Number of patients positive	
	n	%
Psychiatric diagnosis	21	13.3
DSM-III > 6	21	13.3
Nurse report	22	13.9
Self report	35	22.2
Mental status problem (MSP)	36	22.8
MMSE	95	60.1
NEECHAM score		
< 20	23	14.5
≤ 24	62	39.2

weaker correlations were observed with self-report and nurse report (Rho = .44, p < .0001 and .43, p < .0001, respectively). The only indicator that was not significantly correlated with the NEECHAM was psychiatric diagnosis (Rho = .04).

A more detailed analysis was done using cross-tabulations, to see how the NEECHAM related to several of the clinical indicators, in particular, the three primary clinical indicators used in the clinical setting (i.e., the DSM III, the MMSE, and the chart report of mental status problems [MSP]). Over three quarters (78.3%) of the patients with NEECHAM scores below 20 also had a positive DSM-III score; 100% were positive on the MMSE, and 78.3% had a report of a mental status problem (including chronic dementia). Very few of the patients who scored as mildly confused on the NEECHAM had a positive score on the DSM-III (7.7%). More patients classified as mildly confused on the NEECHAM also had a mental status problem (38.5%), and a large number of these had scores below 24 on the Mini-Mental State Exam (84.6%). Nearly all (86.9%) of the patients with NEECHAM scores below 20, 38.5% of those with scores indicating mild confusion (20–24), and only 2.1% of those with scores above 24 had a positive result on two or more of these indicators (see Table 27.4).

To better understand the specific nature of confusion, the NEECHAM groups were compared on the individual items of the DSM-III. These comparisons showed that attention deficits/clouding of consciousness, memory/orientation deficits, and mental status fluctuation distinguished those scoring below 20 on the NEECHAM scale from the normal and mild groups. The DSM-III items that distinguished the group scoring 20–24 on the NEECHAM from the normal group were organic factor, activity disturbance, and sleep disturbance.

TABLE 27.4 Percentage of Patient NEECHAM Groups Who Were Positive on Clinical Indicators of Confusion

	Clinical indicators			
NEECHAM score	DSM-III > 6	MMSE < 24	MSP	2 or more indicators
Severe confusion				
< 20 (n = 23)	78.3	100.0	78.3	86.9
Mild confusion				
20–24 (n = 39)	7.7	84.6	38.5	38.5
Not confused				
> 24 (n = 96)	0.0	40.6	3.1	2.1

NEECHAM scores were not related to the presence of a psychiatric diagnosis. In addition, there was not a strong relationship between the NEECHAM scores and nurse report; less than 50% of those identified as moderately to severely confused by the NEECHAM were also identified by the nurse report. However, on admission, patient self-report of confusion was in good agreement with the NEECHAM for identification of moderate to severe confusion (see Table 27.5).

Because the MSP, MMSE, and DSM-III were the most frequently documented clinical indicators, a positive result on any two or more of these three indicators was used to evaluate the sensitivity and specificity of the NEECHAM. Sensitivity reflects the degree to which an instrument is able to accurately identify those individuals who have an impairment—in this case, confusion. Specificity is the ability of the instrument to correctly identify those who do not have impairment. Each of these indices can range from 0 (0% accuracy) to 100 (perfect accuracy). The NEECHAM was quite successful at identifying patients who were confused. Of the 37 patients who were positive on two or more of the clinical indicators, the NEECHAM correctly identified 35—a sensitivity of 95% [i.e., (35/37) × 100]. Although the NEECHAM was somewhat less accurate at identifying those who were not confused (specificity = 78%), this index was still within an acceptable range. And while the NEECHAM identified some patients as being confused when the clinical indicators did not (false positive rate = 17%), more importantly, it missed only two patients who had been classified as confused by the clinical indicators (false negative rate = 3%) (see Table 27.6).

DISCUSSION

The NEECHAM scores strongly correlated with other clinical indicators of acute confusion. Because it uses data derived during routine nursing assessment, the NEECHAM places a minimal response burden on the patient, in contrast to standard mental status examinations, and it can be repeated at frequent intervals to monitor changes in the patient's status. Although the DSM-III criteria identify patients experiencing severe confusion/delirium, in the ill elderly these criteria have several limitations: (1) they emphasize extreme, overt behaviors—the "delirious state"; (2) they undervalue the milder manifestations that help early diagnosis; and (3) they include several items that are frequently present in the very ill (sleep/wake disturbances, organic-related causes, reduced level of consciousness). Lastly, both patient reports of confusion and positive nurse reports were elicited in this study; the frequency of positive reports from these indicators may be less in the absence of a structured

TABLE 27.5 NEECHAM Groups By Selected Clinical Indicators of Confusion

	Percentage positive		
NEECHAM score	Psychiatric diagnosis	Nurse report	Self-report
Severe confusion			
< 20 (n = 23)	17.4	47.8	78.3
Mild confusion			
20–24 (n = 39)	12.8	20.5	18.0
Not confused			
> 24 (n = 96)	12.5	3.1	10.4

TABLE 27.6 Clinical Indices for Predicting Confusion from the NEECHAM

	Two or more clinical indicators (DSM III, MMSE, MSP)		
	Positive	Not positive	Total
NEECHAM	n	n	n
Severe or mild confusion (≤ 24)	35	27	62
Not confused (> 24)	2	94	96
Total	37	121	158

Clinical indices:

Sensitivity [(35/37) × 100]	95%
Specificity [(94/121) × 100]	78%
Predictive value [(35/62) × 100]	57%
False positive [(27/158) × 100]	17%
False negative [(2/158) × 100]	3%

request for such data. Patient self-report is an easily evaluated indicator on admission, but only a little over half of the patients who were confused were able or willing to acknowledge such feelings.

ACKNOWLEDGMENTS

The authors acknowledge Kathy Moore, M.S.N., Barbara Trapp-Moen, M.S.N., Karen MacMillan, B.S.N., Madelyn Ashley, M.S.N., Carolyn Edmonds, M.S.N., and Pat Sappenfield, M.S.N. Special thanks also go to our clinical liaisons and consultants from the University of North Carolina Hospitals, particularly Fran Ross, R.N., B.S.N., Chair, Department of Nursing. Finally, we have been blessed in our study of confusion by the suggestions, encouragement, and criticisms of Mary Opal Wolanin, M.S.N. This study was partially supported by a grant from the National Center for Nursing Research, National Institutes of Health (NR013390), and by the Biomedical Research Support Grant Program, Division of Research Resources, NIH (BRSG 2S07 RR07072).

REFERENCES

American Psychiatric Association. (1980). Organic mental disorders: Delirium. *The diagnostic and statistical manual* (3rd Ed.). Washington, DC: American Psychiatric Association.

Champagne, M. T., Neelon, V. J., McConnell, E. S., & Funk, S. G. (1987). The NEECHAM Confusion Scale: Assessing acute confusion in the hospitalized and nursing home elderly. *The Gerontologist, 27*(3A). (Abstract).

Duke University Center for the Study of Aging and Human Development. (1978). *Multidimensional functional assessment: The OARS methodology* (2nd. Ed.).

Engel, G. L., & Romano, J. (1959). Delirium: A syndrome of cerebral insufficiency. *Journal of Chronic Diseases, 9*, 260–277.

Folstein, M. F., Folstein, S. F., & McHugh, P. (1975). Mini-Mental State Examination. *Journal of Psychiatric Research, 12*, 189–198.

Gillick, M. R., Serrell, N. A., & Gillick, L. S. (1982). Adverse consequences of hospitalization in the elderly. *Social Science and Medicine, 16*, 1033–1038.

Johnson, K. (1984). A practical approach to patient classification. *Nursing Management, 15*(6), 39–46.

Katz, S. L., Ford, A. G., Moskowitz, R. W., Jackson, B. A., & Jaffe, M. W. (1963). Studies of illness in the aged. *Journal of the American Medical Association, 186*, 914–919.

Knaus, W. S., Wagner, D. P., & Draper, E. A. (1985). Relationship between acute physiologic derangement and risk of death. *Journal of Chronic Diseases, 38*, 295–300.

Levkoff, S. E., Besdine, R. W., & Wetle, T. (1986). Acute confusional states in hospitalized elderly. *Annual Review of Gerontology and Geriatrics, 6*, 1–26.

Levkoff, S. E., Safran, C., Cleary, P. D., Gallop, J., & Phillips, R. S. (1988). Identification of factors associated with the diagnosis of delirium in elderly hospitalized patients. *Journal of the American Geriatrics Society, 36*, 1099–1104.

Lipowski, Z. J. (1983). Transient cognitive disorders (delirium, acute confusional states) in the elderly. *American Journal of Psychiatry, 140*, 1426–1436.

Neelon, V. J., & Champagne, M. T. (1988). *Acute confusion in hospitalized elderly: Patterns and factors.* Unpublished grant proposal (NIH-NCNR-NR01-1339).

Neelon, V. J., Funk, S. G., Carlson, J. R., & Champagne, M. R. (1989). The NEECHAM Confusion Scale: Relationship to clinical indicators of acute confusion in hospitalized elders. *The Gerontologist, 29* (Abstract).

Rabins, P. V., & Folstein, M. F. (1982). Delirium and dementia: Diagnostic criteria and fatality rates. *British Journal of Psychiatry, 140,* 149–153.
Weddington, W. W. (1982). The mortality of delirium: An underappreciated problem? *Psychosomatics, 23,* 1232–1235.
Williams, M. A., Campbell, E. G., Raynor, W. J., Musholt, M. A., Mlynarcyk, S. M., & Crane, L. F. (1985). Predictors of acute confusional states in elderly patients with hip fractures. *Research in Nursing and Health, 8,* 31–40.
Wolanin, M. O., & Phillips, L. R. (1981). *Confusion: Prevention and care.* St. Louis: C. V. Mosby.

[28]

The Predictive Value of the NEECHAM Scale

Georgene C. Siemsen, Judy Miller, Annette H. Newman, and Colleen M. Lucas

This study examined the incidence and severity of acute confusion, or delirium, among elderly patients on a medical unit and evaluated the clinical utility of the NEECHAM Scale in assessing confusion in hospitalized elderly patients. Of particular interest were (1) the reliability of the NEECHAM when used by several raters, that is, the percentage of agreement in scoring by different nurses independently observing the same patient at approximately the same time; and (2) the accuracy (predictive validity) of the NEECHAM as a screening tool for confusion, as compared to the more widely used Mini-Mental State Exam (MMSE).

To put it another way, the aim was to determine what percentage of the patients who were rated as confused according to the MMSE also had NEECHAM scores that indicated they were confused; and what percentage of patients who were not confused according to the MMSE also had NEECHAM scores that indicated they were not confused. An additional goal was to determine the accuracy of patient self report in identifying confusion.

For the purposes of the study, acute confusion or delirium was defined as an organic brain syndrome characterized by transient, global cognitive impairment of abrupt onset and relatively brief duration accompanied by diurnal fluctuation of simultaneous disturbances of the sleep–wake cycle, psychomotor behavior, attention, and affect (Foreman, 1986). This definition was chosen for its congruence with the *Diagnostic and Statistical Manual of Mental Disorders*, 3rd edition (DMS III-R) (American Psychiatric Association, 1987).

METHOD

The study was conducted with a convenience sample of patients over age 65 admitted to a general medicine unit over a 4-month period. The study unit was selected because there was a relatively large percentage of elderly patients on the unit, including people documented at high risk for delirium; further, the staff nurses had identified delirium as a clinical problem and were interested in the development of interventions to prevent or delay its occurrence.

Criteria for entry into the study were age over 65, absence of primary or secondary diagnosis of a psychiatric disorder (excluding dementia), admission to the study unit, and consent to participate. Over one third of potential subjects did not enter the study owing to inability to give consent because of cognitive impairment.

Twenty-nine patients entered the study. Fifty-five percent were female; the average age was 79 years (range 65–100). A majority were admitted from their own home and the others from foster care, retirement facilities, assisted living, or nursing homes.

Measures

The data-collection instruments were the NEECHAM Confusion Scale, the Folstein Mini-Mental State Exam (MMSE), and self-report of perceived mental clarity.

NEECHAM Confusion Scale The primary measure of cognitive functioning was the NEECHAM scale, which was developed to measure disturbances in information processing and acute confusional states in hospitalized elderly patients (Neelon, Funk, Carlson, & Champagne, 1989). The NEECHAM tool has a strong positive correlation with the Folstein Mini Mental State Exam (MMSE) (.78), a tool widely used to detect alteration in mental function in older adults, including those with dementia. The NEECHAM scale has been tested in over 1,000 observations of elderly subjects in hospital and nursing home settings (V. J. Neelon, personal communication, 1990). Although not initially developed for use with patients who have an underlying dementia, it has been used with such individuals. The NEECHAM tool involves both observation and the physiologic measurement of vital sign stability, oxygen saturation stability, and urinary continence control. Oxygen saturation is measured using noninvasive pulse oximetry. NEECHAM scores range from 0 (minimal responsiveness) to 30 (normal function). NEECHAM scores can be classified into three levels of confusion: Level III (not confused), scores of 25–30; Level II (mild–early confusion), scores of 20–24; and Level I (severe confusion), scores of 0–19. Interrater reliability has been reported to be high ($r = .96$), as has test-retest reliability ($r = .98$) in stable, elderly subjects (Champagne, Neelon, McConnell, & Funk, 1987).

In the current study the NEECHAM was used to measure confusion in elderly subjects from admission throughout their hospitalization. In order to detect the diurnal fluctuations in cognitive function that may occur among elderly hospitalized persons, the instrument was administered once during the morning and again in the afternoon or early evening by members of the research team. The NEECHAM scale takes less than 20 minutes to administer and even less time when combined with caregiving. The NEECHAM places a limited response burden on patients, and therefore frequent administration was not viewed as problematic for the patients.

Folstein Mini-Mental State Exam To address the concurrent validity of the NEECHAM tool, mental status was measured intermittently using the MMSE. The MMSE was selected as the reference standard because it is well known and widely used as a structured screening tool for cognitive impairment. The MMSE takes approximately 5-10 minutes to administer and focuses on the cognitive aspects of mental function (Folstein, Folstein, & McHugh, 1975). The MMSE measures orientation, registration, attention and calculation, recall, and language ability. Completion of all items requires that the subject be able to see and communicate verbally and in writing. The MMSE was not administered to eight subjects (30%) who were too ill or otherwise unable to cooperate with the response requirements.

Self-Perceived Mental Clarity Three questions were asked of the patient about his or her self-perceived mental clarity and presence of disturbing dreams. These questions were included because of the importance of perception for behavior (Lawton, 1982). It was recognized that older patients might be reluctant to reveal problems with mental functioning, and the questions were therefore phrased in a manner to avoid causing distress. The three questions were deleted from the interview for only one subject, who had expressed great concern about her mental status and feared involuntary commitment to an institution.

Procedure

Research assistants for the study were five clinically experienced registered nurses. A 7-hour multiphasic program provided instruction in the research protocol and practice in using the NEECHAM, MMSE, and other assessment tools in videotaped and live patient settings. Prior to data collection, the percentage agreement for all raters scoring one practice subject using the NEECHAM was 67%. The total score assigned by raters differed by no more than one point. All raters agreed on scoring for six of the nine NEECHAM items and disagreed by one point on three items.

A midstudy reliability check of five raters using the NEECHAM to assess four subjects found excellent interrater correlation (.99). However, the percent agreement on total scores, a more conservative measure of reliability, was 70%. Raters varied by as many as four points on total scores for one subject.

Thirty paired observations made by two raters over a 3-week period were highly correlated for the NEECHAM total scores (Pearson's product moment correlation, $r = .97$, $p < .001$). This is consistent with reported interrater reliability (Champagne et al., 1987). The percentage agreement was 100% in relation to the cut-off score of 24 or less indicating confusion. For all but one item, scoring agreement was good, ranging from $r = .78$ to $r = 1.00$. The correlations tended to be at the lower end of the range for those items that involved the observation of patient behaviors. The most problematic item was "Performance/appearance, hygiene" with an interrater correlation of $r = .62$. The lower correlation on performance items may have been due to the greater subjective judgment required to score performance and the tendency of less experienced raters to award points for the best observed behavior rather than for the most impaired (V. J. Neelon, personal communication, December 10, 1990).

The interrater agreement for the MMSE prior to data collection was good (94%). Six paired assessments during the study had a high correlation (Pearson product moment, $r = .97$, $p < .001$), comparing favorably with the reported reliability of this instrument (Folstein et al., 1975).

Because the same raters administered both the NEECHAM and the MMSE, there was some potential for bias (criterion contamination). In an effort to avoid bias, the NEECHAM (which requires assignment of a rating according to degrees of behavior observed for six of nine items) was always administered before the MMSE (which is composed of dichotomous items). Also, scores were not totalled until all data for the study were collected.

RESULTS

Incidence of Confusion

Forty-five percent of the elderly patients were found to have cognitive impairment on the initial NEECHAM assessment. However, because of the difficulty in obtaining consent to participate from patients admitted with confusion, it is likely that the actual incidence of confusion was greater than found in this sample.

The number and percentage of patients whose level of confusion was stable over two assessments during hospitalization were examined in relation to the level of confusion on admission (see Table 28.1). Patients admitted with early/mild confusion (Level 2) were far less stable than those admitted with no confusion. Figure 28.1 presents examples of the confusion trajectories for elderly persons admitted with early/mild confusion. At discharge, approximately 75% of the patients were at the same level of confusion as when they were admitted to the study. Thirteen percent left the hospital more confused than they were at admission, and 12% improved in their level of mental clarity from admission.

The NEECHAM As a Screening Tool

The concurrent validity of the NEECHAM, which constitutes a form of criterion-related validity, was examined using Folstein's MMSE as the reference criterion. The purpose was to determine to what extent the total NEECHAM scores correctly identified subjects as being either

TABLE 28.1 Stability by Admitting Levels of Confusion over Hospitalization

Admitting level of confusion (NEECHAM)	Number of patients in level on admission (n)	Number and percentage of patients whose level changed over hospitalization	
		n	%
Level 1—severe (scores of 0–19)	3	2	66.7
Level 2—mild/early (scores of 20–24)	10	9	90.0
Level 3—not confused (scores of 25–30)	16	6	37.5

confused or not confused, as determined by the MMSE total scores obtained at approximately the same time.

Both sensitivity and specificity of the NEECHAM were examined. Sensitivity is the ability of the NEECHAM to correctly identify individuals who are confused, and specificity is the ability to correctly identify individuals who are not confused. NEECHAM scores of 24 or less indicate confusion, while MMSE scores of 23 or less indicate cognitive impairment. Using the MMSE as the reference criterion, this study found the sensitivity of the NEECHAM to be 30% and specificity to be 92% (see Table 28.2). This differs considerably from the reported sensitivity of 95% and specificity of 78% of the NEECHAM (Neelon et al., 1989). The differences, however, may be due to the small sample size in the current study and the use of different raters, or it may be due to the use by Neelon et al. (1989) of a different subject population and different reference criteria. The MMSE has certain limitations as a reference criterion. It is itself a screening test, not a diagnostic test, and educational level has been shown to influence MMSE scores. In addition, lower cut-off scores have been recommended when the MMSE is given to hospitalized patients. Thus the disagreement between the NEECHAM and the MMSE may thus have been a function of a problem with the MMSE.

The predictive value of a positive test is the probability that when a test is positive, confusion is truly present. The predictive value of a positive test was 81% in this study; the predictive value of a negative test was 53%. Because the greater personal risk to the patient lies in not identifying confusion and properly treating its causes, it is preferable that the screening tool identify a higher percentage of those who have

Figure 28.1. Trajectory of three subjects admitted with Level 2 confusion.

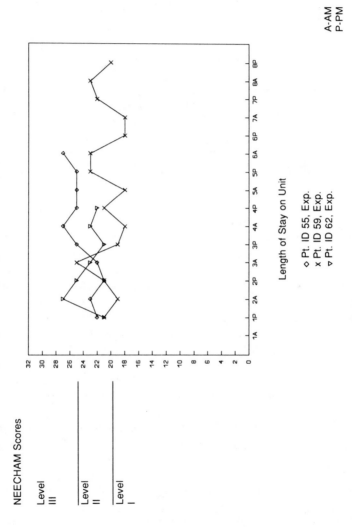

NEECHAM Scores

A-AM
P-PM

Length of Stay on Unit

◇ Pt. ID 55, Exp.
× Pt. ID 59, Exp.
▽ Pt. ID 62, Exp.

295

TABLE 28.2   Sensitivity and Specificity of the NEECHAM in Predicting MMSE
Results

	MMSE		
NEECHAM	Confused ≤ 23	Not confused 24+	Total
Confused (score ≤ 24)	9	2	11
Not confused (score ≥ 25)	21	24	45
Total	30	26	56

Clinical indices:	
Sensitivity [(9/30) × 100]	30%
Specificity [(24/26) × 100]	92%
Predictive value of a positive test [(9/11) × 100]	81%
Predictive value of a negative test [(24/45) × 100]	53%

confusion, or some degree of cognitive impairment (risk having more false positives) than to set the cutoff to obtain a higher specificity (fewer false positives). Neelon (personal communication, April 13, 1991) has noted that subjects with NEECHAM scores of 27 or higher on admission do not develop confusion unless there is some catastrophic occurrence. In this study, use of a NEECHAM cutoff score of 26 or less for confusion, with the MMSE as the only reference criterion, would have yielded a sensitivity of 53% and a specificity of 88%, with the predictive validity of a positive test 84% and the predictive validity of a negative test 62%. This change in cutoff score would have resulted in fewer false negative NEECHAM scores.

The accuracy of two of the three self-report items on perceived mental clarity—the reports of confusion and disturbing dreams—was determined through comparison with the NEECHAM. The third item, which asked the elderly subject to rate his mental clarity compared to the previous assessment period, was not included because patients tended to respond that they were either better or the same. NEECHAM Level 1 or 2 was used as the reference criterion for the presence of confusion. As shown in Tables 28.3 and 28.4, the sensitivity of self-report of confusion, or the ability of patients to accurately identify whether or not they were confused, was only 26%, and the sensitivity of report of troubling dreams was only 16%. Seven subjects were unable to answer the question on confusion. If it is assumed that individuals who were not able to answer were limited because of altered mental status, then sensitivity increases to 36%. Using the same assumption with the

TABLE 28.3 Relationship of Patient Self Report of Confusion to the NEECHAM

Self report of confusion	NEECHAM		Total
	Confused (score ≤ 24) n	Not confused (score ≥ 25) n	
Yes	10	7	17
No	29	21	50
Total	39	28	67

Clinical indices:	
Sensitivity	26%
Specificity	75%
Predictive value of a positive test	59%
Predictive value of a negative test	42%

TABLE 28.4 Relationship of Patient Self Report of Disturbing Dreams to the NEECHAM

Self report of disturbing dreams	NEECHAM		Total
	Confused (score ≤ 24)	Not confused (score ≥ 25)	
Yes	7	3	10
No	37	24	61
Total	44	27	71

Clinical indices:	
Sensitivity	16%
Specificity	89%
Predictive value of a positive test	70%
Predictive value of a negative test	39%

dream question results in a sensitivity of 24% (five subjects were unable to respond). The specificities, or ability of the questions to identify the absence of confusion, were 75% and 89%, respectively. The predictive value of a positive response (i.e., the percentage of the time when self-report questions correctly identified confusion when it was present) was 59% for the confusion questions, and 70% for disturbing dreams (not including those who were unable to respond). Thus, when subjects reported confusion or disturbing dreams they were quite likely to be confused; however, as the low sensitivity indicates, many subjects who were confused did not report either confusion or disturbing dreams.

DISCUSSION

The nurses on the study unit assessed patients' mental status using level of orientation and alertness. On numerous occasions, nurses were not aware that a patient was experiencing significant confusion until informed by the research assistant. The fluctuations in mental status that occur with elderly patients and the development of confusion in patients who are not confused upon admission make the adoption of a nursing assessment tool of major importance.

The NEECHAM does not impose a response burden on the patient and it is not time-consuming to administer because it can be incorporated into usual nursing activities. The low sensitivity observed early in this study appeared to be the result of the research assistants' limited practice in NEECHAM use with impaired persons, resulting in high scores. Retraining during the data-collection period seemed to have corrected this problem; but unfortunately, no further interrater checks were done. As noted earlier, the mismatch between the NEECHAM and the MMSE seen in this study may not be a function of problems with the validity of the NEECHAM but may reflect problems with the MMSE. The nature of the mismatch is interesting—it may be that the two instruments measure different things. It would be desirable to compare NEECHAM scores with chart notations on mental status since clinical judgments have been found to correlate very highly with this tool. However, the absence of even minimal chart documentation of mental status found during this study made that impossible. This is clearly an area where nurses can improve care for patients by consistently documenting their assessments.

The overall reliability of the NEECHAM for determining level of confusion is very good. However, the scale requires nursing judgment and discrimination of observed behaviors, and it should be administered by experienced clinical nurses who have had sufficient training and practice in using the tool to ensure consistent scores (intra- and interrater). This is especially important if treatment decisions are to be based on NEECHAM results. It is recommended that clinical trials be implemented to determine what type and degree of training are necessary for nurses in the clinical setting to use the NEECHAM. The length of the training program developed for the research assistants in this study would be unfeasible for staff nurses, but much of the training might be unnecessary.

The two questions on the patient's self-perception of confusion and disturbing dreams should be routinely used in nursing practice. They were not distressing or time-consuming. Although they are limited in sensitivity, the questions provide more information about confusion than the current assessment practices of the nurses on the study unit. It is probable that structured assessments of confusion, such as the NEECHAM, can provide the most accurate information for planning care when combined with data such as the patients' and caregivers' perceptions of mental status.

REFERENCES

American Psychiatric Association. (1987). *Diagnostic and statistical manual of mental disorders* (3rd ed.). Washington, DC: Author.

Champagne, M., Neelon, V., McConnell, E., & Funk, S. (1987). The NEECHAM Confusion Scale: Assessing acute confusion in the hospitalized and nursing home elderly. *The Gerontologist, 27* (October, special issue), 4A.

Folstein, M. F., Folstein, S. E., & McHugh, P. R. (1975). "Mini-Mental State": A practical method for grading the cognitive state of patients for the clinician. *Journal of Psychiatric Research, 12,* 189–198.

Foreman, M. (1986). Acute confusional states in hospitalized elderly. A research dilemma. *Nursing Research, 35,* 34–38.

Lawton, M. (1982). Competence, environmental press, and the adaptation of older people. In M. Lawton, P. Windley, & T. Byerts (Eds.), *Aging & the environment: Theoretical approaches.* New York: Springer.

Neelon, V. J., Funk, S. F., Carlson, J. T., & Champagne, M. T. (1989). The NEECHAM Confusion Scale: Relationship to clinical indicators of acute confusion in hospitalized elders. *The Gerontologist, 29,* 65A.

[29]

Cognitive and Emotional Function of Stroke Patients

Rebecca A. Sisson

Stroke survival has increased as a result of better management of hypertension, but this increased survival has created new problems since many survivors are left with mental and physical disabilities. Cognitive impairment and depression may increase stroke victims' difficulty with mobility, self-care, and communication, yet traditionally the major focus in stroke rehabilitation has been on physical function. Although it has long been known that emotional changes occur following stroke, until recently few efforts were made to examine or deal with the mental status of stroke victims. Robinson and colleagues (1985) at Johns Hopkins, who have done extensive research on mood following stroke, have found that depression is frequent in stroke victims, both in the acute phase and at 3–6 month follow-up. Though earlier it was thought that left hemisphere lesions were most likely to produce post-stroke depression, it has now been found that mood disorders occur after a stroke regardless of the hemisphere involved (Stein, Hier, & Caplan, 1985; Wade, Wood, & Hewer, 1985).

Cognitive changes following stroke have been studied least of all, and most of the research has been done in England, looking at memory impairment. Evidence of other possible cognitive changes after stroke was collected in the National Stroke Data Bank study (Bronstein et al., 1986), which identified psychosocial problems and difficulty in returning to previous lifestyle, both thought to be emotionally or cognitively based. Dependence in activities of daily living was most problematic for the stroke victims. A study by Ahlsio, Britton, Murray, and Theorell (1984) also found that dementia, memory and concentration problems, as well as poorer quality of life due to dependence in ADL, were present in stroke survivors for up to 2 years after the stroke.

Since cognitive function may influence the ability of stroke victims to gain functional recovery of daily physical activities, Wade and colleagues (1985) have suggested that rehabilitative therapy should concentrate less on physical function and more on cognitive function. However, Holbrook (1982) notes that no disability scale for stroke patients includes cognitive problems, nor is there a scale that includes items on self-perception and self-appraisal. The purposes of this study, therefore, were to evaluate emotional and cognitive function after stroke and determine whether these were related to functional activity status.

METHOD

To explore the relationships between emotional and cognitive status and functional status, as assessed by activities of daily living, patients were interviewed at three points: Time 1: 10 days following the stroke; Time 2: 4 weeks later; Time 3: 3 months later.

The sample was a convenience sample recruited from four hospitals in a large West Coast metropolitan area. Criteria for inclusion were documented stroke from chart and CT scan, ability to respond verbally or in writing or by sign, stable condition noted on the chart, no more than 10 days post-stroke, and availability for follow-up. Fifty-three subjects participated in the study.

Two instruments were used for data collection—the Neurobehavioral Rating Scale (NRS) (Levin et al., 1987) and the Barthel Functional Index (BFI) (Mahoney & Barthel, 1965). The NRS is a 27-item Likert scale that asks about such problems as anxiety, depression, memory deficit, decreased initiative, and comprehension deficit (see Figure 29.1). Items are rated on a 7-point scale according to severity, from not present to extremely severe. To be considered reflective of a deficit, a rating of mild or greater is required. An interview guide was developed for the NRS to gather information on memory, self-report of symptoms, reasoning, focused attention, and self-appraisal. Ratings on the NRS were made based on the patient's response to questions and his or her behavior during the interview. The level of severity of each item (rating) was determined following the interview and out of the patient's presence. All subjects were interviewed by the researcher or a trained research assistant (an RN graduate student). Interrater reliability of the NRS was established at .90 ($p = .001$) during development of the scale.

The BFI is a reliable instrument for scoring ability to carry out activities of daily living. Feeding, dressing, toileting, and ambulation are scored

FIGURE 29.1 Neurobehavioral Rating Scale.

NEUROBEHAVIORAL RATING SCALE
H.S. Levin, J.E. Overall, K.E. Goethe, W. High, R.A. Sisson

DIRECTIONS Place an X in the appropriate box to represent level of severity of each symptom

	Not Present	Very Mild	Mild	Moderate	Mod. Severe	Severe	Extremely Severe
1. **INATTENTION/REDUCED ALERTNESS**—fails to sustain attention, easily distracted, fails to notice aspects of environment, difficulty directing attention, decreased alertness	☐	☐	☐	☐	☐	☐	☐
2. **SOMATIC CONCERN**—volunteers complaints or elaborates about somatic symptoms (e.g. headache, dizziness, blurred vision), and about physical health in general	☐	☐	☐	☐	☐	☐	☐
3. **DISORIENTATION**—confusion or lack of proper association for person, place, or time	☐	☐	☐	☐	☐	☐	☐
4. **ANXIETY**—worry, fear, overconcern for present or future	☐	☐	☐	☐	☐	☐	☐
5. **EXPRESSIVE DEFICIT**—word-finding disturbance, anomia, pauses in speech, effortful and agrammatic speech, circumlocution.	☐	☐	☐	☐	☐	☐	☐
6. **EMOTIONAL WITHDRAWAL**—lack of spontaneous interaction, isolation, deficiency in relating to others	☐	☐	☐	☐	☐	☐	☐
7. **CONCEPTUAL DISORGANIZATION**—thought processes confused, disconnected, disorganized, disrupted, tangential social communication, perseverative	☐	☐	☐	☐	☐	☐	☐
8. **DISINHIBITION**—socially inappropriate comments and/or actions, including aggressive/sexual content, or inappropriate to the situation, outbursts of temper.	☐	☐	☐	☐	☐	☐	☐
9. **GUILT FEELINGS**—self-blame, shame, remorse for past behavior.	☐	☐	☐	☐	☐	☐	☐

302

FIGURE 29.1 *Continued*

10. **MEMORY DEFICIT**—difficulty learning new information, rapidly forgets recent events, although immediate recall (forward digit span) may be intact. □ □ □ □ □ □

11. **AGITATION**—motor manifestations of overactivation (e.g., kicking, arm flailing, picking, roaming, restlessness, talkativeness.) □ □ □ □ □ □

12. **INACCURATE INSIGHT AND SELF-APPRAISAL**—poor insight, exaggerated self-opinion, overrates level of ability and underrates personality change in comparison with evaluation by clinicians and family. □ □ □ □ □ □

13. **DEPRESSIVE MOOD**—sorrow, sadness, despondency, pessimism. □ □ □ □ □ □

14. **HOSTILITY/UNCOOPERATIVENESS**—animosity, irritability, belligerence, disdain for others, defiance of authority. □ □ □ □ □ □

15. **DECREASED INITIATIVE/MOTIVATION**—lacks normal initiative in work or leisure, fails to persist in tasks, is reluctant to accept new challenges. □ □ □ □ □ □

16. **SUSPICIOUSNESS**—mistrust, belief that others harbor malicious or discriminatory intent. □ □ □ □ □ □

17. **FATIGABILITY**—rapidly fatigues on challenging cognitive tasks or complex activities, lethargic. □ □ □ □ □ □

18. **HALLUCINATORY BEHAVIOR**—perceptions without normal external stimulus correspondence. □ □ □ □ □ □

19. **MOTOR RETARDATION**—slowed movements or speech (excluding primary weakness). □ □ □ □ □ □

20. **UNUSUAL THOUGHT CONTENT**—unusual, odd, strange, bizarre thought content. □ □ □ □ □ □

21. **BLUNTED AFFECT**—reduced emotional tone, reduction in normal intensity of feelings, flatness. □ □ □ □ □ □

22. **EXCITEMENT**—heightened emotional tone, increased reactivity. □ □ □ □ □ □

23. **POOR PLANNING**—unrealistic goals, poorly formulated plans for the future, disregards prerequisites (e.g., training), fails to take disability into account. □ □ □ □ □ □

FIGURE 29.1 Continued

24. **LABILITY OF MOOD**—sudden change in mood which is disproportionate to the situation. ☐ ☐ ☐ ☐

25. **TENSION**—postural and facial expression of heightened tension, without the necessity of excessive activity involving the limbs or trunk. ☐ ☐ ☐ ☐

26. **COMPREHENSION DEFICIT**—difficulty in understanding oral instructions on single or multistage commands. ☐ ☐ ☐ ☐

27. **SPEECH ARTICULATION DEFECT**—misarticulation, slurring or substitution of sounds which affect intelligibility (rating is independent of linguistic content.) ☐ ☐ ☐ ☐

Note: From "The Neurobehavioral Rating Scale: Assessment of the Behavioral Sequelae of Head Injury by the Clinician," by H. S. Levin, W. M. High, K. E. Goethe, R. A. Sisson, J. E. Overall, H. M. Rhoades, H. M. Eisenberg, Z. Kalisky, & H. E. Gary, 1987, *Journal of Neurology, Neurosurgery and Psychiatry, 50,* pp. 183–193. Copyright 1987 by the British Medical Association. Reprinted by permission.

according to degree of ability, from intact to null. The BFI was scored based on data in the chart or collected from the patient's caregiver. Both instruments were scored by the same person at each data collection time; however, to reduce researcher bias, the same person did not always interview the patient at every time.

RESULTS

The size of the sample at Time 1 was 53, with ages ranging from 25 to 89 (mean = 67); 33 subjects were male and 20 female. The majority (n = 31) had a right hemisphere stroke. At Time 2, 48 subjects were interviewed (5 were lost to follow-up). As a result of the death of 4 subjects and the critical condition of one other, the final sample at Time 3 was 43. All analyses were done using this final sample.

The patient's functional ability to carry out activities of daily living was determined at all three data-collection times using the Barthel Functional Index (BFI). At Time 1, 8 patients (15%) were totally dependent, 16 (30%) were dependent for most functions, 18 (34%) required a helper to function, and 11 (21%) could provide most self-care (see Table 29.1). By Time 2 most patients were in a rehabilitation program and 28 (58%) of the subjects were doing most of their own care. However, 20 patients were still dependent on a caregiver. By Time 3, 79% were independent, 14% partially dependent, and only 7% dependent.

While poor planning abilities and inability to accurately appraise oneself were frequent at Time 1, the deficits occurring most frequently at all three data-collection times were memory deficit, depression, anxiety, mental fatigue, conceptual disorganization, and inattention. Interestingly, anxiety was present in over half of the sample at all three times, and depression increased over time. Both mental fatigue and inattention were sustained over time, and memory deficits also remained constant over time (see Table 29.2).

A principal components factor analysis of the items from the Neurobehavioral Rating Scale (NRS) produced two factors: (1) behavior disturbance/emotional lability and (2) cognitive dysfunction. Items included in Factor 1 were anxiety, blunted affect, disinhibition, agitation, depressive mood, and excitement. Factor 2 included disorientation, conceptual disorganization, memory deficit, and comprehension deficit.

Scores on the two factors of the NRS were correlated with functional status scores from the BFI at Time 3 to examine the relationship between emotional and cognitive functioning and functional activity status.

TABLE 29.1 Functional Ability

	Time 1		Time 2		Time 3	
Functional ability	*n*	%	*n*	%	*n*	%
Totally dependent	8	15	0	0	0	0
Mostly dependent	16	30	10	21	3	7
Partially dependent	18	34	10	21	6	14
Independent	11	21	28	58	43	79

Cognitive dysfunction and functional status scores were significantly related [$R^2(1,41) = .55$, $p < .001$], but emotional and functional status were not.

DISCUSSION

The increase seen in depression over time among these patients and the sustained memory deficits are significant problems for stroke survivors; they have also been identified as problems by other researchers. The major finding of this study, however, was the positive relationship between cognitive status and functional activity status. There was no correlation between emotional status and functional status, though it is often thought that functional status may affect emotional status.

The positive correlation seen between cognitive status and functional status has major implications for practice. Because of the cost of rehabilitation programs, only patients who are likely to benefit can be selected for them. Rehabilitation must also be timed appropriately to be effective. Clearly, assessment of a stroke patient's mental status (both emotional and cognitive components) is important when planning for rehabilitation. Cognitive function is a vital part of a person's readiness for and ability to learn, and deficits in cognition, especially in memory and the ability to sustain attention, can be deterrents to rehabilitation. Therefore, before appropriate placement and referrals can be made, the stroke patient's cognitive ability must be evaluated.

Both the NRS and the BFI can show patient change over time. They can be used to document observed behaviors, emotions, thinking ability, and functional ability. The BFI has been used for a number of years in rehabilitation settings to document patients' ability to carry out activities of daily living. While the NRS is a new instrument and is still being tested with stroke patients, it can be used by experienced clinicians to

TABLE 29.2 Most Frequently Reported Deficits at Times 1, 2, and 3[a]

Deficit	Time 1 (%)	Time 2 (%)	Time 3 (%)
Poor planning	70	35	2
Inaccurate insight and self-appraisal	67	43	11
Memory deficit	60	58	63
Depressive mood	59	72	76
Blunted affect	57	59	32
Anxiety	54	73	62
Fatigability (mental fatigue)	54	52	56
Conceptual disorganization	50	39	38
Inattention/reduced alertness	45	44	37
Expressive deficit	43	23	23
Somatic concern	38	48	62
Disorientation	34	12	7
Decreased initiative/motivation	31	35	49

[a]Percentages are reported for ratings that were "mild" or more severe than that for at least one third of the sample at any time point.

assess emotional and cognitive changes over time. Both of the instruments are subjectively scored and should be administered and interpreted by the health care team working together.

Nurses have the knowledge and skill to evaluate stroke patients' emotional and cognitive function over time and should assume this responsibility as part of their practice. They can then plan with the family for the patient's discharge and rehabilitation, thus ensuring the appropriateness of placement, retraining activities, and referrals.

ACKNOWLEDGMENTS

This study was partially supported by a grant from the Academic Senate, University of California, San Francisco.

REFERENCES

Ahlsio, B., Britton, M., Murray, V., & Theorell, T. (1984). Disablement and quality of life after stroke. *Stroke, 15,* 886–890.

Bronstein, K., Murray, P., Licata-Gehr, E., Banko, M., Kelly-Hayes, M., Fast, S., & Kunitz, S. (1986). The Stroke Data Bank Project: Implications for nursing research. *Journal of Neuroscience Nursing, 18,* 132–134.

Holbrook, M. (1982). Stroke: Social and emotional outcome. *Journal of Royal College of Physicians of London, 16*(20), 100–104.

Levin, H. S., High, W. M., Goethe, K. E., Sisson, R. A., Overall, J. E., Rhoades, H. M., Eisenberg, H. M., Kalisky, Z., & Gary, H. E. (1987). The neurobehavioral rating scale: Assessment of the behavioral sequelae of head injury by the clinician. *Journal of Neurology, Neurosurgery, and Psychiatry, 50,* 183–193.

Mahoney, F. L., & Barthel, D. W. (1965). Functional evaluation: Barthel index. *Maryland State Medical Journal, 14,* 61–65.

Robinson, R. G., Book Starr, L., Lipsey, J. R., Rao, K., & Price, T. R. (1985). A two-year longitudinal study of poststroke mood disorders. *Journal of Nervous and Mental Disease, 173,* 221–226.

Stein, R. W., Hier, D. B., & Caplan, L. R. (1985). Cognitive and behavior deficits after right hemisphere stroke. *Current Concepts in Cerebrovascular Disease, XX,* 1–5.

Wade, D. T., Wood, V. A., & Hewer, R. L. (1985). Recovery after stroke—the first three months. *Journal of Neurology, Neurosurgery and Psychiatry, 48,* 7–13.

[30]

Decreasing Caregiver Assistance with Older Adults with Dementia

Cornelia Beck, Patricia Heacock, Susan Mercer, and Chris Walton

Older adults with dementia often have decreased ability to perform activities of daily living (ADLs). As ADL ability decreases, these older adults can experience loss of control and self-esteem; and caregivers who provide assistance to them experience frustration and often an overwhelming burden. The extent to which ADL dependence is related to actual physical and cognitive impairment or is environmentally induced is unknown. However, creation of dependency in elderly nursing home residents is a widely reported phenomenon (Baltes & Zerbe, 1976; Barton, Baltes, & Orzech, 1980; Miller, 1985; Sperbeck & Whitbourne, 1981). Some researchers have found that nursing home staff reinforce dependency to increase resident manageability and treatability (Barton et al., 1980; Kane & Kane, 1978).

Other researchers have found that nursing home residents with dementia can become more independent in performing ADLs. McEvoy and Patterson (1986), for example, implemented an ADL teaching program for residents with dementia and concluded that they can reacquire ADL skills. Tappen (1988) found that a training group approach could increase self-care levels of demented older adults. Coyne (1988) found that the use of directed verbal prompts and positive reinforcement was related to improved eating independence in nursing home residents with dementia.

Clinical research on increasing independence in dementia patients is scarce, perhaps because of the difficulties of working with patients whose cognitive features vary widely from each other and from one time to another. This study confronted those difficulties by individualizing an intervention to support each subject's disabilities and by encouraging the use of remaining abilities.

The study took a behavioral approach to increasing independence during dressing. This approach recognizes that though the neuropathologic changes of dementia cannot be arrested, environmental alterations and behavioral strategies may influence behavior. The study examined the amount of dressing assistance that subjects required before and after receiving the interactional behavioral strategies entitled Strategies for Promoting Independence in Dressing (SPID).

METHOD

Subjects

Subjects were selected according to the following criteria:

1. Their primary diagnosis was dementia, either dementia of the Alzheimer's type (DAT), multi-infarct dementia (MID), dementia post–cerebral vascular accident, or dementia secondary to organic brain syndrome (OBS).
2. They had no past history of physical violence.
3. They had no physical impairments that prevented them from participating in dressing activities.
4. They were not independent in dressing themselves prior to the study, as indicated by a score of 1 or less on the Beck Dressing Performance Scale.

Initially a fifth criterion was that subjects score 10 or above on the Mini-Mental State Exam (MMSE) (Folstein, Folstein, & McHugh, 1975); this was designed to ensure that subjects' cognitive abilities were high enough for them to improve in dressing independence. However, this criterion was not followed because the majority of subjects who met all the other criteria scored 10 or below on the MMSE. Also, a low MMSE score did not coincide with decreased dressing abilities; in fact, one potential subject scored a 0 on the MMSE because of aphasia, yet was completely independent in dressing himself.

The convenience sample included 15 subjects with dementia in a long-term care unit at a Department of Veterans' Affairs Hospital. Written consent was obtained from the guardian or a family member.

Preintervention Assessment

Subjects were videotaped during dressing twice during the first week to desensitize the subjects and caregivers. Next, baseline data were collected by videotaping subjects dressing twice a week for 2 weeks. Videotapes of subjects were analyzed using the Beck Dressing Performance Scale (Beck, 1988) to determine the level of caregiver assistance required during dressing. The Beck Scale breaks dressing performance down into 34 components. For example, the components of putting on pants include picking up the pants, positioning the pants, putting the right leg in the pants, putting the left leg in the pants, pulling the pants to the waist, zipping the pants, and snapping or buttoning the pants.

On the Beck Scale, types of dressing assistance are arranged into a hierarchy of categories ranging from no assistance to stimulus control, initial verbal prompting, repeated verbal prompting, gestures or modeling, occasional physical guidance, complete physical guidance, to complete assistance. Numerical values range from 0 (no assistance) to 7 (complete assistance). Levels of assistance are defined in Table 30.1. A total score is obtained by adding the rating on each component and dividing by the number of components performed. The content validity of the scale was established by a geropsychiatric nurse during 26 observations of dressing performance. To evaluate interrater reliability, two master's-prepared gerontologic nurses scored five caregiver–subject dressing interactions in the current study, using these 34 components; interrater reliability was .80.

Prior to videotaping the subjects, the Neurobehavioral Cognitive Status Exam (NCSE) (Northern California Neurobehavioral Group, 1988) and the Cognitive Skills for Dressing Assessment (CSDA) (Heacock, Beck, Mercer, Speck-Kern, & Walton, 1991) were administered. In addition, the MMSE provided descriptive data on the subjects that allowed us to compare our sample with those of other studies. The NCSE uses independent tests to evaluate functioning in eight major ability areas: level of consciousness, orientation, attention, language, construction, memory, calculations, and reasoning. Language is broken down into three subareas—comprehension, repetition, and naming. Reasoning is broken down into similarities and judgment. Points given for correct responses are summed within each cognitive ability area to provide independent scores rather than a single overall score. The NCSE has been shown to be more sensitive than either the MMSE or the Cognitive Capacity Screening Examination in detecting cognitive dysfunction in a neurosurgical population (Schwamm, Van Dyke, Kiernan, Merrin, & Mueller, 1987).

The CSDA was developed to determine a subject's ability to use daily

TABLE 30.1. Definition of Levels of Caregiver Assistance and Scoring for the Beck Dressing Performance Scale (BDPS)

Score	Levels of assistance
0	No Assistance: The subject is able to perform the component of dressing without assistance from a caregiver. The caregiver may be present but does not speak or have any contact with the subject or clothing items.
1	Stimulus Control: The subject is able to perform the component of the dressing task if the caregiver controls the environment—for example, laying clothes out in the correct order.
2	Initial Verbal Prompt: The subject is able to perform the component of the dressing task if the caregiver gives an initial one-step command—for example, "Pull up your pants."
3	Repeated Verbal Prompts: The subject is able to perform the component of the dressing task if he or she is verbally prompted more than once to initiate or complete the behavior.
4	Gestures or Modeling: The subject is able to complete the component of the dressing task if the caregiver points out significant parts of the correct behavior or demonstrates how to perform the behavior.
5	Occasional Physical Guidance: The subject is able to complete the component of the dressing task if the caregiver provides occasional touching, physical prompting, or guiding—for example, guiding the subject's arm into a sleeve and releasing the arm to permit the subject to complete the action.
6	Complete Physical Guidance: The subject is able to complete the component of the dressing task if the caregiver provides constant touch and guidance.
7	Complete Assistance: The caregiver completes the component of the dressing task. The subject does not use his hands or complete any actions that would assist with the component of the dressing task.

skills and thus to bridge the gap between neuropsychological assessment and development of interventions in extended care facilities. The CSDA evaluates functioning in five major ability areas: language, sensory perception, body schema, motor movements, and reasoning/judgment. In contrast to the NCSE, which is more general, the CSDA contains items specific to the task of dressing and other necessary skills, such as face recognition, moving a body part on command, and requesting help. Points given for correct responses are summed within each cognitive ability area to provide independent scores. Reliability of the CSDA was assessed with 15 older adults with dementia using interclass correlation coefficients. Interrater reliability was high ($r = .95$, $p < .001$), and test–retest reliability was also high ($r = .95$, $p < .001$).

In this study, dressing strategies were individualized to each subject based on the scores on the NCSE and the CSDA. In each of these tests, certain cognitive abilities and motor skills are needed to complete a task in each assessed area. A graph incorporating these abilities and skills was developed, to provide a means of plotting emerging patterns of abilities or deficits. For example, comprehension and repetition are two of the four major areas assessed under language skills; the following abilities are involved in comprehension of a verbal command to complete an action: oral language comprehension, fine motor skills, pointing and hand control, body awareness or general proprioception, tactile perception or touch, sequencing, acting on an immediate memory cue, the ability to initiate an action, and the ability to continue an action.

Other cognitive areas assessed by the NCSE and the CSDA require many of the same or slightly differing abilities, such as visual pattern recognition, visual contrast discrimination, or abstract cognitive skills. When these abilities were present or absent, a pattern emerged on the graph. Strategies then could be implemented to match remaining abilities or compensate for disabilities. For example, if a subject had a pattern that indicated a receptive language disability, but sensory perception and body schema abilities were present, then physical guidance, gestures, and modeling were used to assist in dressing.

Intervention

The clinical treatment Strategies for Promoting Independence in Dressing (SPID) includes environmental and interactional strategies. An example of an environmental strategy is the reduction of external stimuli for subjects who have problems with attention. An example of an interactional strategy is the use of modeling for subjects who do not recognize clothing items. SPID is designed to be taught to caregivers, who then implement the treatment with subjects. In this study SPID was taught to caregivers in eight 1-hour sessions, using several different teaching methods. Behavioral strategies and techniques for prompting behavior were reviewed and demonstrated. A videotape was shown that put the strategies into action, with scenes of four different persons with dementia based on actual case histories. The abilities and disabilities of each of the patients in the study were then reviewed, and handouts listing behavioral strategies designed to promote the use of the remaining abilities of each subject were given to caregivers and reviewed. Interventions were individualized to each subject's abilities and disabilities. At the end of the teaching sessions, caregivers demonstrated the use of SPID by dressing research team members, who acted out roles based on actual residents with various abilities and disabilities.

In addition to instructing caregivers to implement SPID, the teaching sessions were designed to help caregivers improve their ability to cope with stress, increase their understanding of the physiologic reasons for the behavior of dementia patients, and improve their communication with the residents. The sessions incorporated lectures, slide and videotape presentations, discussions, and role-playing.

Postintervention Assessment

After the clinical intervention SPID was taught to caregivers, the caregivers received reinforcement for 6 weeks regarding the implementation of the individualized behavioral strategies, and progressively incorporated these strategies into their routine care. During this time, caregivers were videotaped twice a week during dressing interactions, and these videotapes were reviewed to assure that caregivers were implementing the strategies. At the end of this 6-week period, feedback and encouragement were stopped, and data collection continued twice a week for 2 more weeks. Data collection then was stopped for 3 weeks, and after that period, follow-up data were collected twice a week for 1 week. Videotapes were randomized, and using the Beck Scale, each dressing interaction was rated for the level of caregiver assistance by two master's-prepared gerontologic nurses, who were blind to the time sequence of the videotapes.

RESULTS

Because of the small sample, findings are presented as group data, then two individual case studies are presented.

Twelve caregivers participated in the study, including four aides, six LPNs, and two RNs, one with a diploma and one with a BSN. The 15 subjects, all male veterans, had a primary diagnosis of dementia or Alzheimer's disease. Their mean age was 71.56 (SD = 7.66), and their mean MMSE score was 10.06 (SD = 13.15), indicating severe cognitive impairment.

Mean scores on the Beck Dressing Performance Scale (BDPS) were calculated for the four baseline observations, the four observations following 6 weeks of treatment, and the two follow-up observations. The significance of changes in the mean BDPS over time was assessed by the paired t-test.

Mean BDPS scores showed that level of caregiver assistance decreased from 6.26 (SD = 1.49)—complete physical guidance—at baseline, to 4.93 (SD = 1.63)—occasional physical guidance—following 6 weeks of treatment [$t(13) = 3.76$, $p = .002$]; the level decreased further to 4.71 (SD = 1.47) at follow-up [$t(14) = 3.96$, $p = .001$]. A Wilcoxon sign rank test confirmed the significance of the decreases, indicating greater dressing independence of subjects following the use of Strategies for Promoting Independence in Dressing.

Case Study I

Mr. C., a 68-year-old Caucasian male, had a primary diagnosis of dementia and a mean score of 5 on the MMSE. After reviewing Mr. C.'s scores on the NCSE and the CSDA, it was determined that he could dress himself with only minimal caregiver assistance. The strategies prescribed for him included laying out clothes, occasional verbal prompts, and positive reinforcement. From the baseline to treatment videotapes, Mr. C. showed dramatic improvement. During the treatment period his mean caregiver assistance score decreased from 6.48—needing occasional physical guidance, to 1.52—needing only stimulus control. The score decreased again to 1.22 during follow-up observations.

Case Study II

Mr. G., a 78-year-old Caucasian male, had a primary diagnosis of dementia and scored 3 on the MMSE. After reviewing Mr. G.'s scores on the NCSE and the CSDA, it was determined that he could dress himself if caregivers handed him clothes in the correct position, and gave physical and verbal prompts and positive reinforcement. From baseline to treatment videotapes, Mr. G. showed great improvement. His mean caregiver assistance score decreased from 7.00—needing complete assistance, to 2.81—needing only verbal prompts during the treatment period. When follow-up observations were made, however, Mr. G. had an injury to his left arm, and caregiver assistance increased to 4.11.

Discussion

A severe level of cognitive impairment in older nursing home residents, as indicated by a very low MMSE score, does not mean that they require a great deal of caregiver assistance during dressing. Subjects in this study had very low MMSE scores but were able to complete items on the

NCSE and CSDA, and were able to increase their level of dressing independence. These findings provide evidence that caregiver assistance can decrease if the caregiver implements specific strategies to promote independence.

The decreases in caregiver assistance did show a good deal of fluctuation over time. There seems to be some variability in what subjects with dementia are able to do from one day to the next, and this may have led to the fluctuations. Also, the fluctuations may have been attributable to the fact that different caregivers assisted the subjects in dressing. Some of the caregivers were able to incorporate the interventions more quickly than others. Also, some caregivers simply had better rapport with some subjects. Caregivers usually did not work with the same subjects throughout the study because of the scheduling system in the institution. The hours caregivers worked and their days off varied, which led to a lack of consistency for subjects. If greater caregiver consistency could be obtained, subjects might show less fluctuation in level of independence.

This study indicates that simply providing custodial care for dementia residents no longer can be considered adequate. Nurses who assess demented older adults and initiate individualized interventions can play a crucial role in improving their lives. The assessment and strategies developed for this study can be simplified for use in clinical practice. The first part of the assessment involves determining what the resident already is doing to dress himself or herself. This assessment can be done by using the BDPS and observing the patient during dressing three or four times. We suggest three or four observations because, unless you videotape the subject dressing, it is difficult to observe and record everything that is happening simultaneously. This initial assessment provides baseline information from which goals can be derived.

The second part of the assessment involves setting up a hypothetical situation in which the resident is asked to accomplish a task. This part of the assessment should begin with simple tasks such as asking the resident to raise his or her arm or touch his or her nose. The assessment then should progress to more complex tasks such as buttoning buttons and zipping zippers. The assessor should record the tasks the patient is able to complete.

If the resident is unable to complete a task, the assessor should assist the resident by using these strategies, in the following order: repeated verbal prompts, modeling, physical prompts, and physical guidance. The assistance the resident requires also should be recorded. Additional data that should be included in the assessment are hearing and vision problems. Also, note how alert the resident is and whether he or she is attentive or easily distracted.

TABLE 30.2. Behavioral Strategies for Dressing

Specific Behavioral Strategies

I. Interactional
  A. Verbal
     1. Use one-step verbal commands. Keep sentences simple; use one or two words if possible.
     2. Ask yes/no questions.
     3. Be concrete; tell the resident exactly what you want him or her to do.
     4. Give verbal praise after completing each step.
     5. Give praise regarding appearance after completion of dressing.
  B. Nonverbal
     1. Dress bottom half, then top half of body. (This eliminates the confusion of moving back and forth from the upper to lower body.)
     2. Hand clothing items to the resident in the correct position.
     3. Place shoes beside the foot the resident will put them on.
     4. Use gestures to indicate what you want the resident to do (i.e., point to the item of clothing you want the resident to put on).
     5. Use modeling to indicate what you want the resident to do (i.e., show the resident how to pull up pants by making the motion of pulling up pants).
     6. Use physical touch to indicate to the resident which body part you want moved or used.
     7. Use physical guidance to start the resident's movement, then allow the resident to complete the action without help.
     8. Use reverse chaining (graduated physical guidance) by allowing the resident to finish the dressing step, and decrease assistance as the resident is able to do more.
     9. Stop perseveration and replace with dressing activity.
    10. Use touch by giving the resident a pat on the back or a hug after completing each dressing step.

II. Environmental
  A. Prepare a consistent environment
     1. Use a dark-color bedspread to contrast with clothing.
     2. Lay clothes face down in the order they will be put on.
     3. Cluster matching outfits on hangers.
     4. Introduce clothing one item at a time.
     5. Reduce the number of clothing options. (Let the resident choose from only two clothing items.)
     6. Provide an incentive for completing dressing.
  B. Reduce external stimuli
     1. Turn off radio or TV.
     2. Reduce number of people in room.
     3. Provide privacy.

TABLE 30.2. *Continued*

General Behavioral Strategies
I.   Interactional
     1. Restrict conversation to dressing.
     2. Speak in a calm voice.
     3. Keep pitch of voice low.
     4. Speak clearly.
     5. Call resident by name.
     6. Keep sentences simple, using one or two words when possible.
     7. Consistently use the same word for the same thing (shirt/blouse).
II. Environmental
     1. Make up the bed.
     2. Minimize clutter of nonclothing items in the area.
     3. Put other clothing out of resident's sight (range of vision).
     4. Increase lighting.
     5. Eliminate improper clothing options (i.e., place dirty clothes in hamper).

From the assessment you can determine which behavioral strategies can help an individual patient (see Table 30.2).

This study shows great promise for improving the lives of demented older adults by beginning to identify interventions that promote independence. In the past, caregivers have been found to reinforce dependency to increase the manageability of nursing home residents (Barton et al., 1980; Kane & Kane, 1978). In the future, caregivers can be taught independence-promoting strategies to replace those strategies that encourage dependency.

REFERENCES

Baltes, M. M., & Zerbe, M. B. (1976). Independence training in nursing home residents. *The Gerontologist, 16,* 428–432.

Barton, E., Baltes, M. M., & Orzech, M. J. (1980). Etiology of dependence in older nursing home residents during morning care: The role of staff behavior. *Journal of Personality and Social Psychology, 38,* 423–431.

Beck, C. (1988). Measurement of dressing performance in persons with dementia. *American Journal of Alzheimer's Care and Related Disorders and Research, 3*(3), 21–25.

Coyne, M. L. (1988). The effects of directed verbal prompts and positive reinforcement on the level of eating independence of elderly nursing home clients with dementia. *Dissertation Abstracts International,* Section B (1990, Feb.), *5*(8), 3396.

Folstein, M. F., Folstein, S. E., & McHugh, P. R. (1975). Mini-mental state: A practical method for grading the cognitive state of patients for the clinician. *Journal of Psychiatric Research, 12,* 189–198.

Heacock, P., Beck, C., Mercer, S. O., Speck-Kern, B., & Walton, C. (1991). *The development of cognitive skills in dressing assessment.* Paper presented at The Sixth Annual Phyllis J. Verhonick Nursing Research Conference, University of Virginia, Charlottesville, VA.

Kane, R. L., & Kane, R. A. (1978). Care of the aged: Old problems in need of new solutions. *Science, 200*(4344), 913–919.

McEvoy, C. L., & Patterson, R. L. (1986). Behavioral treatment of deficit skills in dementia patients. *The Gerontologist, 26,* 475–478.

Miller, A. (1985). A study of the dependency of elderly patients in wards using different methods of nursing care. *Age and Ageing, 14,* 132–138.

Northern California Neurobehavioral Group Inc. (1988). *Manual for the neurobehavioral cognitive status exam.* Fairfax, CA: Author.

Schwamm, L. H., Van Dyke, C., Kiernan, R. J., Merrin, E. L., & Mueller, J. (1987). The Neurobehavioral Cognitive Status Examination: Comparison with the cognitive capacity screening examination and the Mini-Mental State Examination in a neurosurgical population. *Annals of Internal Medicine, 107,* 486–491.

Sperbeck, D. J., & Whitbourne, S. K. (1981). Dependency in the institutional setting: A behavioral training program for geriatric staff. *The Gerontologist, 21,* 268–275.

Tappen, R. (1988). *Revitalization: A study of the effectiveness of a specific training group approach to raising and maintaining self-care levels of cognitively impaired older adults* (Report, Grant No. 10831). Princeton, NJ: The Robert Wood Johnson Foundation.

[31]

Alzheimer's Disease: Stressors and Strategies Associated with Caregiving

Brenda L. Cleary

Alzheimer's disease is a cruel disease, for it is a thief of minds, destroyer of personalities, wrecker of family finances, and filler of nursing homes (American Association of Retired Persons, 1986). There is at present no known cause or cure. Alzheimer's disease is now the fourth leading cause of death in the United States; however, "so serious is the impact of this disorder on both patient and caregiver that death is often met by a sense of relief" (Hutton, 1987, p. 4).

Reviewing the literature on family caregiving in general, Ory (1985) noted that the vast majority of older people with functional limitations remain noninstitutionalized. It has been documented that caregiving responsibilities fall primarily on one family member, often a female (Stone, Cafferata, & Sangl, 1987). In addition to interpersonal support, family caregivers provide a wide range of services for impaired elders, such as personal care, housekeeping, supervision, and meal preparation. The physical and emotional stresses for family members providing care at home for individuals with Alzheimer's disease can be overwhelming (Fisk, 1983). Although subjective burden does not always directly reflect the objective caregiving situation, there are clearly unique problems in giving care to Alzheimer's patients, including behavioral disturbances, wandering, suspiciousness, aggressive behavior, and the need for constant repetition of verbal communications (Chenoweth & Spencer, 1986; George & Gwyther, 1986; Given, Collins, & Given, 1988; Gonzalez-Lima & Gonzalez-Lima, 1987; Morycz, 1985; Rabins, Mace, &

Lucas, 1982; Stewart-Dedmon, 1988; Zarit, Reever, & Bach-Peterson, 1980).

The demands of caring for a family member with Alzheimer's disease have been well documented. Few studies, however, have systematically documented caregiving stresses and strategies for coping throughout the course of the disease. The purpose of this exploratory study, therefore, was to identify the stressors perceived by family member caregivers of individuals with Alzheimer's disease and to determine the coping strategies they perceived as useful in ameliorating these stressors. Stressors, strategies, and the global burden perceived by caregivers were examined at different stages of the disease. Coping strategies were categorized as either palliative (emotion-focused) or instrumental (problem-focused) or a combination of the two (Lazarus & Folkman, 1984).

METHOD

Since Alzheimer's disease is a lengthy, progressively debilitating illness with three characteristic stages (mild, moderate, and severe), it may be assumed that the stresses of caregiving change over time. Therefore, a sample reflecting the three major stages of the illness was solicited through the Alzheimer's Association.

Arrangements were made for interviews to take place in subjects' homes at their convenience, with two exceptions. One caregiver's husband was newly diagnosed, and although he was willing for her to meet for an interview, he was not comfortable enough to have the interview in their home. One other interview with a male caregiver took place in a car outside the beauty shop where his wife was having her hair done; he had requested this arrangement as it was one of the few times he could be free of disruptions. Participation in the interview process was entirely voluntary. Interviews generally lasted about an hour, although some of the sessions were over 3 hours in duration.

During the initial phase of the interview, the approximate stage of Alzheimer's disease of the family member being cared for at home was assessed. To evaluate the stage of disease, selected items from the Functional Rating Scale for Symptoms of Dementia (Hutton & Christians, 1985) were administered. Caregivers were questioned about ill family members' functioning in the areas of eating, dressing, grooming, continence, communication, orientation, and memory for names and events. The information gathered through these questions corresponded to symptom descriptions that Reisberg (1984) gives as characterizing the major stages of Alzheimer's disease. On the basis of the assessment, five family members were evaluated as in the mild stage of disease, five in the moderate stage, and five in the severe stage. The sample of caregivers included five wives, three husbands, five daughters, one daughter-in-law, and one son-in-law.

Caregivers were asked to think about a typical day of providing care and respond to questions about stressors and strategies of caregiving. They were asked to describe daily challenges associated with the role of caregiving as well as strategies perceived as useful in dealing with the challenges. This portion of the interview was audiotaped for transcription and content analysis. In addition, caregivers provided background information and were also asked to evaluate, on a scale from 1 to 10, their perception of the global burden of providing care, with 1 representing little burden and 10 representing extreme burden. The investigator summarized the findings at the close of each interview for validation purposes. Subjects were also provided the investigator's phone number, and one subject did indeed telephone with additional information she wanted to share.

RESULTS

Mild or Early Alzheimer's Disease

Stressors and strategies identified during the mild or early stage of Alzheimer's disease are summarized in Table 31.1. Caregivers indicated that adjusting to the diagnosis was the major stressor, followed by the patient's forgetfulness. All five caregivers noted that these were major problems, not only for themselves but for the affected family member as well. Forgetfulness led to frustration and agitation on the part of the ill family member and to frustration and impatience on the part of the caregiver, as a result of the necessity for constant repetition of routines. The majority of problem-focused coping strategies revolved around minimizing deficits and maximizing independence. Providing memory cues and pursuing financial and legal arrangements were important coping strategies. Emotion-focused coping strategies that emerged at this time and remained helpful included maintaining a sense of humor and spirituality. It became necessary to view television programs selectively, as intricate plots were frustrating for the patient. Interestingly, television was found to provoke or reinforce delusions and hallucinations as the disease progressed.

Moderate or Middle Alzheimer's Disease

Stressors and strategies associated with the middle or moderate stage of Alzheimer's disease are summarized in Table 31.2. The caregiving stres-

TABLE 31.1   Mild or Early Alzheimer's Disease: Stressors and Strategies

Stressors identified by caregivers in order of priority[a]	Related strategies
Adjustment to illness and change in lifestyle	Establish power of attorney; maintain sense of humor and spirituality[b]; show love and patience[b]
Short-term memory loss; repetition	Provide clues; keep written records
Agitation and irritability	Maximize independence where possible; follow routines, use medication as last resort; watch television (game shows best)
Loss of personal items	Keep personal items in specific place
Spatial disorientation	Avoid patient driving or at least driving alone
Avoidance by friends and even family	Find other reliable support systems and alternative outlets

[a]Priority determined by frequency of occurrence and stated importance.
[b]Noted as important throughout illness.

sors identified were in many ways extensions of stressors experienced in the early stage of the illness. Agitated and inappropriate patient behaviors increased (noted by all five caregivers), in some cases to the point of aggression and acting out (noted by three caregivers). Problem-focused coping strategies employed by caregivers during this stage focused on management of the myriad problem behaviors demonstrated by the patient. It was at this stage that caregivers resorted to the use of tranquilizers. Either Haldol or Mellaril was administered by all five caregivers of patients in this stage, as compared to only two caregivers of patients in the early or mild stage of disease. Offspring felt the impact of a marked role reversal, while spousal caregivers felt the loss of their life partners. Safety issues became critical and houseproofing was necessary. Learning to avoid "sweating the small stuff" and finding respite and support services were identified as emotion-focused coping mechanisms.

Severe or Late Alzheimer's Disease

Stressors and strategies associated with late-stage, severe Alzheimer's disease are summarized in Table 31.3. In many ways, late-stage Alzheimer's disease resembles any condition that requires complete

TABLE 31.2   Moderate or Middle Alzheimer's Disease: Stressors and Strategies

Stressors identified by caregivers in order of priority[a]	Related strategies
Parent–child relationship (role reversal, spousal grieving)	Only exert control where necessary, but limit choices; use time out or respite
Increased agitation; confusion, particularly at night (sundowning); wandering	Follow more structured routine; provide safe items to arrange and manipulate; take long rides in automobile; change sleeping arrangements (within earshot)
Suspiciousness	Make references to reality, but remember that arguing is useless
Violence and acting out behavior	Use medications (major tranquilizers); give wine at bedtime
Decreased ability to carry out activities of daily living, e.g., eating, dressing, toileting	Have four small meals and eliminate distractions; serve milkshakes with nutritional supplement; use disposable undergarments
Safety concerns, e.g., medications, use of appliances, falls	Try houseproofing
Financial burdens	Establish power of attorney if not already established; assess financial resources; use support system, e.g., family, friends, church, support group (if support system fails, identify alternatives); address issue of nursing home placement

[a]Priority determined by frequency of occurrence and stated importance.

care. The major stressors associated with providing care to a family member in this stage were the pervasiveness of the demands of total care and cumulative fatigue; these were noted by all five caregivers in this group. Particular concerns included complete incontinence of bowel and bladder; constipation; progressive immobility and potential skin breakdown; and difficulties in assuring adequate nutrition. Problem-focused coping strategies were aimed at finding ways to provide food and fluids and generally avoid the hazards of immobility. Tranquilizers were used less, although one patient remained on Haldol and another received a hypnotic. Emotionally, caregivers tried to maintain

TABLE 31.3 Severe or Late Alzheimer's Disease: Stressors and Strategies

Stressors identified by caregivers in order of priority[a]	Related strategies
Fatigue associated with complete care	Reflect on having moved through previous stages to a more "peaceful" stage
Concerns about nutrition	Give nutritional supplements
Elimination/incontinence	Use washable protective pads and infant disposable diapers adapted for adult use
Immobility; skin breakdown, concerns about comfort	Use adaptive clothing (with matching mittens); keep clean, dry, and positioned
Financial burdens	Take cost-containment measures
Preparing for eventual death	Maintain connection with patient through touch and other personal activities

[a]Priority determined by frequency of occurrence and stated importance.

some kind of connectedness to ill family members as death eventually approached.

Perceptions of Overall Burden

Despite the limitations of a small sample for making inferences, the perceptions of global burden in the different stages of Alzheimer's disease were interesting. With one exception, caregivers with family members in late-stage Alzheimer's perceived their burden to be less (mean burden score = 3.4) than those with family members in earlier stages. Caring for family members in the middle stage was perceived as the most burdensome (mean = 7.2), and the early stage seemed to pose a moderate burden (mean = 5.2) (see Table 31.4). An analysis of variance revealed differences in perceived burden to be significant [$F(2,12)$ = 2.98, $p < .089$; given the small sample size, an alpha of .10 was used to determine significance].

Caregivers of late-stage Alzheimer's patients also made comments that reflected diminished burden, as compared to earlier stages. For example, caregiving demands, although heavy because of the complete care required in late Alzheimer's disease, were more predictable and thus more controllable. As a result, caregivers felt less burden.

TABLE 31.4   Caregivers' Perceived Global Burden in Different Stages of Alzheimer's Disease

| Stage of Alzheimer's | Perceived burden[a] | | | | |
| | Mild (1–3) | Moderate (4–7) | Extreme (8–10) | | |
	n	n	n	Mean	SD
Mild or early (n = 5)	0	5	0	5.2	1.30
Moderate (n = 5)	1	0	4	7.2	2.39
Severe or late (n = 5)	4	0	1	3.4	3.29

[a]Scale 1–10.

DISCUSSION

A comparison of burden across the stages of Alzheimer's disease using a large sample is warranted. In the meantime, family caregivers could benefit from learning that the demands of caregiving do not necessarily intensify as the illness progresses; in fact, care may be perceived as more manageable in the late stage of the illness because of greater control and predictability.

The stressors and strategies derived from this study could be used to develop a checklist both for further research and for clinical practice. Caregivers could select and prioritize stressors and strategies that applied to their situation, and an "other" category could also be included. The information provided on the checklist could be used to focus the information provided to families on what to expect as the disease progresses, and to teach them coping strategies deemed useful by experienced caregivers.

The search for a cause and a cure for Alzheimer's disease continues. Treatment remains highly experimental. Therefore, the development of nursing interventions to ease the burden of this illness for both patients and families is a major challenge for our profession. As one caregiver in this study eloquently stated, "It's kinda like the Lord gave me a mountain this time, but I've lived with the man for nearly 43 years and he's special and precious and I hate to see this happening to him, but we'll go through it together."

ACKNOWLEDGMENT

This research was supported through a National Research Service Award, National Center for Nursing Research, NIH.

REFERENCES

American Association of Retired Persons. (1986). *Coping & caring: Living with Alzheimer's disease*. Washington, DC: AARP.

Chenoweth, B., & Spencer, B. (1986). Dementia: The experience of family caregivers. *The Gerontologist, 26*, 267–272.

Fisk, A. (1983). Alzheimer's disease: A five-article symposium (Introduction). *Postgraduate Medicine, 73*, 204–205.

George, L., & Gwyther, L. (1986). Caregiver well-being: A multidimensional examination of family caregivers of demented adults. *The Gerontologist, 26*, 253–259.

Given, C. W., Collins, C. E., & Given, B. A. (1988). Sources of stress among families caring for relatives with Alzheimer's disease. *Nursing Clinics of North America, 23*, 69–82.

Gonzalez-Lima, E., & Gonzalez-Lima, F. (1987). Sources of stress affecting caregivers of Alzheimer's disease patients. *Health Values, 11*(6), 3–10.

Hutton, J. T. (1987, January). Alzheimer's disease. *Texas Medicine, 83*, 4–5.

Hutton, J. T., & Christians, B. (1985, November). *Functional rating scale for symptoms of dementia*. Paper presented at the Alzheimer's Disease Conference, University of Texas at Austin.

Lazarus, R., & Folkman, S. (1984). *Stress, appraisal, and coping*. New York: Springer.

Morycz, R. (1985). Caregiving strain and the desire to institutionalize family members with Alzheimer's disease. *Research on Aging, 7*, 329–361.

Ory, M. G. (1985). The burden of care. *Generations, 10*, 14–17.

Rabins, P., Mace, N., & Lucas, M. (1982). The impact of dementia on the family. *Journal of the American Medical Association, 248*, 333–335.

Reisberg, B. (1984). Stages of cognitive decline. *American Journal of Nursing, 84*, 225–228.

Stewart-Dedmon, M. (1988). Strain and strategy. *Nursing Times, 84*(17), 39–41.

Stone, R., Cafferata, G. L., & Sangl, J. (1987). Caregivers of the frail elderly: A national profile. *The Gerontologist, 27*, 616–626.

Zarit, S., Reever, K., Bach-Peterson, J. (1980). Relatives of the impaired elderly: Correlates of feelings of burden. *The Gerontologist, 20*, 649–655.

[32]

The Clinical Assessment of Mutuality and Preparedness in Family Caregivers to Frail Older People

Patricia G. Archbold, Barbara J. Stewart, Merwyn R. Greenlick, and Theresa A. Harvath

This chapter presents new measures for nurses to use in assessing mutuality and preparedness in family members who provide care to frail older people. We define mutuality as the positive quality of the relationship between a family caregiver and a care receiver. Based on the results of a qualitative study with family caregivers and receivers, we conceptualize mutuality as having four dimensions: love and affection, shared pleasurable activities, shared values, and reciprocity. Previous work by other investigators such as Cantor (1983), Horowitz and Shindleman (1983), and Motenko (1989) indicates that the quality of the relationship between the caregiver and care receiver is an important aspect of caregiving situations. Our own thinking about mutuality has been influenced by the work of Hirschfeld (1983), who found that caregivers reporting high levels of mutuality tolerated caregiving for a demented relative longer than did caregivers who experienced low levels of mutuality.

We define preparedness as how well prepared the caregiver believes he or she is for the tasks and stress of the caregiving role. Our original notion of preparedness was derived from role theory, in which anticipatory socialization to a role—that is, what the person learns about the role before entering it—is very important to role enactment and performance (Burr, Leigh, Day, & Constantine, 1979). Qualitative data from caregivers in our early work, however, suggested that for the most part, caregivers learned the caregiving role while in it (Harvath, Archbold, Lucas, & Stewart, 1986). Thus, we have focused on caregivers' appraisal of how well-prepared they are, no matter when they learned the role.

Few investigators have examined preparedness or any similar concept. Haley and his colleagues (Haley, Levine, Brown, & Bartolucci, 1987) have examined the self-efficacy of caregivers in managing specific caregiving tasks; they found that caregivers who reported higher levels of self-efficacy also reported lower levels of depression. Lawton and his colleagues (Lawton, Kleban, Moss, Rovine, & Glicksman, 1989) found support for a factor called "mastery" in their analysis of new measures of caregiving variables. However, although Haley's work comes closest to our concept of preparedness, neither Haley nor Lawton has examined the effects of preparedness on caregiver role strain.

We define caregiver role strain as the felt difficulty in performing the caregiver role. Our early qualitative work led us to view caregiver role strain as a multidimensional construct. We measured nine aspects of strain: strain from direct care, worry, role conflict, increased tension, feelings of being manipulated, mismatched expectations, lack of resources, economic burden, and global strain. We developed new measures for seven of these dimensions of role strain, but used Montgomery and Borgatta's (undated) scales to measure strain from feelings of being manipulated and strain from increased tension.

Previous studies of the predictors of negative consequences of family caregiving for the caregiver (e.g., caregiver role strain or stress) have focused on (1) the gender of the caregiver (e.g., Fitting, Rabins, Lucas, & Eastham, 1986); (2) whether the caregiver is a spouse or nonspouse (e.g., George & Gwyther, 1986); (3) the cognitive and physical impairment of the care receiver (e.g., Deimling & Bass, 1986); and (4) the amount of direct care done by the caregiver for the care receiver (Montgomery, Gonyea, & Hooyman, 1985). While the understanding of such relationships is important, it does not provide the nurse with an avenue for intervention in the majority of family caregiving situations— those in which the caregiver wants to continue caregiving despite the strain involved in the situation. In our last study (Archbold, Stewart, Greenlick, & Harvath, 1990), therefore, we wanted to find variables that predict caregiver role strain and are amenable to nursing intervention.

In a paper published in 1990 in *Research in Nursing and Health*, we presented findings indicating that after controlling for five variables— gender of the caregiver, whether the caregiver was a spouse or nonspouse, the cognitive and physical impairment of the care receiver, and the amount of direct care the caregiver gave to the care receiver—

mutuality and preparedness for caregiving were strongly predictive of the *lack* of caregiver role strain in family caregivers for post-hospitalized older persons. This chapter presents our measures of mutuality and preparedness for caregiving. While the two scales have been used as research instruments, the clinical utility of the scales has not been formally assessed. However, we think that these measures will have clinical utility for nurses in home health and clinics, and for discharge planners or any nurse who conducts assessments of family caregiving situations.

METHOD

The instruments described here have been used in three studies of family caregiving—an instrument evaluation study (Archbold, Stewart, Harvath, & Lucas, 1986), a longitudinal correlational study of family caregiving to older persons who had recently been discharged from the hospital (Archbold & Stewart, 1988), and a survey of caregivers for older persons with Alzheimer's disease (Stewart & Archbold, 1991). This chapter focuses on results from the longitudinal study.

The sample included 103 dyads (a caregiver and a care receiver) who participated in an interview 6 weeks after the care receiver had been discharged from the hospital. At 9 months after discharge, 78 of the dyads participated in a second in-home interview. To qualify for the study, the care receiver had to be 65 years of age or older and require assistance from a family member or friend in one or more of the following areas: (1) medications or injections; (2) bathing, shampooing, or dressing; (3) walking, shopping, or errands; or (4) household chores such as cleaning. Family caregivers had to be 18 years of age or older and able to speak English. Details of the sample are reported elsewhere (Archbold et al., 1990).

The instrument used in the study was the Family Caregiving Inventory developed by Archbold and Stewart (1986). This inventory contains the Mutuality Scale, the Preparedness for Caregiving Scale, and nine scales measuring caregiver role strain.

Mutuality Scale

The Mutuality Scale contains 15 items and is self-administered in a paper-and-pencil format. Items are answered using a 1 to 4 response format; for example, 1 = *not at all*, and 4 = *a lot*. A caregiver's overall score is computed by averaging her responses to the 15 items so that the scores for the scale range from 1.00 to 4.00. Caregivers who have high scores on the Mutuality Scale report that their relationship with the care receiver is characterized by a great deal of love, shared pleasurable activities, common values, and reciprocity. The Mutuality Scale is designed to be self-administered, because this method reduces the effect of social desirability on responses. In our study, more than 90% of caregivers were able to read and answer the scale on their own; the remaining 10% gave their answers orally.

The scale and the descriptive statistics for the items on the scale are presented in Table 32.1. In the study reported here the internal consistency reliability (Cronbach's alpha) of the scale was .91 at both the 6-week and 9-month interviews. Most caregivers reported fairly high levels of mutuality. Mean scores were 3.21 (SD = .56, n = 101) at 6-weeks and 3.11 (SD = .56, n = 78) at 9 months. The range of scores for the sample was 1.60 to 4.00.

Multiple regression analyses were performed to examine the relationship between mutuality and caregiver role strain. After taking into account five variables usually associated with greater strain—for example, the level of impairment of the care receiver and the amount of direct care done by the caregiver—we found that caregivers reporting low mutuality reported higher levels of strain than would be expected. Low mutuality was associated with greater strain in six areas: feelings of being manipulated, global strain, mismatched expectations, tension in the relationship, role conflict, and strain from direct care. Thus, caregivers who have a poor relationship with the care receiver may experience levels of strain that are elevated above what would be expected from the objective caregiving situation. Conversely, caregivers with high mutuality who are in objectively difficult caregiving situations are likely to report less strain than would be expected based on their situation.

Although researchers in the area of family caregiving to older persons view the concept of mutuality as important, they may have greatly underestimated its beneficial effects. The clinical significance of mutuality was reflected in our regression analyses by the magnitude of the statistically significant increments in variance explained by mutuality. These increments ranged from 4 to 24%, with a median value of 12%. Such values are substantial. It is likely that caregivers who have a positive relationship with the care receiver experience less strain because they find caregiving inherently meaningful. We would like to point out, however, that mutuality does not provide universal protection against strain. In our longitudinal study, three aspects of strain were not alleviated by mutuality: strain from lack of resources (for example, being too tired emotionally), economic burden, and worry.

TABLE 32.1 The Mutuality Scale with Response Frequencies, Means, and Standard Deviations[a]

Item			n	Mean	SD
1.	How close do you feel to him/her?			3.57	.65
	Not close at all	1	0		
	Somewhat close	2	9		
	Pretty close	3	25		
	Very close	4	67		
	Missing		2		
2.	How much do you and he/she enjoy talking about the "good old days"?			3.06	.86
	None	1	4		
	Some	2	22		
	Quite a bit	3	39		
	A great deal	4	36		
	Missing		2		
3.	How much does he/she express feelings of appreciation for you and the things you do?			3.13	.93
	Not very much	1	8		
	Some	2	14		
	Quite a bit	3	36		
	A great deal	4	43		
	Missing		2		
4.	To what extent do you and he/she see eye to eye?			3.10	.78
	Not at all	1	3		
	A little	2	17		
	Some	3	48		
	A lot	4	33		
	Missing		2		
5.	How attached are you to him/her?			3.78	.50
	Not at all	1	0		
	A little	2	4		
	Some	3	14		
	A lot	4	83		
	Missing		2		
6.	How much does he/she help you?			2.61	1.09
	None	1	18		
	A little	2	32		
	Some	3	22		
	A lot	4	29		
	Missing		2		

Instructions to respondents

Now we would like you to let us know how you and _____ feel about each other. Please read the following questions and circle the number corresponding to the appropriate answer.

TABLE 32.1 *Continued*

Item		n	Mean	SD
7.	How much do you like to sit and talk with him/her?		3.28	.80
	Not at all _____ 1	1		
	A little _____ 2	19		
	Some _____ 3	32		
	A lot _____ 4	49		
	Missing	2		
8.	How much love do you feel for him/her?		3.66	.67
	Not very much _____ 1	2		
	Some _____ 2	5		
	Quite a bit _____ 3	18		
	A great deal _____ 4	76		
	Missing	2		
9.	To what extent do you and he/she share the same values?		3.45	.66
	None _____ 1	1		
	A little _____ 2	6		
	Some _____ 3	41		
	A lot _____ 4	53		
	Missing	2		
10.	When you really need it, how much does he/she comfort you?		3.13	.91
	Not at all _____ 1	8		
	A little _____ 2	12		
	Some _____ 3	40		
	A lot _____ 4	41		
	Missing	2		
11.	How much do you and he/she laugh together?		3.16	.76
	Not at all _____ 1	1		
	A little _____ 2	19		
	Some _____ 3	44		
	A lot _____ 4	37		
	Missing	2		
12.	How much do you confide in him/her?		2.96	.97
	None _____ 1	9		
	A little _____ 2	22		
	Some _____ 3	34		
	A lot _____ 4	36		
	Missing	2		

TABLE 32.1 *Continued*

Item		*n*	Mean	SD
13. How much emotional support does he/ she give you?				
Not very much _____ 1		13	2.74	1.02
Some _____ 2		29		
Quite a bit _____ 3		30		
A great deal _____ 4		29		
Missing		2		
14. To what extent do you and he/she enjoy the time you spend together?				
Not at all _____ 1		0	3.55	.58
A little _____ 2		4		
Some _____ 3		38		
A lot _____ 4		59		
Missing		2		
15. How often does he/she express feelings of warmth toward you?				
Rarely _____ 1		8	2.95	.97
Sometimes _____ 2		26		
Much of the time _____ 3		30		
Nearly always _____ 4		37		
Missing		2		

[a]Results based on *N* = 103 caregivers from Caregiver Relief Study, Archbold and Stewart, (1988).

Clinical Relevance of Mutuality   We think that reports of low mutuality should be taken very seriously by the nurse, because caregiving situations characterized by low mutuality place the caregiver at risk for strain. We recommend that the nurse use the Mutuality Scale to assess for low mutuality in two ways.

First, an average score below 2.50 on the scale indicates the need for further assessment of the caregiving situation. We selected this value of 2.50 as a cutoff point in part because to obtain an overall score on the Mutuality Scale this low, the caregiver would have to answer at least half of the items with response options of 2 or lower. For most of the items, a value of 2 corresponds to the response option of *a little* and the value of 1 to the response option of *not at all*. Such responses reflect aspects of the relationship between caregiver and care receiver that are greatly lacking in mutuality and may contribute to higher levels of caregiver role strain.

Second, if the caregiver reports extremely low mutuality by respond-ing with a 1 or a 2 on the items asking about closeness to the care receiver, attachment to the care receiver, or love for the care receiver, a more extensive assessment of the quality of the relationship is also indicated. We think these three items may most accurately reflect the enduring quality of the relationship and the caregiver's commitment to it. A low score on these items may thus be especially revealing of a vulnerable caregiving situation.

Information about low mutuality may assist the nurse in targeting interventions—for example, caregivers expressing extremely low mutuality may be ones who should be advised to find alternative methods for providing care for the older person (e.g., another family member, an institution, day care, etc.). In contrast, caregivers with high strain and high mutuality may be candidates for instruction about how to do caregiving activities more efficiently and competently.

Preparedness for Caregiving Scale

The Preparedness for Caregiving Scale contains five items, which may be administered in a paper-and-pencil or interview format. Items are answered using a 1 to 4 response format; for example 1 = *not at all prepared*, and 4 = *very well prepared*. A caregiver's overall score is computed by averaging responses to the five items, so that scores for the scale range from 1.00 to 4.00.

Descriptive statistics for the items are presented in Table 32.2. In our study, the internal consistency reliability (Cronbach's alpha) for the scale was .72 at the 6-week interview and .71 at the 9-month interview. The mean scores on the scale were 3.00 (SD = .52, n = 102) at 6 weeks and 3.08 (SD = .48, n = 77) at 9 months. The range of scores for this sample was 2.00 to 4.00. Although the overall level of preparedness was relatively high, about a third of the caregivers in our study did not feel well prepared to provide some aspect of care or handle the stress of caregiving. Caregivers felt less well prepared to take care of the emotional needs of the care receiver and arrange for needed services than to take care of physical needs.

Clinical relevance of preparedness   Caregivers who think that they are not well prepared to manage the caregiving situation are at risk for strain. In our regression analyses, after taking into account five variables usually associated with strain as well as the variable of mutuality, we found that caregivers who scored low on preparedness reported higher levels of strain than would be expected except in the areas of economic burden and role conflict. Conversely, caregivers scoring high on preparedness, but who were in objectively difficult caregiving situations, reported less strain than would be expected based on their difficult situation. The statistically significant increments in explained variance due to preparedness ranged from 3 to 16%, with a median value of 6%.

Further assessment by the nurse is indicated if a caregiver responds to any item on the preparedness scale that she feels "not at all prepared" or "not too well prepared." This assessment should be directed toward

TABLE 32.2 The Preparedness for Caregiving Scale with Response Frequencies, Means, and Standard Deviations[a]

Item		n	Mean	SD
1. How well prepared do you think you are to take care of his/her physical needs? Would you say you are:				
Not at all prepared _____ 1		3	3.18	.69
Not too well prepared _____ 2		8		
Pretty well prepared _____ 3		60		
Very well prepared to take care of his/her physical needs _____ 4		32		
2. How well prepared do you think you are to take care of his/her emotional needs? Would you say you are:				
Not at all prepared _____ 1		4	2.84	.75
Not too well prepared _____ 2		26		
Pretty well prepared _____ 3		54		
Very well prepared to take care of his/her emotional needs _____ 4		18		
Missing		1		
3. How well prepared do you think you are to find out about and set up services for him/her? Would you say you are:				
Not at all prepared _____ 1		12	2.72	.94
Not too well prepared _____ 2		27		
Pretty well prepared _____ 3		41		
Very well prepared to find out about and set up services for him/her _____ 4		22		
Missing		1		
4. How well prepared do you think you are for the stress of caregiving? Would you say you are:				
Not at all prepared _____ 1		5	2.95	.96
Not too well prepared _____ 2		26		
Pretty well prepared _____ 3		50		
Very well prepared for the stress of caregiving _____ 4		13		
Or that caregiving is not stressful _____ 5[b]		9		

TABLE 32.2 Continued

Item		n	Mean	SD
5. Overall, how well prepared do you think you are to care for him/her? Would you say you are:				
Not at all prepared ——————————— 1		0	3.21	.55
Not too well-prepared ——————————— 2		7		
Pretty well-prepared ——————————— 3		67		
Very well-prepared to care for				
him/her ——————————— 4		28		
Don't know		1		
6. If Q.5 = 1, 2, or 3, ASK: Please explain. What kinds of things did you feel unprepared for?				

---

[a]Results based on $N = 103$ caregivers from Caregiver Relief Study, Archbold and Stewart (1988).
[b]5 is recoded to 4 in computing score for Preparedness Scale.

eliciting more detailed information from the caregiver about the areas of care or stress management that she does not feel well prepared to handle. Such information will help identify areas for needed intervention.

Traditionally, nurses have prepared everyone from new mothers caring for their infants to diabetics monitoring their own blood sugar and self-administering insulin. Thus, increasing the caregiver's preparedness to do caregiving tasks is a natural extension of the traditional role of the nurse. Although it is currently being done to some degree, it needs to receive increased attention from nurses in all settings. Responses to the five items on the Preparedness Scale provide the nurse with an idea of which areas of caregiving are problematic for the caregiver. Interventions then can be developed and targeted to increase preparation for providing physical or emotional care, finding out about and obtaining services, and managing the stress of caregiving.

CONCLUSION

The results of our longitudinal study indicate that higher levels of mutuality and preparedness are strongly predictive of lower levels of some, but not all, aspects of caregiver role strain. Although the Mutuality and Preparedness Scales performed well, we are continuing to refine both scales. In our current work, we are examining a 5-point response format for the Mutuality Scale and a slightly revised wording for the response options on the Preparedness Scale. Clinicians and researchers who are interested in using our scales should contact either Archbold or Stewart to obtain information about revisions in the scales and updated psychometric documentation.

We think that our new measure of mutuality provides a way to screen family caregivers for early detection of those who may experience high levels of strain. Our preparedness scale also should assist the nurse in identifying areas of potential intervention. Ultimately, we think that an understanding of mutuality and preparedness will help the nurse prevent or reduce caregiver role strain.

At present, we also are developing a set of nursing interventions designed, in part, to increase the caregiver's preparation for caregiving and enhance mutuality. These interventions will be used by home health nurses who provide care to family members assisting older persons recently discharged from the hospital.

ACKNOWLEDGMENT

This research was supported by the National Center for Nursing Research, NIH, Grant #5R01 NU 01140.

REFERENCES

Archbold, P. G., & Stewart, B. J. (1986). *Family caregiving inventory*. Unpublished manuscript, Oregon Health Sciences University, School of Nursing, Department of Family Nursing, Portland.

Archbold, P. G., & Stewart, B. J. (1988). *Final report: The effects of organized caregiver relief* (Grant No. 5R01 NU 01140). Washington, DC: National Center for Nursing Research, NIH.

Archbold, P. G., Stewart, B. J., Greenlick, M. R., & Harvath, T. A., (1990). Mutuality and preparedness as predictors of caregiver role strain. *Research in Nursing and Health, 12*, 375–384.

Archbold, P. G., Stewart, B. J., Harvath, T. A., & Lucas, S. A. (1986). *New measures of concepts central to an understanding of caregiving*. Unpublished manuscript, Oregon Health Sciences University, School of Nursing, Department of Family Nursing, Portland.

Burr, W. R., Leigh, G. K., Day, R. D., & Constantine, J. (1979). Symbolic interaction and the family. In W. R. Burr, R. Hill, F. I. Nye, & I. L. Reiss (Eds.), *Contemporary theories about the family: Vol. 2* (pp. 42–111). New York: Free Press.

Cantor, M. H. (1983). Strain among caregivers: A study of experience in the United States. The *Gerontologist, 23*, 597–604.

Deimling, G. T., & Bass, D. M. (1986). Symptoms of mental impairment among elderly adults and their effects on family caregivers. *Journal of Gerontology, 41*, 778–784.

Fitting, M., Rabins, P., Lucas, M. J., & Eastham, J. (1986). Caregivers for dementia patients: A comparison of husbands and wives. *The Gerontologist, 26*, 248–252.

George, L. K., & Gwyther, L. P. (1986). Caregiver well-being: A multi-dimensional examination of family caregivers of demented adults. *The Gerontologist, 26*, 253–259.

Haley, W. E., Levine, E. G., Brown, S. L., & Bartolucci, A. A. (1987). Stress, appraisal, coping, and social support as predictors of adaptational outcome among dementia caregivers. *Psychology and Aging, 2*, 323–330.

Harvath, T. A., Archbold, P. G., Lucas, S. A., & Stewart, B. J. (1986, October). Measurement of caregiver role acquisition. In P. G. Archbold & B. J. Stewart (conveners), *An evaluation of new measures of family caregiving*. Symposium conducted at the 39th Annual Scientific Meeting of the Gerontological Society of America, Chicago, IL.

Hirschfeld, M. (1983). Homecare versus institutionalization: Family caregiving and senile brain disease. *International Journal of Nursing Studies, 20*, 23–32.

Horowitz, A., & Shindleman, L. W. (1983). Reciprocity and affection: Past influences on current caregiving. *The Journal of Gerontological Social Work, 5*, 5–20.

Lawton, M. P., Kleban, M. H., Moss, M., Rovine, M., & Glicksman, A. (1989). Measuring caregiving appraisal. *Journal of Gerontology, 44*, P62–P71.

Montgomery, R., & Borgatta, E. F. (Undated). Interview schedules. Family support project, Institution on Aging, Long-Term Care Center, University of Washington, Seattle, WA.

Montgomery, R., Gonyea, G., & Hooyman, N. (1985). Caregiving and the experience of subjective and objective burden. *Family Relations, 34*, 19–26.

Motenko, A. K. (1989). The frustrations, gratifications, and well-being of dementia caregivers. *The Gerontologist, 29*, 166–172.

Stewart, B. J., & Archbold, P. G. (1991). [Evaluation of measures to be used with family caregivers of persons with Alzheimer's disease.] Unpublished raw data.

[33]

Research on Cognitive Impairment: Implications for Practice

Mary T. Champagne and Ruth A. Wiese

The term "delirium" was probably introduced into the medical literature by Celsus in the first century A.D. The word has always been ambiguous. For most of history it was a general term for insanity yet it also referred specifically to a "transient acute mental disorder associated mostly with febrile diseases" (Lipowski, 1990, p. 4). Similarly, over the years, there have been numerous and confusing shifts in the terminology used to describe the two major syndromes of cognitive impairment in the elderly. Today the semantic muddle has cleared somewhat: now we speak of acute confusional states or delirium and chronic cognitive impairments such as dementias of the Alzheimer's type.

As noted in Chapter 24, "Managing Cognitive Impairment," acute confusion or delirium (the two terms are often used interchangeably) is a disturbance in information processing resulting from diffuse impairment of higher cortical function. This is a global impairment characterized by disordered cognition, including disturbances in perception, thinking, and memory; by dysfunction of the reticular activating system, including disturbances in attention and wakefulness; and by dysfunction of the autonomic nervous system, including psychomotor (hypo and hyper) disturbances and alterations in regulatory functions manifested by abnormalities in vital signs. The pathogenesis of delirium appears to have a final common pathway at the neuronal level involving an impairment in cellular oxidative metabolism and/or neurotransmitter deficiencies. Like many clinical syndromes, the presentation of acute confusion may vary—as Fothergill (1874) pointed out a century ago, "Each differs somewhat from every other case, and there are peculiarities in each and every one" (p. 400).

340

More importantly, acute confusion differs from chronic or progressive cognitive impairments such as dementias of the Alzheimer's type by its rapid onset (developing in hours, days, or weeks), its fluctuating manifestations, the abrupt deterioration of present mental status, and the potential for reversibility. What is key is that the syndrome has the potential for reversibility if the underlying problem is treated. Potential outcomes for patients who develop acute confusion include full recovery, progression to stupor and coma, and progression to an irreversible mental syndrome with global or focal cognitive deficits (Lipowski, 1990). Given this range of possible outcomes, it is imperative to clearly identify acute confusional states and initiate treatment immediately.

In contrast, chronic cognitive impairments such as dementias of the Alzheimer's or multi-infarct type develop more slowly and are progressive. These two dementias, which are the most common dementias in the elderly, are not reversible. (Other types of dementias may be static or remitting.) Dementias are characterized by impairments in short- and long-term memory, impaired thinking, and judgment and other disturbances of higher cortical functions. Often the individual has associated personality changes or behavioral problems.

Perhaps because the two syndromes share global cognitive impairments, they are often not differentiated. Distinguishing these syndromes from each other is especially difficult in the elderly as acute confusion and dementia can and often do coexist in the same patient. Labeling all global cognitive impairments in the elderly "dementia" is particularly harmful, however, as the underlying reversible cause of acute confusion may then be ignored and treatment not provided, causing adverse outcomes for the patient.

The chapters in this book highlight the very real problem of acute confusion, particularly in the hospitalized elderly. Neelon and colleagues report a prevalence of acute confusion on admission to the hospital of 39%; and Foreman, in two studies, reports the incidence of acute confusion developed after admission as 38% and 48%, respectively. These figures are consistent with other reports, and they are very disturbing: acute confusion is a costly problem associated with increased length of hospital stay, increased treatments such as sedatives and restraints, increased mortality, and increased readmissions to the hospital within 6 months of discharge. Acute confusion is also a frightening problem for patients and for their families.

Interestingly, the chapters by Neelon et al., Vermeersch, and Siemsen and colleagues indicate that acute confusion may vary in severity. This is an important finding, as it raises the possibility of early identification of a prodromal or mild confusion followed by interventions to prevent the development of full-blown delirium. Yet acute confusion is frequently underdiagnosed and undertreated. Neelon et al. found that nurses, even when asked specifically to document acute confusion, identified less than 50% of those who were moderately to severely confused. This problem of underdiagnosis by health care professionals, including physicians and nurses, has also been documented in the literature. We are not systematically assessing the cognitive status of elderly patients on admission to the hospital or during hospitalization.

We should be doing such systematic assessments. Foreman's study of the clinical features observed in acute confusion documented that alertness and orientation, two assessments most commonly made by clinicians, are not sufficient to identify the syndrome. A more comprehensive assessment is needed to identify cognitive impairment; further, a history should be taken from the family when cognitive impairment is present on admission. Patients with acute confusional states will have a history of recent and rapid onset of cognitive deterioration. In contrast, the onset of a dementia is typically insidious. A history can thus help to distinguish the two.

The chapters in this book suggest at least four instruments that can be used to assess cognitive status in elderly patients. Foreman, Neelon et al., and Siemsen et al. all used the Mini-Mental State Exam (MMSE) (Folstein, Folstein & McHugh, 1975) to assess cognitive function. This is a good screening instrument for cognitive impairment: its reliability and validity are well established, it takes only 5 to 10 minutes to administer, and it is easily scored. The MMSE is well recognized and its scores are understood by physicians and other health care professionals—it is perhaps the most widely used cognitive screening instrument in this country today. However, the MMSE is not specific for acute confusional states and, furthermore, there are some problems with it. Some items require patients to be literate, and to be able to see, hear, and/or write. Thus, it may be difficult to administer the instrument to ill elderly patients who are uneducated or have sensory or mobility impairments. In these cases scoring adjustments have to be made. There is also an educational bias—patients whose educational level is eight grades or less tend to score lower and may be rated as "false positives" (Anthony et al., 1982). In these cases an adjusted cut score for normal may need to be used. Finally, the MMSE does cause some patient-response burden—repeating the exam over and over again each shift or every day would not be pleasant and thus might not be successful if patients refused to cooperate. The best way to use the MMSE is to administer it on admission and observe for cognitive and behavioral changes during hospitalization. Should changes occur, the MMSE is repeated. Changes in the patient's score, particularly below the normal level, would suggest the development of acute confusion.

The diagnostic criteria for delirium in the DSM-III-R (APA, 1987) are specific for delirium or acute confusion, are behaviorally based, and place little response burden on the patient. In addition, these criteria are used by other health care professionals, notably psychiatrists. There are some difficulties in using the DSM-III-R criteria to identify acute confusion, however. Some of the behaviors listed are common in hospitalized ill elderly. More importantly, the DSM-III-R criteria identify only patients who have full-blown delirium. They will not identify those with prodromal or early, mild confusion that might be treated.

The NEECHAM Confusion Scale described by Neelon et al., and tested by Siemsen et al., is an observational scale that can be completed during the usual care of a patient. It can be repeated frequently because it has little patient response burden. Most importantly, the NEECHAM identifies patients with early or mild symptoms of an acute confusional state. The reliability and validity of the scale compared to other clinical indicators are good. Siemsen et al. report that among five clinical raters, the interrater reliability overall was good, and except for one item, "performance/appearance, hygiene," scoring agreement was good.

Siemsen et al. report that compared to the MMSE (using a traditional cut score of 24/23 on the MMSE), the NEECHAM failed to identify a considerable percentage of those who were confused. This differs from the findings of Neelon et al., however, who compared the results of the NEECHAM to three clinical indicators—the MMSE, the DSM-III, and chart report of mental status problems. Anthony et al. (1982), in a sample of 97 patients admitted to a general medical ward, reported that the MMSE had a false positive ratio of 39.4%. The false positive group had a greater proportion of older and poorly educated individuals. Thus the difference reported by Siemsen may be due to the inexperience of raters as she suggests, or to the educational bias of the MMSE. The NEECHAM Confusion Scale is ready for clinical trials by nurses interested in testing a measure of acute confusion in their setting.

A final instrument for measuring acute confusion reported in this book is Vermeersch's Clinical Assessment of Confusion (CAC) scale, forms A and B. The CAC-A is a 25-item observational checklist developed from nurses' descriptions of confusion behavior. The CAC-B is an expanded and modified version of the CAC-A. Vermeersch suggests that the CAC-A might be used to screen for the presence of acute confusion and the CAC-B used to grade its severity. Both scales require little training to use and put little response burden on the patient. Their content validity and reliability are good. These scales are also ready for clinical trials.

We know it is important to assess cognitive status, and instruments now exist that can be used to systematically make that assessment. Let's think for a moment about how you would get a busy staff to try any assessment of mental status or acute confusion. You might begin by educating staff about the problem and telling them what others have found about its incidence and prevalence. This could be done through inservice programs, posting articles on the unit or in the chart of a patient who is acutely confused, having an expert round on patients, or holding grand rounds or a case study of a "severe case," that is, a patient who has full-blown delirium. Once the interest is high, conduct a study to see if acute confusion is common in your setting. Select an instrument that assesses acute confusion and use it with all elderly patients for a period of 2–3 months, then evaluate your results. If acute confusion is common in the elderly patients on your unit, you need to adopt a permanent way of assessing cognitive function. You may need to modify the instrument in order for it to work in your setting. Retain the key elements of the assessment, however, and be sure to go beyond orientation and attention. Assessment will open the door to interventions to prevent or reverse the acute confusion.

The chapters in this book also point out ways to think about interventions for those who are acutely confused or at risk for acute confusion. Once the syndrome is present, the key is to locate and treat the underlying cause or causes and provide good general supportive nursing care. Foreman identifies a number of metabolic abnormalities in the development of acute confusion. In the elderly, it is likely that more than one factor will be related to the development of this syndrome. Neelon and Champagne suggest that a careful review of environmental, physiological, and metabolic systems and challenges is needed to identify factors related to acute confusion. The key then is to not only treat the causes but also protect vulnerable systems that have little reserve. For example, for those with low cognitive reserve (dementias), decrease the challenge to that system by structuring the environment to facilitate the use of information; for those with low metabolic reserve, carefully monitor hydration, electrolyte balance, nutrition, and drug use. Careful clinical thinking and experimentation as well as case study reports will greatly enrich our knowledge of this problem and offer guidance about which interventions should be validated through clinical trials.

One chapter in this book addressed problems experienced by patients with dementias of the Alzheimer's type. Working with severely cognitively impaired patients in a nursing home, Beck showed how caregivers can be taught to provide appropriate cues that facilitate greater independence in dressing. This is a powerful study: it demonstrates that contrary to common clinical belief, severe cognitive impairment does not mean total functional dependence. Independence can be promoted when caregiver assistance is matched to the abilities of the patient.

Beck's chapter provides clear guidance on the assessments needed to determine areas of ability and shows how to structure a task to optimize the use of those abilities. This approach holds promise for promoting independence in a variety of self-care activities in the cognitively impaired. As Beck notes, custodial care is no longer acceptable and the dignity of our patients will be better maintained when we promote independence rather than encouraging dependence.

Sisson explores the relationship between cognitive, functional, and emotional status in her chapter on the rehabilitation potential of stroke patients. She found a positive correlation between cognitive status and functional status: patients who were experiencing cognitive problems such as mental fatigue, memory deficit, conceptual disorganization, and inattention required greater assistance with activities of daily living. Sisson therefore recommends assessment of cognitive function in stroke patients, particularly in planning for rehabilitation. Timing the rehabilitation referral or designing retraining activities without attention to cognitive abilities may result in inadequate matching of the task with the patient's abilities. Both the studies by Beck and Sisson illustrate that function is best maximized through careful assessment of abilities and matching of tasks with those abilities.

Cleary's chapter focuses on the population often called the "second patient" of the nurse caring for Alzheimer's disease patients—the caregiver. Her report that the stressors and coping strategies used by caregivers vary with the stage of the disease provides direction for assessment and intervention with caregivers. For example, the most burdensome phase described by Cleary's caregivers was the middle or moderate stage of the disease, when caregivers had to deal with more behavioral problems, including agitated or aggressive acting-out behaviors. Caregivers may need increased support and help in learning how to care for the patients during this phase. Cleary's work shows that anticipatory guidance for families must be based on the recognition that different problems may occur at different stages of the illness. And it suggests that careful assessment of actual stressors is essential if we are to intervene effectively.

Archbold and colleagues' chapter examines caregiver strain in those caring for frail elderly patients post hospitalization. Archbold et al. looked at two positive constructs—mutuality and preparedness for caregiving and their relationship to caregiver strain. They found that higher levels of mutuality and preparedness for caregiving predicted lower strain in some aspects of the caregiver role. The Mutuality Scale helps identify those at high risk for caregiver strain (those with low mutuality); the Preparedness for Caregiving Scale identifies how prepared caregivers feel to provide different aspects of care. Use of these scales will help clinicians in many settings, from hospitals to homes and nursing homes, target interventions to help caregivers.

The chapters in this book on cognitive impairment help us view the cognitively impaired elderly in a different light. They remind us that assessment is the key to successful treatment and that many of our long held beliefs about cognitive and functional performance in the elderly are beliefs and little more. Clearly, nurses can do much to alleviate the problems of acute confusion in hospitalized elderly, functional dependence in Alzheimer's patients, and the burden of caregiving.

REFERENCES

American Psychiatric Association. (1987). *Diagnostic and statistical manual of mental disorders*, 3rd Ed., Revised, Washington, DC: Author.

Anthony, J. C., LeResche, L., Niaz, U., Von Korff, M. R., Michael, R., Folstein, M. F., & Marshal, F. (1982). Limits of the "Mini-Mental State" as a screening test for dementia and delirium among hospital patients. *Psychological Medicine, 12*, 397–408.

Folstein, M. F., Folstein, S. E., & McHugh, P. R. (1975). "Mini-Mental State": A practical method for grading the cognitive state of patients for the clinician. *Journal of Psychiatric Research, 12*, 189–198.

Fothergill, J. M. (1874). The management of delirium. *The Practitioner, 13*, 400–408.

Lipowski, Z. (1990). *Delirium: Acute confusional states.* New York: Oxford University Press.

Index

Index